T0258583

Encyclopedia of Tuberculosis: Mycobacterium Tuberculosis Roots

Volume II

Encyclopedia of Tuberculosis: Mycobacterium Tuberculosis Roots

Volume II

Edited by **Morris Beckler**

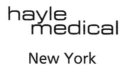

New York

Published by Hayle Medical,
30 West, 37th Street, Suite 612,
New York, NY 10018, USA
www.haylemedical.com

Encyclopedia of Tuberculosis: Mycobacterium Tuberculosis Roots
Volume II
Edited by Morris Beckler

International Standard Book Number: 978-1-63241-203-4 (Hardback)

Printed in the United States of America.

Contents

Preface

Every book is a source of knowledge and this one is no exception. The idea that led to the conceptualization of this book was the fact that the world is advancing rapidly; which makes it crucial to document the progress in every field. I am aware that a lot of data is already available, yet, there is a lot more to learn. Hence, I accepted the responsibility of editing this book and contributing my knowledge to the community.

This book is an attempt to explain the degree to which the bacilli evolve in accordance with its host and its final objective. It covers discussions by experts on the manipulation of immune response to attain novel prophylactic. The book will be a valuable source of reference to students and clinicians.

While editing this book, I had multiple visions for it. Then I finally narrowed down to make every chapter a sole standing text explaining a particular topic, so that they can be used independently. However, the umbrella subject sinews them into a common theme. This makes the book a unique platform of knowledge.

I would like to give the major credit of this book to the experts from every corner of the world, who took the time to share their expertise with us. Also, I owe the completion of this book to the never-ending support of my family, who supported me throughout the project.

Editor

Manipulating the Immune Responses to Favor the Host

Immune Responses Against *Mycobacterium tuberculosis* and the Vaccine Strategies

Toshi Nagata[1] and Yukio Koide[2]

[1]*Department of Health Science, Hamamatsu University School of Medicine, Hamamatsu*
[2]*Department of Infectious Diseases, Hamamatsu University School of Medicine,
Hamamatsu
Japan*

1. Introduction

Tuberculosis (TB) is an infectious disease caused by *Mycobacterium tuberculosis* (Mtb). Robert Koch identified Mtb as a causative agent of TB at 1882 (Sakula, 1983). Since then, TB has been one of the most important infectious diseases for human being. According to the WHO report regarding the global burden of TB in 2009, there were 9.4 million incident cases of TB with approximately one third of the world total population being infected (World Health Organization, 2010). Especially, coinfection of Mtb and HIV is a serious issue in sub-Sahara Africa area. Distribution of multi-drug-resistant TB or extensively drug-resistant TB has been another issue in TB.

The epidemiological studies revealed that only 10 to 30% of people who exposed Mtb are infected with Mtb and that 90% or more of the infected people do not develop TB. Only 5% shows the symptoms within 1 year and 95% of the infected individuals are considered to remain infected latently for the long time. Further, only 5% of individuals who have persistently infected Mtb show internal reactivation, i.e., show the overt symptoms the long time later (North and Jung, 2004). These facts indicate that immune responses that are necessary to contain Mtb are induced in the majority of Mtb-infected individuals. Induction of appropriate immune responses against protective Mtb antigens in appropriate stages is necessary for preventing TB. In this chapter, we review the aspect of immune responses and the vaccine strategies against Mtb.

2. Protective immunity against Mtb

2.1 Immune cell effectors against Mtb

Mtb is a facultative intracellular bacterium that survives in phagosomes of alveolar macrophages. In general, effective immune responses against intracellular pathogens are based on the cellular arm (T cells), not on the humoral arm (antibodies) of immune responses (reviewed in Stenger & Modlin, 1999; Kaufmann, 2003). The followings are effective cell subsets that have been considered to be important for protection against Mtb infection.

2.1.1 CD4[+] T cells

Intracellular bacteria in phagosomes including Mtb are processed via major histocompatibility complex (MHC) class II-mediated antigen processing pathway and antigens of the bacteria are presented to CD4+ helper T cells (reviewed in Kaufmann, 2003; Flynn & Chan, 2001; Cooper, 2009). Therefore, CD4+ T cells are considered to be the principal effectors against Mtb. Mice that have a deletion in MHC class II or CD4 gene have been shown to be succumbed against Mtb challenge infection (Ladel et al., 1995; Caruso et al., 1999). CD4+ T cells are divided to mainly two subsets depending on the difference of cytokines produced, type 1 helper T cells (Th1) and type 2 helper T cells (Th2). Th1 produces interferon (IFN)-γ, tumor necrosis factor (TNF)- α, and/or interleukin (IL)-2, and contribute to macrophage activation or granuloma formation through effects of these cytokines. IFN-γ has been reported to be the most critical for the protective immunity through analyses of mice or humans which have a deletion in genes encoding IFN-γ or the receptor (Cooper et al., 1993; Flynn et al., 1993; Ottenhoff et al., 1998). Therefore, Th1 has been considered to play a pivotal role for protection against Mtb infection. IFN-γ amounts or the number of IFN-γ producing T cells has been considered to be a relevant marker for induction of a protective immunity against Mtb (Ellner et al., 2000; Walzl et al., 2011), although it is not the unique marker (Agger & Anderesn, 2001). This cytokine is also able to induce inflammation in the lesion, possibly to help aggravating the disease. Th2 produce IL-4, IL-5, and/or IL-10 and contribute to antibody-mediated immune responses or type 1 allergy development. Therefore, Th2 are considered to have inhibitory effects for protective immunity against Mtb.

2.1.2 CD8[+] T cells

Theoretically, CD4+ T cells are major effecter cells against phagosome-localized pathogens. However, CD8+ T cells also have been shown to play an important role in protective immunity against Mtb by analysis of Mtb infection experiments to mice that have deficiency in β2-microglobulin gene critical for MHC class I expression (Flynn et al., 1992; Ladel et al., 1995). Mtb are reported to be cross-presented to CD8+ T cells via MHC class I antigen presentation pathway. Kaufmann's group reported that Mtb-infected macrophages induce apoptotic process and then cross-presentation via apoptotic vesicles (Winau et al., 2006). The process may lead to induction of antigen-specific CD8+ T cells. van Pinxteren and colleagues (2000) reported that CD8+ T cells are particularly important in protective immunity at the latent phase of TB.

CD8+ T cells contribute to protective immunity against Mtb in the following mechanisms (Smith & Duckrell, 2000; Kaufmann & Flynn, 2005). (1) Secretion of cytokines such as IFN-γ and TNF-α. IFN-γ production is essential for CD8+ T-cell mediation of protective immunity against Mtb (Tascon et al., 1998). (2) Lysis of infected host cells through perforin and granzyme B secretion. (3) Direct killing of bacteria infected through granulysin secretion (Stenger et al., 1997). Stegelmann and colleagues (2005) showed that a subset of CD8+ T cells coordinately expresses CC chemokine ligand 5 (CCL5, RANTES), perforin and granulysin, attracts Mtb-infected macrophages and kill the intracellular Mtb (Stegelmann et al., 2005).

2.1.3 Th17 cells

Th17 is a subtype of CD4+ T cells and produce IL-17. Th17 promote migration of Th1, neutrophils, and monocytes to TB lesion in the presence of chemokines and contribute to protective immunity against Mtb (Khader et al., 2007).

2.1.4 CD1-restricted T cells

A subset of T cells is antigen-presented through CD1 molecules, not through conventional MHC class I (Ia) or II molecules. Genes encoding CD1 molecules are mapped outside of MHC and are less polymorphic than conventional MHC genes. CD1-restricted T cells have been reported to recognize glycolipids in mycobacterial cell wall such as mycolic acid (Beckman et al., 1994).

2.1.5. γδ T cells

Most CD4+ and CD8+ T cells express T-cell receptors of α and β protein chains. A minor subset of T cells expresses T-cell receptor of γ and δ protein chains (γδ T cells). γδ T cells tend to distribute in epithelial tissues and contribute to early protection against pathogens invading through epithelium. The phosphoantigen-specific γδ T cells (Vγ2Vδ2+) displayed major expansion during BCG infection and a clear memory-type response after BCG reinfection in a macaque model (Shen et al., 2002)..

2.1.6 NK cells

NK cells have been associated with early resistance against Mtb (Junqueira-Kipnis et al., 2003). NK cells increased in the lung after aerosol infection of Mtb and produce IFN-γ and perforin. But in vivo NK cell depletion experiment had no influence on bacterial load within the lungs in mouse system, suggesting that NK cells do not play essential roles in early stage of Mtb infection.

2.1.7 Regulatory T cells

Regulatory T cells (Treg) are composed of a subset of T cells that express Foxp3 transcription factor and inhibit effector T-cell responses by both cell-to-cell direct contact and secretion of inhibitory cytokines such as IL-10 or transforming growth factor (TGF)-β. They also constitutively express CD25 molecule, α chain protein of the high affinity IL-2 receptor. So, this T-cell subset can be deleted in vivo with injection of anti-CD25 monoclonal antibody and the depletion experiments confirmed that it has been shown to be critical for prevention of autoimmunity and graft rejection. Treg have been reported to be induced in Mtb-infected mice and humans and this cell subset is considered to be important for the persistence of Mtb infection (Kursar et al., 2007).

2.1.8 Antibodies

In general, humoral immunity does not contribute to induction of the protective immunity against Mtb. However, antibodies specific for heparin-binding haemagglutinin (HBHA) and arabinomannan are reported to contribute to reduce the bacterial load in lung (Teitelbaum et al., 1998; Pethe et al., 2001). Antibodies specific for antigens presented on the surface of Mtb may have some effect to prevent invading Mtb into the host cells.

2.2 Protective antigens of Mtb

The analysis of genome of Mtb H37Rv strain reveals that 3,985 open reading frames exist in the genome (Cole et al., 1998). Since the report, DNA vaccines are possible to be constructed through the genome information. Information of mycobacterial genes and proteins is available from several comprehensive databases (e.g., The Pasteur Institute TubercuList [http://genolist.pasteur.fr/tuberculist/], The Institute for Genomic Research (TIGR) Comprehensive Microbial Resource (CMR) [http://cmr.tigr.org/tigr-scripts/CMR/CmrHomePage.cgi]). The most important issue in developing effective TB vaccines is to clarify which genes or gene products are important for the protective immunity against Mtb. The fact that viable Mtb, but not killed Mtb, can induce the protective immunity (Orme, 1988) leads to the speculation that mainly secretory proteins would be the protective antigens. In fact, the majority of the target antigens of the cellular arm of immunity has been reported to be secretory or cell-membrane proteins (Andersen, 1994). Representative protective antigens of Mtb have been clarified by analyses of T-cell responses against protein fractions separated with the electrophoresis analyses (Belisle et al., 2005). The followings are the representative protective antigens of Mtb reported.

2.2.1 Antigen 85 complex proteins

Antigen 85 (Ag85) complex proteins are mycobacterial major secreted proteins of 30 to 32 kDa. The proteins have mycolyl transferase function that is necessary for synthesis of lipid components of mycobacterial cell wall and fibronectin-binding function (Wiker & Harboe, 1992; Belisle et al., 1997). Ag85 complex proteins are composed of Ag85A (p32A), Ag85B (p30, MPT59, α antigen), and Ag85C protein. These proteins are well conserved in *Mycobacterium* genus. MPT51 protein has some homology to these proteins (Nagai et al., 1991; Ohara et al., 1995) and has been shown to be a protective antigen (Miki et al., 2004).

2.2.2 Low-molecular-mass secretory proteins

Low-molecular-mass proteins (less than 20 kDa) in Mtb culture fluid proteins (CFPs) have been reported to be major antigens that evoke T-cell responses (Boesen et al., 1995; Demissie et al., 1999). Among a variety of low-molecular-mass secreted proteins, early secreted antigenic target 6-kDa protein (ESAT6) and culture fluid protein 10 (CFP10) have been well studied (Berthet et al., 1998). Recently, ESAT6 and CFP10 proteins are widely used in whole blood IFN-γ release assays for TB diagnosis (Andersen et al., 2000) (QuantiFERON® TB Gold; Cellestis, Ltd., Carnegie, Victoria, Australia).

2.2.3 Heat shock proteins

A variety of heat shock proteins have been shown to be targets for antibodies and T cells in murine and human systems. Among them, heat shock protein 65 (Hsp65) is a major stress protein Mtb produces in macrophage cells. Mtb Hsp65 protein has more than 50% homology with *Escherichia coli* GroEL or human Hsp60 protein (Lee & Horwitz, 1995). Heat shock proteins have been shown to be expressed in Mtb in macrophages and induce protective immune responses.

2.2.4 Dormant phase proteins

Aforementioned proteins are expressed mainly in acute phage of TB. A different set of genes are expressed in late infection phase or chronic (dormant) phase of TB. DosR regulon is a unit of genes composed of 48 genes, the expression of which is regulated by DosR (Rv3133c). DosR regulon proteins are the major proteins expressed in chronic (dormant) phase of TB (Karalousis et al., 2004). HspX protein (Rv2031c) is one of the immunodominant antigens belong to DosR regulon proteins. It plays an important role in slowing the growth of Mtb as *hspX* gene-deleted Mtb mutants showed increased growth both in mice and in macrophages (Hu et al., 2006). T-cell responses specific for HspX were found in latent Mtb infection (Demissie et al., 2006). In addition, mycobacterial DNA-binding protein-1 (MDP1) has been shown to be expressed in the late phase of TB and induce humoral and cellular immune responses (Matsumoto et al., 2005; Suzuki et al., 2010). Analysis of dormant phase proteins is critical for development of therapeutic TB vaccines against persistent Mtb infection.

2.3 T-cell epitopes of Mtb proteins

T-cell epitopes are the peptides in antigenic proteins that bind to MHC molecules on antigen-presenting cells. In other words, T-cell epitopes are the peptides that stimulate T cells through the MHC-T-cell receptor interaction.

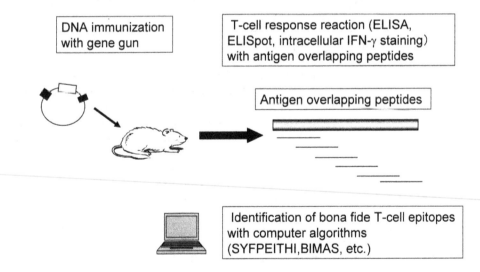

Fig. 1. Shematic diagram for identification of T-cell with DNa immunization

Identification of T-cell epitopes in Mtb antigens is indispensable for accurate analysis of T-cell responses against Mtb antigens with specific MHC tetramers or intracellular cytokine staining. We realized that DNA immunization with gene gun bombardment is an excellent method for identification of Mtb T-cell epitopes as it is highly reproducible and efficiently

Antigen	Epitope peptide	MHC restriction	Reactive T cells	References
Ag85B	p30-38 (9-mer)	A*0201	CD8	Tang et al., 2011
	p183-192 (10-mer)	A*0201	CD8	Geluk et al., 2000
	p239-247 (9-mer)	A*0201	CD8	Geluk et al., 2000
	p10-27 (18-mer)	DR3, 52, 53	CD4	Mustafa et al., 2000b
	p19-36 (18-mer)	Promiscuous	CD4	Mustafa et al., 2000b
	p91-108 (18-mer)	Promiscuous	CD4	Mustafa et al., 2000b
MPT51	p51-70 (10-mer)	A*0201	CD8	Aoshi et al., 2008
	p191-202 (12-mer)	DR4 (Promiscuous)	CD4	Wang et al., 2009
Hsp65	p369-377 (19-mer)	A*0201	CD8	Charo et al., 2001
	p3-13 (11-mer)	DR3	CD4	Geluk et al., 1992
ESAT6	p72-95 (24-mer)	DR52, DQ2	CD4	Mustafa et al., 2000a
HspX	p21-29 (9-mer)	A*0201	CD8	Caccamo et al., 2002
(16kDa Protein)	p120-128 (9-mer)	A*0201	CD8	Caccamo et al., 2002
(DosR regulon)	p91-105 (15-mer)	A*0201	CD8	Geluk et al., 2007
	p31-50 (20-mer)	DR3	CD4	Geluk et al., 2007
Rv1733c (DosR regulon)	p161-169 (9-mer)	A*0201	CD8	Commandeur et al., 2011
Rv1733c	p181-189 (9-mer)	A*0201	CD8	Commandeur et al., 2011
Rv2029c (DosR regulon)	p161-169 (9-mer)	A*0201	CD8	Commandeur et al., 2011

Table 1. Human T-cell epitopes of Mtb antigens (examples)

induces T-cell responses (Yoshida et al., 2000). Therefore, we have used gene gun DNA immunization method for identification of CD8+ and CD4+ T-cell epitopes of Mtb antigens (Fig. 1). After immunization with plasmid DNA encoding Mtb antigens, immune spleen cells were examined for their IFN-γ responses to overlapping peptides covering full-length Mtb antigens by measuring IFN-γ levels by enzyme-linked immunosorbent assay (ELISA) or by counting the numbers of IFN-γ-secreting cells by enzyme-linked immunospot assay (ELISPOT). We combined these methods with computer algorithms to predict T-cell epitopes. T-cell epitope prediction algorithm programs we used are as follows. They are able to access through their websites. (1) SYFPEITHI Epitope program (http://www.syfpeithi.de/) (Rammensee et al., 1999), (2) the National Institutes of Health Bioinformatics and Molecular Analysis Section (BIMAS) HLA Peptide Binding Predictions (http://bimas.dcrt.nih.gov/cgi-bin/molbio/ken_parker_comboform) (Parker et al., 1994), RANKPEP MHC binding peptide prediction algorithm (http://immunax.dfci.harvard.edu/Tools/rankpep.html) (Reche et al., 2004), and (4) ProPred HLA-DR binding peptide prediction algorithm (http://www.imtech.res.in/raghava/propred/) (Singh & Raghava, 2001). These programs are helpful for narrowing down the amino acid regions of T-cell epitopes. However, the algorithms are still not perfect for exact identification of bona fide T-cell epitopes. A peptide that shows the highest score in these algorithms is not necessarily the best T-cell epitope. Experimental validation is definitely necessary to determine actual T-cell epitopes. A variety of

T cell epitopes of Mtb antigens have been reported. A comprehensive analysis of T-cell epitope data regarding *Mycobacterium* genus in the immune epitope database (IEDB; http://immuneepitope.org) was performed (Blythe et al., 2007). Huygen and colleagues have reported identification of murine T-cell epitopes of Ag 85 family proteins (Ag85A, Ag85B, and Ag85C) (Denis et al., 1998, D'Souza, et al., 2003) using intramuscular DNA immunization. We have used gene gun DNA immunization method for identification of murine CD8+ and CD4+ T-cell epitopes of Mtb antigens including MPT51 (Suzuki et al., 2004), MDP1 (Suzuki et al., 2010), and low-molecular-mass secretory antigens (CFP11, CFP17, and TB18.5) (Eweda et al., 2010).

In addition to murine T-cell epitopes, human T-cell epitopes have been reported (some examples are shown in Table 1). HLA-A02 is the most frequent HLA molecule in Caucasians and HLA-A*0201 represents the most frequent allele. HLA-A*0201-restricted CD8+ T-cell epitopes have been identified in a variety of antigens including those derived from cancers, viruses, bacteria, and protozoan. Mtb-derived HLA-A*0201-restricted CD8+ T-cell epitopes have been reported, including epitopes in Ag85A (Smith et al., 2000), Ag85B (Geluk et al., 2000), ESAT6 (Lalvani et al., 1998), and Hsp65 (Charo et al., 2001).

T-cell epitope (10-mer)	Position 1 2 3 4 5 6 7 8 9 10										
Anchor residues	L, M					L, V, I					
MPT51 p53-62	T	L	A	G	K	G	I	S	V	V	Aoshi et al., 2008
Ag85B p143-152	F	I	Y	A	G	S	L	S	A	L	Geluk et al., 2000
T cell epitope (9 mer)	Position 1 2 3 4 5 6 7 8 9										
Anchor residues	L, M					L,V, I					
Ag85B p30-38	G	L	A	G	G	A	A	T	A		Tang et al., 2011
Ag85B p183-192	K	L	V	A	N	N	T	R	L		Geluk et al., 2000
Ag85B p239-247	G	L	A	G	G	A	A	T	A		Geluk et al., 2000
Hsp65 p369-337	K	L	A	G	G	V	A	V	I		Charo et al., 2001
HspX (DosR reg) p13-21	L	F	A	A	F	P	S	F	A		Caccamo et al., 2002
HspX (DosR reg) p120-128	G	I	L	T	V	S	V	A	V		Caccamo et al., 2002
Rv1733c (DosR reg) p161-169	I	A	D	A	A	L	A	A	L		Commandeur et al., 2011
Rv1733c (DosR reg) p181-189	A	L	L	A	L	T	R	A	I		Commandeur et al., 2011
Rv2029c (DosR reg) p314-322	E	L	A	A	E	P	T	E	V		Commandeur et al., 2011

Table 2. HLA-A*0201-restricted T-cells epitopes od Mtb antigens (examples)

Most HLA-A*0201-restricted T-cell epitopes were nonamer peptides (Falk et al., 1991, Parker, 1994), but some epitopes were decamer peptides. We reported an immunodominant HLA-A*0201-restricted T-cell epitope in MPT51 antigen (Aoshi et al., 2008; Tables 1, 2). Main anchor amino acid positions are, position 2 (Leu) and position 9 (Val), which were conserved in MPT51 p53-62 (TLAGKGISVV) (Table 2). MPT51 p53-62 decamer peptide was capable of binding to HLA-A*0201 and of stimulating CD8[+] T cells of HLA-A*0201-transgenic mice, but MPT51 p53-61 nonamer was not. The conformational and electrostatic differences between the nonamer and the decamer would affect their binding affinity to HLA-A*0201 molecule and following T-cell responses. Ruppert and colleagues (1993) studied in detail the role of different amino acid residues on each position of nonamer or decamer peptides for binding to HLA-A*0201 molecule. They suggested that nonamer or decamer peptide has different preference of amino acid residues for binding to HLA-A*0201 molecule. They showed that, for example, Tyr, Phe, Trp residues at positions 1, 3, and 5 in nonamer peptides, Gly residues at positions 4 and 6 in decamer peptides are preferable for binding to HLA-A*0201. According to their speculation, MPT51 p53-62 peptide seems to have better A*0201 binding features than MPT51 p53-61 peptide (Gly residues at positions 4 and 6 in MPT51 p53-62 peptide are suggested to be associated with good A*0201 binding). Interestingly, MPT51 p21-29 peptide (FLAGGPHAV) was not immunogenic in terms of IFN-γ production and cytolytic ability although the peptide showed high affinity to HLA-A*0201 as predicted by MHC binding algorithms (Aoshi et al., 2008). Previous reports showed a strong association between immunodominance and HLA binding affinity (Geluk et al., 1998). But, binding of peptides to the restricted MHC molecules is a prerequisite for T-cell epitopes, but all the peptides which show high affinity binding for MHC molecules are not necessarily immunodominant epitopes.

3. Vaccine strategies against Mtb

3.1 Recombinant BCG vaccines

Mycobacterium bovis bacillus Calmette-Guérin (BCG) is the only approved attenuated live vaccine to date against TB. Original BCG strain was reported approximately ninety years ago (1921) by Calmette and Guérin (Bloom & Fine, 1994). Despite the fact that BCG is among the most widely used vaccine throughout the world since then, TB still poses a serious global health threat. Whereas BCG is believed to protect newborns and young children against early manifestations of TB (Rodgrigues et al., 1993), its efficacy against pulmonary TB in adults is still a subject of debate (Bloom & Fine, 1994; Andersen & Doherty, 2005) and was reported to wane with time since vaccination (Sterne et al., 1998). Variable levels of the protective efficacy ranging from 0 to 80% have been reported in different studies (Fine, 1995). Moreover, the viable nature of BCG makes it partly unsafe in case of immunocompromised people such as HIV-infected individuals. This highlights the need to develop more effective, safe and reliable vaccines against TB (Kaufmann, 2010).

To improve the immunoreactivity of conventional BCG vaccines, a variety of recombinant BCG (rBCG) vaccines have been tried and evaluated for the protective efficacy (Stover et al., 1991). One of the problems of conventional BCG vaccines in induction of protective immune responses is that BCG is not effective for induction of CD8[+] T-cell responses compared with Mtb. BCG is less effective in MHC class I-mediated antigen presentation, which is prerequisite for CD8[+] T-cell induction (Mazzaccaro et al., 1996). To improve CD8[+] T-cell responses of BCG, Kaufmann and colleagues reported recombinant BCG (rBCG) introduced with listeriolysin O (LLO) gene derived from *Listeria monocytogenes* (Hess et al., 1998). *L. monocytogenes* escapes from the phagosomes into the cytoplasm shortly after infection into host macrophage cells. LLO, a thiol-activated cytolysin, has membrane-disrupting capability and plays a pivotal role in this process. The rBCG expressing LLO was reported to improve MHC class I-mediated antigen presentation of co-phagocytosed ovalbumin, suggesting that LLO endows BCG with an improved capacity to stimulate CD8[+] T cells. Further, the same group constructed urease C gene (*ureC*)-disrupted rBCG expressing LLO (Grode et al., 2005). Mycobacterial ureC increases pH value in the phagosome. The ureC deficiency induces low pH value in the phagosome, helping the LLO enzyme activity (to disrupt phagosome membranes), which leads enhancement of MHC class I-mediated CD8[+] T-cell responses.

Another promising rBCG is BCG overexpressing Ag85B protein (Horwitz et al., 2000). Ag85B is a major mycobacterial secreted protein and has been shown to be a protective antigen. Even though BCG does have endogenous Ag85B, overexpression of Ag85B in BCG was further enhanced the protective ability. In addition to these rBCG, attenuated auxotroph strains of Mtb have been examined (Guleria et al., 1996; Sambandamurthy et al., 2006; Larsen et al., 2009).

3.2 DNA Vaccination against TB

Many reports on DNA vaccination against Mtb have been published since 1996 (Huygen et al., 1996, Tascon et al., 1996). So far, a variety of Mtb antigen genes have been used for DNA vaccines, which include Hsp 65, Hsp 70, Ag85A, Ag85B, and ESAT6 (reviewed in Huygen, 2003 for early studies). DNA immunization with genes encoding dormancy regulon-encoded proteins has also been examined (Roupie et al., 2007). DNA immunization with naked DNA has been shown to efficiently induce cellular as well as humoral immune responses. DNA vaccines in most of these reports use needle injection through intramuscular or intradermal routes although some studies used gene gun (Sugawara et al., 2003). The DNA immunization with needle injection tends to raise predominant Th1 responses which are indispensable for induction of the protective immunity. On the other hand, gene gun DNA immunization is apt to produce "mixed type" (Th1 and Th2; producing IFN-γ and IL-4) T-cell responses which is not necessarily adequate for induction of the protective immunity (Tanghe et al., 2000). The difference is considered to be mainly due to the difference in the amount of antigen produced from the plasmids (high amounts in needle injection and low amounts in gene gun bombardment). Therefore, DNA vaccination with gene gun will need additional factors such as adjuvants for eliciting protective immunity against Mtb (D'Souza et al., 2002; Tollefsen et al., 2002; Li et al., 2006; Zhang et al., 2007).

Naked DNA vaccines have been evaluated as therapeutic TB vaccines as well as prophylactic TB vaccines. Lowrie and colleagues (1999) showed that intramuscular injection of mice with Hsp65 and MPT70 DNA vaccines reduced Mtb numbers in spleens and lungs after Mtb challenge by 1 to two log_{10} order compared with untreated mice. Further, they showed that three intramuscular injection of Hsp65 DNA vaccine eliminated residual Mtb after chemotherapy (isoniazid and pyrazinamid treatment) and immunosupprssive corticosteroid treatment. However, Orme's group reported that Ag85A DNA vaccine that was shown to induce protective immunity in mice when the vaccine was used as a prophylactic vaccine, could not give any therapeutic effect on the course of the infection in the lungs in mice earlier infected by Mtb aerosol (Turner et al., 2000). Moreover, they reported that vaccination with DNA encoding hsp60 of *Mycobacterium leprae* induced cellular necrosis throughout the lung granulomas when the DNA was given in a mouse immunotherapeutic model (Taylor et al., 2003). Repique and colleagues (2002) also reported that vaccination with a DNA vaccine cocktail containing ten Mtb antigen genes which had showed significant protective responses in mice could not prevent reactivation of disease in a murine latent TB model. These reports indicate that therapeutic TB vaccines still have room for further studies in terms of safety.

3.3 Improvement in immunization regimen: prime-boost immunization

Evaluation of vaccination has indicated that the repeated injection of the same vaccine has a limitation in terms of its overall immunological effects. Especially, DNA immunization has been reported to induce considerably strong immunological responses in the rodents, but not in the primates including human (Li et al., 1993). Instead of the repeated injection of the same vaccine, the heterologous prime-boost regimen including DNA vaccination, which is primed with naked DNA vaccination and boosted with recombinant viral vectors such as vaccinia virus and adenovirus, has been shown to evoke superior levels of immunity to DNA vaccine or recombinant virus alone (Ramshaw & Ramsay, 2000). The relatively low-level but persistent expression of immunogenic proteins in vivo by naked DNA vaccines has been suggested to be important for priming immunological responses and inducing enhanced cellular immunity (Ramshaw & Ramsay, 2000).

A variety of prime-boost regimens have been examined for Mtb infection (McShane & Hill, 2005). Many investigators examined the regimens in which priming with DNA vaccines and boosting with other immunization strategies. Feng and colleagues (2001) showed that priming with Ag85B DNA vaccine and boosting with BCG vaccine strengthened protective immunity against Mtb induced by BCG vaccine alone in mice. Skinner and colleagues (2003) also reported that priming with ESAT6 andAg85A DNA vaccines and boosting with BCG vaccine enhanced specific IFN-γ production from immune splenocytes compared with that by the DNA vaccine or BCG vaccine alone in mice. Ferraz and colleagues (2004) used DNA vaccines encoding mycobacterial Hsp70, Hsp65, and Apa antigens as priming vaccine and showed that the DNA vaccines enhanced BCG boosting effects. Romano and colleagues (2006) showed that immunization of BALB/c mice with Ag85A DNA vaccine first and boosting with BCG vaccine induced stronger protective immunity against Mtb challenge than that by Ag85A DNA vaccine alone. These results demonstrated that DNA vaccine priming and BCG vaccine boosting enhanced immune responses induced by BCG vaccine alone.

The regimens in which BCG vaccine was used as a priming vaccine also have been tried. As the BCG vaccine has been injected to people all over the world, this regimen seems to be reasonable. Derrick and colleagues (2004) showed that a polyvalent DNA vaccine encoding an ESAT6-Ag85B fusion protein protects mice against a primary Mtb infection and boosts BCG-induced protective immunity. Priming with BCG vaccine and intranasal boosting with MVA85A in mice enhanced Ag85A-specific CD4+ and CD8+ T-cell responses and strengthened protective immunity against aerosol Mtb challenge infection in mice (Goonetilleke et al., 2003). This regimen was reported in humans. McShane and colleagues

(2004) reported that in volunteers who had been vaccinated 0.5 to 38 years previously with BCG, vaccination with MVA85A induced substantially higher levels of antigen-specific IFN-γ-secreting T cells and that at 24 weeks after vaccination, these levels were 5 to 30 times greater than in vaccinees administered a single BCG vaccination.

3.4 Ongoing tuberculosis vaccine projects

A variety of TB vaccines have been evaluated (reviewed in Hoft, 2008; Kaufmann, 2010a, 2010b). WHO have showed a list of TB vaccine candidates (TB vaccine pipeline: http://www.stoptb.org/retooling/). These TB vaccine strategies are based on the prime-boost regimens and the vaccine candidates are categorized into three vaccine groups, namely, (1) priming vaccines, (2) boosting vaccines, and (3) therapeutic vaccines after Mtb infection. Some of vaccine candidates that have been ongoing are shown in Table 3.

Vaccine	Source	Explanation	References
Priming Vaccines			
rBCG30	UCLA (M. Horwitz)/NIAID	Ag85B recombinant BCG	Horwitz et al., 2000
rBCG ΔureC:Hly (VPM1002)	Max Planck Inst. (S. Kaufmann) /VPM/TBVI	Listeriolysin O (LLO) recombinant BCG	Grode et al., 2005, Tchilian et al., 2009
mc²6220, 6221, 6222, 6231	Albert Einstein College of Med.	ΔlysAΔpanCD (lysin/pantothetic acid-erquiring attenuated *M. tuberculosis*	Sambandamurthy et al., 2006
Booster Vaccines			
MVA85A/AERAAS-485	Oxford/Isis/Aeras/Ermergent	Ag85A recombinant Vaccinia Virus	McShane et al., 2001, Goonetilleke et al., 2003, McShcane et al., 2004, Scriba et al., 2010
AERAS-402/Crucell Ad35	Crucell/Aeras	Ag85A, Ag85B, TB10.4 recombinant Adenovirus type 35	Radošević et al., 2007 Abel et al., 2010
GSK M72	GSK/Aeras	PPE family protein Rv1196-Rv0125 fusion protein + AS01 adjuvant	Skeikey et al., 2004
SSI Hybrid I	Statens Serum Inst. (SSI)	Ag85B-ESAT6 fusion protein+IC31 adjuvant	Olsen et al., 2004 Aagaard et al., 2011
SSI HyVac 4/AERAS-404	SSI/Sanori Pasteur/ Intercell/Aeras	Ag85B-TB10.4 fision protein+IC31 adjuvant	Dietrich et al., 2005, Skeikey et al., 2010
rBCG30	UCLA (M. Horwitz)/NIAID	Ag85B recombinant BCG	Horwitz et al., 2000
HVJ-liposome/ Hsp65 DNA+IL-12 DNA	Kinki-chuo Chest Medical Center (Okada)	Hsp65 DNA+IL-12 DNA + HVJ-liposome	Yoshida et al., 2006
Therapeutic Vaccines			
MVA85A	Oxford	Ag85A recombinant Vaccinia Virus	McShane et al., 2001, Goonetilleke et al., 2003, McShcane et al., 2004
Hsp65 DNA vaccine	Cardiff Univ. (D. Lowrie)	hsp65 DNA Vaccine	Lowrie et al., 1999

Table 3. TB vaccine candidates (According to WHO TB Vaccine Pipeline)

BCG vaccines and rBCG vaccines are considered to be priming vaccines. For priming vaccines, BCG overexpressing Ag85B (rBCG30) and *ureC*-deleting BCG expressing lysteriolysin O (ΔureC hly⁺ BCG) have been evaluated. For booster vaccines, Ag85A recombinant vaccinia virus (MVA85A), Ag85B-ESAT6 fusion protein with adjuvant (SSI Hybrid I), and Ag85B-TB10.4 fusion protein with adjuvant (SSI HyVac4/AERAS-404) have been examined. MVA85A and Hsp65 DNA vaccine are candidate TB vaccine are candidate therapeutic TB vaccines. Human studies using the prime-boost regimens by these TB vaccine candidates have been publishing. Tchilian and colleagues (2009) reported that priming with ΔureC hly⁺ BCG and boosting with MVA85A induced protective immunity against Mtb infection in mice. The protective effects were much higher in ΔureC hly⁺ BCG vaccination than that in parental BCG vaccination. MVA85A boost immunization enhanced

Ag85A-specific T-cell responses, but did not affect bacterial numbers in the lung after Mtb aerosol infection. Scriba and colleagues (2010) reported that vaccination with MVA85A in healthy adolescents and children from a TB endemic region, who received BCG at birth, is safe and induces polyfunctional CD4$^+$ T cells co-expressing IFN-γ, TNF-α, and IL-2. Further, Abel and colleagues (2010) reported that vaccination with AERAS-402 (Adenovirus type 35 expressing a fusion protein created from the sequences of Ag85A, Ag85B, and TB10.4) is safe and immunogenic in healthy South African BCG-vaccinated adults.

4. Conclusion

Mtb, a causative agent of TB, is a unique facultative intracellular bacterium. The cellular immunity is essential for protection against Mtb. The main effectors are type 1 CD4$^+$ T cells and CD8$^+$ T cells. IFN-γ produced from them has been considered to be important as biomarker of TB. Induction of appropriate immune responses against protective Mtb antigens in appropriate stages is necessary for preventing TB. Identification of protective Mtb antigens and the T-cell epitopes are critical for clarification of kinetics of TB and development of effective TB vaccines. A variety of TB vaccine strategies have been examined including rBCG and DNA vaccines. Prime-boost strategies with combination of different TB vaccines are promising for prophylactic TB vaccines. Therapeutic TB vaccines for latent TB have also been examined.

5. References

Aagaard C, Hoang T, Dietrich J, Cardona PJ, Izzo A, Dolganov G, Schoolnik GK, Cassidy JP, Billeskov R, Andersen P. (2011). A multistage tuberculosis vaccine that confers efficient protection before and after exposure. *Nature Medicine*, Vol.17, No. 2, (February 2011), pp. 189-194, ISSN 1078-8956

Abel, B., Tameris, M., Mansoor, N., Gelderbloem, S., Hughes, J., Abrahams, D., Makhethe, L., Erasmus, M., de Kock, M., van der Merwe, L., Hawkridge, A., Veldsman, A., Hatherill, M., Schirru, G., Pau, M. G., Hendriks, J., Weverling, G.J., Goudsmit, J., Sizemore, D., McClain, J.B., Goetz, M., Gearhart, J., Mahomed, H., Hussey, G. D., Sadoff, J. C. & Hanekom, W. A. (2010). The novel tuberculosis vaccine, AERAS-402, induces robust and polyfunctional CD4$^+$ and CD8$^+$ T cells in adults. *American Journal of Respiratory and Critical Care Medicine*, Vol. 181, No. 12, (June 2010), pp. 1407-1417, ISSN 1073-449X

Agger, E. M. & Andersen, P. (2001). Tuberculosis subunit vaccine development: on the role of interferon-γ. *Vaccine*, Vol. 19, No. 17-19, (March 2001), pp. 2298-2302, ISSN 0264-410X

Andersen, P. (1994). Effective vaccination of mice against *Mycobacterium tuberculosis* infection with a soluble mixture of secreted mycobacterial proteins. *Infection and Immunity*, Vol. 62, No. 6, (June 1994), pp. 2536-2544, ISSN 0019-9567

Andersen, P & Doherty, T.M. (2005). The success and failure of BCG — implications for a novel tuberculosis vaccine. *Nature Reviews Microbiology*, Vol.3, No. 8, (August 2005), pp. 656-662, ISSN 1740-1526

Andersen, P., Munk, M. E., Pollock, J. M. & Doherty, T. M. (2000). Specific immune-based diagnosis of tuberculosis. *Lancet*, Vol. 356, (September 2000), pp. 1099-1104, ISSN 0140-6736

Aoshi, T., Nagata, T., Suzuki, M., Uchijima, M., Hashimoto, D., Rafiei, A., Suda, T., Chida, K. & Koide, Y. (2008). Identification of an HLA-A*0201-restricted T-cell epitope on the MPT51 protein, a major secreted protein derived from *Mycobacterium tuberculosis*, by MPT51 overlapping peptide screening. *Infection and Immunity*, Vol.76, No. 4, (April 2008), pp. 1565-1571, ISSN 0019-9567

Beckman, E. M., Porcelli, S. A., Morita, C. T., Behar, S. M., Furlong, S. T. & Brenner, M. B. (1994). Recognition of a lipid antigen by CD1-restricted αβ+ T cells. *Nature*, Vol. 372, No. 6507, (December 1994), pp. 691-694, ISSN 0028-0836

Belisle, J. T., Braunstein, M., Rosenkrands, I. & Andersen, P. (2005). The proteome of *Mycobacterium tuberculosis*. In: *Tuberculosis and the tubercle bacillus*, S. T. Cole, K. D. Eisenach, D. N. McMurray & W. R. Jacobs Jr (Eds.), pp. 235-260, ASM Press, ISBN 1-55581-295-3, Washington, DC.

Belisle, J. T., Vissa, V. D., Sievert, T., Takayama, K., Brennan, P. J. & Besra, G. S. (1997). Role of the major antigen of *Mycobacterium tuberculosis* in cell wall biogenesis. *Science*, Vol.276, No. 5317, (May 1997), pp. 1420-1422, ISSN 0036-8075

Berthet, F. X., Rasmussen, P. B., Rosenkrands, I., Andersen, P. & Gicquel, B. (1998). A *Mycobacterium tuberculosis* operon encoding ESAT-6 and a novel low-molecular-mass culture filtrate protein (CFP-10). *Microbiology*, Vol. 144, (November 1998), pp. 3195-3203, ISSN 0026-2617

Bloom, B.R. & Fine, P.E.M. (1994). The BCG experience: implications for future vaccines against tuberculosis. In: *Tuberculosis: pathogenesis, protection, and control*, Bloom (Ed.), pp. 531-557, ASM Press, ISBN 1-55581-072-1, Washington, DC.

Blythe, M. J., Zhang, Q., Vaughan, K., de Castro Jr, R., Salimi, N., Bui, H. H., Lewinsohn, D. M., Ernst, J. D., Peters, B. & Sette, A. (2007). An analysis of the epitope knowledge related to Mycobacteria. *Immunome Research*, Vol. 3, No. 10, (December 2007), online, ISSN1745-7580.

Boesen, H., Jensen B. N., Wilcke, T. & Andersen, P. (1995). Human T-cell responses to secreted antigen fractions of *Mycobacterium tuberculosis*. *Infection and Immunity*, Vol. 63, No. 4, (April 1995), pp. 1491-1497, ISSN 0019-9567

Caccamo, N., Milano, S., Sano, C., Cigna, D., Ivanyi, J., Krensky, A. M., Dieli, F. & Salerno, A. (2002). Identification of epitopes of *Mycobacterium tuberculosis* 16-kDa protein recognized by human leukocyte antigen-A*0201 CD8+ T lymphocytes. *Journal of Infectious Diseases*, Vol. 186, No. 7, (October 2002), pp. 991-998, ISSN 0022-1899

Caruso, A. M., Serbina, N., Klein, E., Triebold, K., Bloom, B. R. & Flynn J. L. (1999). Mice deficient in CD4 T cells have only transiently diminished levels of IFN-γ, yet succumb to tuberculosis. *Journal of Immunology*, Vol. 162, No. 9, (May 1999), pp. 5407-5416, ISSN 0022-1767

Charo, J., Geluk, A., Sundbäck, M., Mirzai, B., Diehl, A. D., Malmberg, K.-J., Achour, A., Huriguchi, S., van Meijgaarden, K. E., Drijfhout, J.-W., Beekman, N., van Veelen, P., Ossendorp, F., Ottenhoff, T. H. M. & Kiessling, R. (2001). The identification of a common pathogen-specific HLA class I A*0201-restricted cytotoxic T cell epitope encoded within the heat shock protein 65. *European Journal of Immunology*, Vol.31, No. 12, (December 2001), pp. 3602-3611, ISSN 0014-2980

Cole, S. T., Brosch, R., Parkhill, J., Garunier, T., Churcher, C., Harris, D., Gordon, S. V., Eiglemeier, K., Gas, S., Barry III, C. E., Tekaia, F., Badcock, K., Basham, D., Brown, D., Chillingworth, T., Connor, R., Davies, R., Devlin, K., Feltwell, T., Gentles, S.,

Hamlin, N., Holroyd, S., Hornsby, T., Jagels, K., Krogh, A., McLean, J., Moule, S., Murphy, L., Oliver, K., Osborne, J., Quail, M. A., Rajandream, M.-A., Rogers, J., Rutter, S., Seeger, K., Skelton, J., Squares, R., Squares, S., Sulston, J. E., Taylor, K., Whitehead, S. & Barrell, B. G. (1998). Deciphering the biology of *Mycobacterium tuberculosis* from the complete genome sequence. *Nature*, Vol.393, No. 6707, (November 1998), pp. 537-544, ISSN 0028-0836

Commandeur, S., Lin, M. Y., van Meijgaarden, K. E., Friggen, A. H., Franken, K. L. M. C., Drijfhout, J. W., Korsvold, G. E., Oftung, F., Geluk, A. & Ottenhoff, T. H. M. (2011). Double- and monofunctional CD4+ and CD8+ T-cell responses to *Mycobacterium tuberculosis* DosR antigens and peptides in long-term latently infected individuals. *European Journal of Immunology*, in press, ISSN 0014-2980

Cooper, M. A. (2009). Cell-mediated immune responses in tuberculosis. *Annual Review of Immunology*, Vol.27, pp. 393-422, ISSN 0732-0582

Cooper, M. A., Dalton, D. K., Stewart, T. A., Griffin, J. P., Russell, D. G. & Orme, I. M. (1993). Disseminated tuberculosis in interferon γ gene-disrupted mice. *Journal of Experimental Medicine*, Vol. 178, No. 6, (December 1993), pp. 2243-2247, ISSN 0022-1007

Demissie, A., Leyten, F. M., Abebe, M., Wassie, L., Aseffa, A., Abate, G., Fletcher, H., Owiafe, P., Hill, P. C., Brookes, R., Rook, G., Zumla, A., Arend, S. M., Klein, M., Ottenhoff, T. H., Andersen, P., Doherty, T. M. & VACSEL Study Group. (2006). Recognition of stage-specific mycobacterial antigens differentiates between acute and latent infections with *Mycobacterium tuberculosis*. *Clinical and Vaccine Immunology*, Vol.13, No. 2, (February 2006), pp. 179-186, ISSN 1556-6811

Demissie, A., Ravn, P., Olobo, J., Doherty, T. M., Eguale, T., Geletu, M., Hailu, W., Andersen, P. & Britton, S. (1999). T-cell recognition of *Mycobacterium tuberculosis* culture filtrate fractions in tuberculosis patients and their household contacts. *Infection and Immunity*, Vol. 67, No. 11, (November 1999), pp. 5967-5971, ISSN 0019-9567

Denis, O., Tanghe, A., Palfliet, K., Jurion, F., van den Berg, T.-P., Vanonckelen, A., Ooms, J., Saman, E., Ulmer, J. B., Content, J. & Huygen, K. (1998): Vaccination with plasmid DNA encoding mycobacterial antigen 85A stimulates a CD4+ and CD8+ T-cell epitopic repertoire broader than that stimulated by *Mycobacterium tuberculosis* H37Rv infection. *Infection and Immunity*, Vol.66, No. 4, (April 1998), pp.1527-1533, ISSN 0019-9567

Derrick, S. C., Yang, A. L. & Morris, S. L. (2004). A polyvalent DNA vaccine expressing an ESAT6-Ag85B fusion protein protects mice against a primary infection with *Mycobacterium tuberculosis* and boosts BCG-induced protective immunity. *Vaccine*, Vol.23, No. 6, (December 2004), pp. 780-788, ISSN 0264-410X

Dietrich, J., Aagaard, C., Leah, R., Olsen, A. W., Stryhn, A., Doherty, T. M. & Andersen, P. (2005). Exchanging ESAT6 with TB10.4 in an Ag85B fusion molecule-based tuberculosis subunit vaccine: efficient protection and ESAT6-based sensitive monitoring of vaccine efficacy. *Journal of Immunology, Vol*.174, No. 10, (May 2005), pp. 6332-6339, ISSN 0022-1767

D'Souza, S., Rosseels, V., Denis, O., Tanghe, A., De Smet, N., Jurion, F., Palfliet, K., Castiglioni, N., Vanonckelen, A., Wheeler, C. & Huygen, K. (2002). Improved tuberculosis DNA vaccines by formulation in cationic lipids. *Infection and Immunity*, Vol.70, No. 7, (July 2002), pp. 3681-3688, ISSN 0019-9567

D'Souza, S., Rosseels, V., Romano, M., Tanghe, A., Denis, O., Jurion, F., Castiglione, N., Vanonckelen, A., Palfiliet, K., Huygen, K. (2003). Mapping of murine Th1 helper T-cell epitopes of mycolyl transferases Ag85A, Ag85B, and Ag85C from *Mycobacterium tuberculosis*. *Infection and Immunity*, Vol.71,No. 1, (January 2003), pp. 483-493, ISSN 0019-9567

Ellner, J. J., Hirsch, C. S. & Whalen, C. C. (2000). Correlates of protective immunity to *Mycobacterium tuberculosis* in humans. *Clinical Infectious Diseases*, Vol.30, Suppl. 3, (June 2000), pp. S279-S282, ISSN 1058-4838

Eweda, G., Suzuki D, Nagata T, Tsujimura K, Koide, Y. (2010). Identification of murine T-cell epitopes on low-molecular-mass secretory proteins (CFP11, CFP17, and TB18.5) of *Mycobacterium tuberculosis*. *Vaccine*, Vol.28, No. 29, (June 2010), pp. 4616-4625, ISSN 0264-410X

Falk, K., Rötzschke, O., Stevanović, S., Jung, G. & H. G. Rammensee, H. G. (1991). Allele-specific notifs revealed by sequencing of self-peptides eluted from MHC molecules. *Nature*, Vol.351, No. 6324, (May 1991), pp. 290-296, ISSN 0028-0836

Feng, C. G., Palendira, U., Demangel, C., Spratt, J. M., Malin, A. S. & Brittion, W. J. (2001). Priming by DNA immunization augments protective efficacy of *Mycobacterium bovis* Bacille Calmette-Guerin against tuberculosis. *Infection and Immunity*, Vol.69, No. 6, (June 2001), pp. 4174-4176, ISSN 0019-9567

Ferraz, J. C., Stavropoulos, E., Yang, M., Coade, S., Espitia, C., Lowrie, D. B., Colston, M. J. & Tascon, R. E. (2004). A heterologous DNA priming-*Mycobacterium bovis* BCG boosting immunization strategy using mycobacterial Hsp70, Hsp65, and Apa antigens improves protection against tuberculosis in mice. *Infection and Immunity*, Vol.72, No. 12, (December 2004), pp. 6945-6950, ISSN 0019-9567

Fine, P. E. M. (1995): Variation in protection by BCG: implications of and for heterologous immunity. *Lancet*, Vol.346, No. 8986, (November 1995), pp. 1339-1345, ISSN 0140-6736

Flynn, J. L. & Chan, J. (2001): Immunology of tuberculosis. *Annual Review Immunology*, Vol.19, pp. 93-129, ISSN 0732-0582

Flynn, J. L., Chan, J., Triebold, K. J., Dalton, D. K., Stewart, T. A. & Bloom, B. R. (1993). An essential role for interferon γ in resistance to *Mycobacterium tuberculosis*. *Journal of Experimental Medicine*, Vol. 178, No. 6, (December 1993), pp. 2249-2254, ISSN 0022-1007

Flynn, J. L., Goldstein, M. M., Triebold, K. J., Koller, B. & Bloom, B. R. (1992). Major histocompatibility complex class I-restricted T cells are required for resistance to *Mycobacterium tuberculosis* infection. *Proceedings of the National Academy of Sciences of the United States of America*, Vol.89, No. 24, (December 1992), pp. 12013-12017, ISSN 0027-8424

Geluk, A., Bloemhoff, W., De Vries, R. R. P. & Ottenhoff, T. H. M. (1992). Binding of a major T cell epitope of mycobacteria to a specific pocket within HLA-DRw17 (DR3) molecules. *European Journal of Immunology*, Vol.22, No. 1, (January 1992), pp. 107-113, ISSN 0014-2980

Geluk, A., Lin, M. Y., van Meijgaarden, K. E., Leyten, E. M., Franken, K. L., Ottenhoff, T. H. & Klein, M. R. (2007). T-cell recognition of the HspX protein of *Mycobacterium tuberculosis* correlates with latent *M. tuberculosis* infection but not with *M. bovis* BCG vaccination. *Infecion and Immunity*, Vol.75, No. 6, (June 2007), pp. 2914-2921, ISSN 0019-9567

Geluk, A., Taneja, V., van Meijgaarden, K. E., Zanelli, E., Abou-Zeid, C., Thole, J. E., de Vries, R. R., David, C. S. & Ottenhoff, T. H. (1998). Identification of HLA class II-restricted determinants of *Mycobacterium tuberculosis*-derived proteins by using HLA-transgenic, class II-deficient mice. *Proceedings of the National Academy of Science of the United States of America*, Vol. 95, No. 18, (September 1998), pp. 10797-10802, ISSN 0027-8424

Geluk, A., van Meijgaarden, K. E., Franken, K. L. M. C., Drijfhout, J. W., D'Souza, S., Neeker, A., Huygen, K. & Ottenhoff, T. H. M. (2000). Identification of major epitopes of *Mycobacterium tuberculosis* AG85B that are recognized by HLA-A*0201-restricted CD8+ T cells in HLA-transgenic mice and humans. *Journal of Immunology*, Vol.165, No. 11, (December 2000), pp. 6463-6471, ISSN 0022-1767

Goonetilleke, N. P., McShane, H., Hannan, C. M., Anderson, R. J., Brooks, R. H. & Hill, A. V. S. (2003). Enhanced immunigenicity and protective efficacy against *Mycobacterium tuberculosis* of bacille Calmette-Guerin vaccine using mucosal administration and boosting with a recombinant modified vaccinia virus Ankara. *Journal of Immunology*, Vol.171, No. 3, (Augsut 2003), pp. 1602-1609, ISSN 0022-1767

Grode, L., Seiler, P., Baumann, S., Hess, J., Brinkmann, V., Eddine, A. N., Mann, P., Goosmann, C., Bandermann, S., Smith, D., Bancroft, G. J., Reyrat, J.-M., van Soolingen, D., Raupach, B. & Kaufmann, S. H. E. (2005). Increased vaccine efficacy against tuberculosis of recombinant *Mycobacterium bovis* bacille Calmette-Guérin mutants that secrete listeriolysin. *Journal of Clinical Investigation*, Vol.115, No. 9, (September 2005), pp. 2472-2479, ISSN 0021-9738

Guleria, I., Teitelbaum, R., McAdam, R. A., Kalpana, G., Jacobs Jr, W. R. & Bloom, B. R. (1996). Auxotrophic vaccines for tuberculosis. *Nature Medicine*, Vol.2, No. 3, (March 1996), pp. 334-337, ISSN 1078-8956

Hess, J., Miko, D., Catic, A., Lehmensiek, V., Russell, D. G. & Kaufmann, S. H. (1998). *Mycobacterium bovis* Bacille Calmette-Guérin strains secreting listeriolysin of *Listeria monocytogenes*. *Proceedings of the National Academy of Sciences of the United States of America*, Vol.95, No. 9, (April 1998), pp. 5299-5304, ISSN 0027-8424

Hoft, D. F. (2008). Tuberculosis vaccine development: goals, immunological design, and evaluation. *Lancet*, Vol. 372, No. 9633, (July 2008), pp. 164-175, ISSN 0140-6736

Horwitz, M. A., Harth, G., Dillon, B. J. & Masleša-Galić, S. (2000). Recombinant bacillus Calmette-Guérin (BCG) vaccines expressing the *Mycobacterium tuberculosis* 30-kDa major secretory protein induce greater protective immunity against tuberculosis than conventional BCG vaccines in a highly susceptible animal model. *Proceedings of the National Academy of Sciences of the United States of America*, Vol.97, No. 25, (December 2000), pp. 13853-13858, ISSN 0027-8424

Hu, Y., Movahedzadeh, F., Stoker, N. G. & Coates, A. R. (2006). Deletion of the *Mycobacterium tuberculosis* α-crystallin-like *hspX* gene causes increased bacterial growth in vivo. *Infection and Immunity*, Vol.74, No. 2, (February 2006), pp. 861-868, ISSN 0019-9567

Huygen, K. (2003). On the use of DNA vaccines for the prophylaxis of mycobacterial diseases. *Infecion and Immunity*, Vol.71, No. 4, (April 2003), pp. 1613-1621, ISSN 0019-9567

Huygen, K., Content, J., Denis, O., Montgomery, D. L., Yawman, A. M., Deck, R. R., DeWitt, C. M., Orme, I. M., Baldwin, S., D'Souza, C., Drowart, A., Lozes, E., Vandenbussche, P., Van Vooren, J.-P., Liu, M. A. & Ulmer, J. B. (1996). Immunogenicity and protective efficacy of a tuberculosis DNA vaccine. *Nature Medicine*, Vol.2, No. 8, (August 1996), pp. 893-898, ISSN 1078-8956

Junqueira-Kipnis, A. P., Kipnis, A., Jamieson, A., Juarrero, M. G., Diefenbach, A., Raulet, D. H., Turner, J. & Orme, I. M. (2003). NK cells respond to pulmonary infection with *Mycobacterium tuberculosis*, but play a minimal role in protection. *Journal of Immunology*, Vol.171, No. 11, (December 2003), pp. 6039-6045, ISSN 0022-1767

Karakousis, R. C., Yoshimatsu, T., Lamichhane, G., Wookwine, S. C., Nuermberger, E. L., Grosset, J. & Bishai, W. R. (2004). Dormancy phenotype displayed by extracellular *Mycobacterium tuberculosis* within artificial granulomas in mice. *Journal of Experimental Medicine*, Vol.200, No. 5, (September 2004), pp. 647-657, ISSN 0022-1007

Kaufmann, S. H. E. (2003). Immunity to intracellular bacteria, In: *Fundamental Immunology, 5th edition*, W. E. Paul (Ed.), pp. 1229-1261, Lippincott Williams & Wilkins Publishers, ISBN 0-7817-3514-9, Philadelphia.

Kaufmann, S. H. E. (2010a). New vaccines for tuberculosis. *Lancet*, Vol. 375, No. 9731, (June 2010), pp. 2110-2119, ISSN 0140-6736

Kaufmann, S.H.E. (2010b). Future vaccination strategies against tuberculosis: Thinking outside the box. *Immunity*, Vol.33, No. 4, (October 2010), pp. 567-577, ISSN 1074-7613

Kaufumann, S.H.E. & Flynn, J.L. (2005). CD8 T cells in tuberculosis. In: *Tuberculosis and the tubercle bacillus*, S. T. Cole, K. D. Eisenach, D. N. McMurray & W. R. Jacobs Jr (Eds.), pp. 465-474, ASM Press, ISBN 1-55581-295-3, Washington, DC.

Khader, S. A., Bell, G. K., Pearl, J. E., Fountain, J. J., Rangel-Moreno, J., Cilley, G. E., Shen, F., Eaton, S. M., Gaffen, S. L., Swain, S. L., Locksley, R. M., Haynes, L., Randall, T. D. & Cooper, A. M. (2007). IL-23 and IL-17 in the establishment of protective pulmonary CD4+ T cell responses after vaccination and during *Mycobacterium tuberculosis* challenge. *Nature Immunology*, Vol.8, No. 4, (April 2007), pp. 369-377, ISSN 1529-2908

Kursar, M., Koch, M., Mittrücker, H. W., Nouailles, G., Bonhagen, K., Kamradt, T. & Kaufmann, S. H. (2007). Regulatory T cells prevent efficient clearance of *Mycobacterium tuberculosis*. *Journal of Immunology*, Vol. 178, No. 5, (March 2007), pp.2661-2665, ISSN 0022-1767

Ladel, C. H., Daugelat, S. & Kaufmann, S. H. E. (1995). Immune response to *Mycobacterium bovis* bacille Calmette Guérin infection in major histocompatibility complex class I- and II-deficient knock-out mice: contribution of CD4 and CD8 T cells to acquired resistance. *European Journal of Immunology*, Vol.25, No. 2, (February 1995), pp. 377-384, ISSN 0014-2980

Lalvani, A., Brookes, R., Wilkinson, R. J., Malin, A. S., Pathan, A. A., Andersen, P., Dockrell, H., Pasvol, G. & Hill, A. V. (1998). Human cytolytic and interferon γ-secreting CD8+ T lymphocytes specific for *Mycobacterium tuberculosis*. *Proceedings of the National Academy of Sciences of the United States of America*, Vol.95, No. 1, (January 1998), pp. 270-275, ISSN 0027-8424

Larsen, M. H., Biermann, K., Chen, B., Hsu, T., Sambandamurthy, V. K., Lackner, A. A., Aye, P. P., Didier, P., Huang, D., Shao, L., Wei, H., Letvin, N. L., Frothingham, R., Haynes, B. F., Chen, Z. W. & Jacobs Jr., W. R. (2009). Efficacy and safety of live attenuated persistent and rapidly cleared *Mycobacterium tuberculosis* vaccine candidates in non-human primates. *Vaccine*, Vol. 27, No. 34, (July 2009), pp. 4709-4717, ISSN 0264-410X

Lee, B.-Y. & Horwitz, M. A. (1995). Identification of macrophage and stress-induced proteins of *Mycobacterium tuberculosis*. *Journal of Clinical Investigation*, Vol. 96, No. 1, (July 1995), pp. 245-249, ISSN 0021-9738

Li, S., Rodrigues, M., Rodriguez, D., Rodriguez, J. R., Esteban, M., Palese, P., Nussenzweig, R. S. & Zavala, F. (1993). Priming with recombinant influenza virus followed by administration of recombinant vaccinia virus induces CD8+ T-cell-mediated protective immunity against malaria. *Proceedings of the National Academy of Science of the United States of America*, Vol. 90, No. 11, (June 1993), pp. 5214-5218, ISSN 0027-8424

Li, Z., Zhang, H., Fan, X., Zhang, Y., Huang, J., Liu, Q., Tjelle, T. E., Mathiesen, I., Kjeken, R. & Xiong, S. (2006). DNA electroporation prime and protein boost strategy enhances humoral immunity of tuberculosis DNA vaccines in mice and non-human primates. *Vaccine*, Vol.24, No. 21, (May 2006), pp. 4565-4568, ISSN 0264-410X

Lowrie, D B., Tascon, R. E., Bonato, V. L. D., Lima, V. M. F., Faccioli, L. H., Stavropoulos, E., Colston, M. J., Hewinson, R. G., Moelling, K. & Silva, C. L. (1999). Therapy of tuberculosis in mice by DNA vaccination. *Nature*, Vol.400, No. 6741, (July 1999), pp. 269-271, ISSN 0028-0836

Matsumoto, S., Matsumoto, M., Umemori, K., Ozeki, Y., Furugen, M., Tatsuo, T., Hirayama, Y., Yamamoto, S., Yamada, T., Kobayashi, K. (2005). DNA augments antigenicity of mycobacterial DNA-binding protein 1 and confers protection against *Mycobacterium tuberculosis* infection in mice. *Journal of Immunology*, Vol. 175, No. 1, (July 2005), pp. 441-449, ISSN 0022-1767

Mazzaccaro, R. J., Gedde, M., Jensen, E. R., van Santen, H. M., Ploegh, H. L., Rock, K. L. & Bloom, B. R. (1996). Major histocompatibility complex class I presentation of soluble antigen facilitated by *Mycobacterium tuberculosis* infection. *Proceedings of the National Academy of Sciences of the United States of America*, Vol.93, No. 21, (October 1996), pp. 11786-11791, ISSN 0027-8424

McShane, H., Brookes, R., Gilbert, S. C. & Hill, A. V. S. (2001). Enhanced immunogenicity of CD4+ T-cell responses and protective efficacy of a DNA-modified vaccinia virus Ankara prime-boost vaccination regimen for murine tuberculosis. *Infection and Immunity*, Vol.69, No. 2, (February 2001), pp. 681-686, ISSN 0019-9567

McShane, H. & A. Hill, A. (2005). Prime-boost immunisation strategies for tuberculosis. *Microbes and Infection*, vol. 7, No. 5-6, (May 2005), pp. 962-967, ISSN 1286-4579

McShane, H., Pathan, A. A., Sander, C. R., Keating, S. M., Gilbert, S. C., Huygen, K., Fletcher, H. A. & Hill, A. V. S. (2004). Recombinant modified vaccinia virus Ankara expressing antigen 85A boosts BCG-primed and naturally acquired antimycobacterial immunity in humans. *Nature Medicine*, Vol.10, No. 11, (November 2004), pp. 1240-1244, ISSN 1078-8956

Miki, K., Nagata, T., Tanaka, T., Kim, Y. H., Uchijima, M., Ohara, N., Nakamura, S, Okada, M. & Koide, Y. (2004). Induction of protective cellular immunity against

Mycobacterium tuberculosis by recombinant attenuated self-destructing *Listeria monocytogenes* strains harboring eukaryotic expression plasmids for antigen 85 complex and MPB/MPT51. *Infection and Immunity*, Vol.72, No. 4, (April 2004), pp. 2014-2021, ISSN 0019-9567

Mustafa, A. S., Oftung, F., Amoudy, H. A., Madi, N. M., Abal, A. T., Shaban, F., Krands, I. R. & Andersen, P. (2000a). Multiple epitopes from the *Mycobacterium tuberculosis* ESAT-6 antigen are recognize by antigen-specific human T cell lines. *Clinical Infectious Diseases* Vol.30 (Suppl. 3), (June 2000), pp. S201-S205, ISSN 1058-4838

Mustafa, A. S., Shaban, F. A., Abal, A. T., Al-Attiyah, R., Wiker, H. G., Lundin, K. E. A., Oftung, F. & Huygen, K. (2000b). Identification and HLA restriction of naturally derived Th1-cell epitopes from the secreted *Mycobacterium tuberculosis* antigen 85B recognized by antigen-specific human CD4+ T-cell lines. *Infection and Immunity*, Vol.68, No. 7, (July 2000), pp. 3933-3940, ISSN 0019-9567

Nagai, S., Wiker, H. G., Harboe, M. & Kinomoto, M. (1991). Isolation and partial characterization of major protein antigens in the culture fluid of *Mycobacterium tuberculosis*. *Infection and Immunity*, Vol.59, No. 1, (January 1991), 372-382, ISSN 0019-9567

North, R. J. & Jung, Y. J. (2004). Immunity to tuberculosis. *Annual Review of Immunology*, Vol.22, pp. 599-623, ISSN 0732-0582

Ohara, N., Kitaura, H., Hotokezaka, H., Nishiyama, T., Wada, N., Matsumoto, S., Matsuo, T., Naito, M. & Yamada, T. (1995). Characterization of the gene encoding the MPB51, one of the major secreted protein antigens of *Mycobacterium bovis* BCG, and identification of the secreted protein closely related to the fibronectic binding 85 complex. *Scandinavian Journal of Immunology*, Vol.41, No. 5, (May 1995), pp. 433-442, ISSN 0300-9475

Olsen, A. W., Williams, A., Okkels, L. M., Hatch, G. & Andersen, P. (2004). Protective effect of a tuberculosis subunit vaccine based on a fusion of antigen 85B and ESAT-6 in the aerosol guinea pig model. *Infection and Immunity*, Vol.72, No. 10, (October 2004), pp. 6148-6150, ISSN 0019-9567

Orme, I. A. (1988). Induction of nonspecific acquired resistance and delayed-type hypersensitivity, but not specific acquired resistance, in mice inoculated with killed mycobacterial vaccines. *Infection and Immunity*, Vol.56, No. 12, (December 1988), pp. 3310-3312, ISSN 0019-9567

Ottenhoff, T. H., Kumamaratne, D. & Casanova, J. L. (1998). Novel human immunodeficiencies reveal the essential role of type-I cytokines in immunity to intracellular bacteria. *Immunology Today*, Vol.19, No. 11, (November 1998), pp. 491-494, ISSN 1471-4906

Parker, K. C., Bednarek, M. A. & Coligan, J. E. (1994). Scheme for ranking potential HLA-A2 binding peptides based on independent binding of individual peptide side-chains. *Journal of Immunology*, Vol.152, No. 1, (January 1994), pp. 163-175.

Pethe, K., Alonso, S., Blet, F., Delogu, G., Brennan, M. J., Locht, C. & Menozzi, F. D. (2001). The heparin-binding haemagglutinin of *M. Tuberculosis* is required for extrapulmonary dissemination. *Nature*, Vol.412, No. 6843, (July 2001), pp. 190-194, ISSN 0028-0836

Radošević, K., Wieland, C. W., Rodriguez, A., Weverling, G. J., Mintardjo, R., Gillissen, G., Vogels, R., Skeiky, Y. A. W., Hone, D. M., Sadoff, J. C., van der Poll, T., Havenga,

M. & Goudsmit, J. (2007). Protective immune responses to a recombinant adenovirus type 35 tuberculosis vaccine in two mouse strains: CD4 and CD8 T-cell epitope mapping and role of gamma interferon. *Infection and Immunity*, Vol.75, no. 8, (August 2007), pp. 4105-4115, ISSN 0019-9567

Ramshow, I. A. & Ramsay, A. J. (2000). The prime-boost strategy: exciting prospects for improved vaccination. *Immunology Today*, Vol.21, No. 4, (April 2000), pp. 163-165, ISSN 0167-5699

Rammensee, H.-G., Bachmann, J., Emmerich, N. P. N., Bachor, O. A. & Stevanović, S. (1999). SYFPEITHI: database for MHC ligands and peptide. *Immunogenetics*, Vol.50, No. 3-4, (November 1999), pp. 213-219, ISSN 0093-7711

Reche, P. A., Glutting, J. P., Zhang, H. & Renherz, E. L. (2004). Enhancement to the RANKPEP resource for the prediction of peptide binding to MHC molecules using profiles. *Immunogenetics*, Vol. 56, No. 6, (September 2004), pp. 405-419, ISSN 0093-7711

Repique, C. J., Li, A., Collins, F. M. & Morris, S. L. (2002). DNA immunization in a mouse model of latent tuberculosis: effect of DNA vaccination on reactivation of disease and on reinfection with a secondary challenge. *Infection and Immunity*, Vol.70, No. 7, (July 2002), pp. 3318-3323, ISSN 0019 9567

Rodrigues, L. C., Diwan, V. K. & Wheeler, J. G. (1993). Protective effect of BCG against tuberculosis meningitis and miliary tuberculosis: a meta-analysis. *International Journal of Epidemiology*, (December 1993), Vol.22, No. 6, pp. 1154-1158, ISSN 0300-5771

Romano, M., D'Souza, S., Adnet, P.-Y., Laali, R., Jurion, F., Palfliet, K. & Huygen, K. (2006). Priming but not boosting with plasmid DNA encoding mycolyl-transferase Ag85A from *Mycobacterium tuberculosis* increases the survival time of *Mycobacterium bovis* BCG vaccinated nice against low dose intravenous challenge with *M. tuberculosis* H37Rv. *Vaccine*, Vol.24, No. 16, (April 2006), pp. 3353-3364, ISSN 0264-410X

Roupie, V., Romano, M., Zhang, L., Korf, H., Lin, M Y., Franken, K. L. M. C., Ottenhoff, T. H. M., Klein, M. R. & Huygen, K. (2007). Immunogenicity of eight dormancy regulon-encoded proteins of *Mycobacterium tuberculosis* in DNA-vaccinated and tuberculosis-infected mice. *Infection and Immunity*, Vol.75, No. 2, (February 2007), pp. 941-949, ISSN 0019-9567

Ruppert, J., Sidney, J., E. Celis, E., Kubo, R. T., Grey, H. M. & Sette, A. (1993). Prominent role of secondary anchor residues in peptide binding to HLA-A2.1 molecules. *Cell*, Vol.74, No. 5, (September 1993), pp. 929-937, ISSN 0092-8674

Sakula, A. (1983). Robert Koch: centenary of the discovery of the tubercle bacillus, 1882. *Canadian Veterinary Journal*, Vol. 24, No. 4, (April 1983), pp. 127-131. ISSN 0008-5286

Sambandamurthy, V. K., Derrick, S. C., Hsu, T., Chen, B., Larsen, M. H., Jalapathy, K. V., Chen, M., Kim, J., Porcelli, S. A., Chan, J., Morris, S. L. & Jacobs Jr., W. R. (2006). *Mycobacterium tuberculosis* ΔRD1 ΔpanCD: A safe and limited replicating mutant strain that protects immunocompetent and immunocompromised mice against experimental tuberculosis. *Vaccine*, Vol.24, No. 37-39, (September 2006), pp. 6309-6320, ISSN 0264-410X

Scriba, T. J., Tameris, M., Mansoor, N., Smit, E., van der Merwe, L., Isaacs, F., Keyser, A., Moyo, S., Brittain, N., Lawrie, A., Gelderbloem, S., Veldsman, A., Hatherill, M., Hawkridge, A., Hill, A. V., Hussey, G. D., Mahomed, H., McShane, H. & Hanekom,

W. A. (2010). Modified vaccinia Ankara-expressing Ag85A, a novel tuberculosis vaccine, is safe in adolescents and children, and induces polyfunctional CD4+ T cells. *European Journal of Immunology*, Vol. 40, No. 1, (January 2010), pp. 279-290, ISSN 0014-2980

Shen, Y., Zhou, D., Lai, X., Simon, M., Shen, L., Kou, Z., Wang, Q., Jiang, L., Estep, J., Hunt, R., Clagett, M., Sehgal, P. K., Li, Y., Zeng, X., Morita, C. T., Brenner, M. B., Letvin, N. L. & Chen, Z. W. (2002). Adaptive immune response of Vγ2Vδ2+ Tcells during mycobacterial infections. *Science*, Vol.295, No. 5563, (March 2002), pp. 2255-2258, ISSN 0036-8075

Singh, H. & Raghava, G.P.S. (2001). ProPred: prediction of HLA-DR binding sites. *Bioinformatics*, Vol.17, No. 12, (December 2001), pp. 1236-1237. ISSN 1367-4803

Skeiky, Y. A. W., Alderson, M. R., Overndale, P. J., Guderian, J. A., Brandt, L., Dillon, D. C., Campos-Neto, A., Lobet, Y., Dalemans, W., Orme, I. M. & Reed, S. G. (2004). Differential immune responses and protective efficacy induced by components of a tuberculosis polyprotein vaccine, Mtb72F, delivered as naked DNA or recombinant protein. *Journal of Immunology*, Vol.172. No. 12, (June 2004), pp. 7618-7628, ISSN 0022-1767

Skeiky, Y. A. W., Diethrich, J., Lasco, T. M., Stagliano, K., Dheenadhayalan, V., Goetz, M. A., Cantarero, L., Basaraba, R. J., Bang, P., Kromann, I., McMclain, J. B., Sadoff, J. C. & Andersen, P. (2010). Non-clinical efficacy and safety of HyVac4:IC31 vaccine administered in a BCG prime-boost regimen. *Vaccine*, Vol.28, No. 4, (January 2010), pp. 1084-1093, ISSN 0264-410X

Skinner, M. A., Ramsay, A. J., Buchan, G. S., Keen, D. L., Ranasinghe, C., Slobbe, L., Collins, D. M., De Lisle, G. W. & Buddle, B. M. (2003). A DNA prime-live vaccine boost strategy in mice can augment IFN-γ responses to mycobacterial antigens but does not increase the protective efficacy of two attenuated strains of *Mycobacterium bovis* against bovine tuberculosis. *Immunology*, vol. 108, No. 4, (April 2003), pp. 548-555, ISSN 0019-2805

Smith, S. M., Brookes, R., Klein, A. S., Malin, A. S., Lukey, P. T., King, A. S., Ogg, G. S., Hill, A. V. & Dockrell, H. M. (2000). Human CD8+ CTL specific for the mycobacterial major secreted antigen 85A. *Journal of Immunology*, Vol. 165, No. 12, (December 2000), pp. 7088-7095, ISSN 0022-1767

Smith, S.M. & Duckrell, H.M. (2000). Role of CD8+ T cells in mycobacterial infections. *Immunology and Cell Biology*, Vol.78, No. 4, (August 2000), pp. 325-333, ISSN 0818-9641

Stegelmann, F., Bastian, M., Swoboda, K., Bhat, R., Kiessler, V., Krensky, A. M., Roellinghoff, M., Modlin, R. L. & Stenger, S. (2005). Coordinate expression of CC chemokine ligand 5, granulysin, and perforin in CD8+ T cells provides a host defense mechanism against *Mycobacterium tuberculosis*. *Journal of Immunology*, Vol. 175, No. 11, (December 2005), pp. 7474-7483, ISSN 0022-1767

Stenger, S., Mazzaccaro, R. J., Uyemura, K., Cho, S., Barnes, P. F., Rosat, J. P., Sette, A., Brenner, M. B., Porcelli, S. A., Bloom, B. R. & Modlin, R. L. (1997): Defferential effects of cytolytic T cell subsets on intracellular infection. *Science*, Vol.276, No. 5319, (June 1997), pp. 1684-1687, ISSN 0036-8075

Stenger, S.R. & Modlin, L. (1999). T cell mediated immunity to *Mycobacterium tuberculosis*. *Current Opinion in Microbiology*, Vol.2, No. 1, (February 1999), pp. 89-93, ISSN 1369-5274

Sterne, J.A.C., Rodrigues, L.C. & Guedes, I.N. (1998). Does the efficacy of BCG decline with time since vaccination? *Internation Journal of Tuberculosis and Lung Disease*, Vol.2, No. 3, pp. 200-207, ISSN 1027-3719

Stover, C. K., de la Cruz, V. F., Fuerst, T. R., Burlein, J. E., Benson, L. A., Bennett, L. T., Bansal, G. P., Young, J. F., Lee, M. H., Hatfull, G. F., Snapper, S. B., Barletta, R. G., Jacobs Jr., W. R. & Bloom, B. R. (1991). New use of BCG for recombinant vaccines. *Nature*, Vol.351, No. 6326, (June 1991), pp. 456-460, ISSN 0028-0836

Sugawara, I., Yamada, H., Udagawa, T. & Huygen, K. (2003). Vaccination of guinea pigs with DNA encoding Ag85A by gene gun bombardment. *Tuberculosis (Edinb)*, Vol.83, No. 6, (June 2003), pp. 331-337, ISSN 1472-9792

Suzuki, D., Nagata, T., Eweda, G., Matsumoto, S., Matsumoto, M., Tsujimura, K. & Koide, Y. (2010). Characterization of murine T-cell epitopes on mycobacterial DNA-binding protein 1 (MDP1) using DNA vaccination. *Vaccine*, Vol.28, No. 8, (February 2010), pp. 2020-2025, ISSN 0264-410X

Suzuki, M., Aoshi, T., Nagata, T. & Koide, Y. (2004). Identification of murine H2-D^d- and H2-A^b-restricted T-cell epitopes on a novel protective antigen, MPT51, of *Mycobacterium tuberculosis*. *Infection and Immunity*, Vol.72, No. 7, (July 2004), pp. 3829-3837, ISSN 0019-9567

Tang, S. T., van Meijgaarden, K. E., Caccamo, N., Guggino, G., Klein, M. R., van Weeren, P., Kazi, F., Stryhn, A., Zaigler, A., Sahin, U., Buus, S., Dieli, F., Lund, O. & Ottenhoff, T. H. (2011). Genome-based in silico identification of new *Mycobacterium tuberculosis* antigens activating polyfunctional CD8+ T cells in human tuberculosis. *Journal of Immunology*, Vol. 186, No. 2, (January 2011), pp.1068-1080, ISSN 0022-1767

Tanghe, A., Denis, O., Lambrecht, B., Motte, V., van den Berg, T. & Huygen, K. (2000). Tuberculosis DNA vaccine encoding Ag85A is immunogenic and protective when administered by intramuscular needle injection but not by epidermal gene gun bombardment. *Infection and Immunity*, Vol.68, No. 7, (July 2000), pp. 3854-3860, ISSN 0019-9567

Tascon, R. E., Colston, M. J., Ragno, S., Stavropoulos, E., Gregory, D. & Lowrie, D. B. (1996). Vaccination against tuberculosis by DNA injection. *Nature Medicine*, Vol.2, No. 8, (August 1996), pp. 888-892, ISSN 1078-8956

Tascon, R. E., Stavropoulos, E., Lukacs, K. V. & Colston, M. J. (1998). Protection against *Mycobacterium tuberculosis* infection by CD8+ T cells requires the production of gamma interferon. *Infecion and Immunity*, Vol.66, No. 2, (February 1998), pp. 830-834, ISSN 0019-9567

Taylor, J. L., Turner, O. C., Basaraba, R. J., Belisle, J. T., Huygen, K. & Orme, I. M. (2003). Pulmonary necrosis resulting from DNA vaccination against tuberculosis. *Infection and Immunity*, Vol.71, No. 4, (April 2003), pp. 2192-2198, ISSN 0019-9567

Tchilian, E. Z., Desel, C., Forbes, E. K., Bandermann, S., Sander, C. R., Hill, A. V. S., McShane, H. & Kaufmann, S. H. E. (2009). Immunogenicity and protective efficacy of prime-boost regimens with recombinant ΔureC hly+ *Mycobacterium bovis* BCG and modified vaccinina virus Ankara expressing *M. Tuberculosis* antigen 85A against murine tuberculosis. *Infection and Immunity*, Vol. 77, No. 2, (February 2009), pp. 622-631, ISSN 0019-9567

Teitelbaum, R., Gratman-Freedman, A., Chen, B., Robbins, J. B., Unanue, E., Casadevall, A. & Bloom, B. R. (1998). A mAb recognizing a surface antigen of *Mycobacterium tuberculosis* enhances host survival. *Proceedings of the National Academy of Science of the United States of America*, Vol. 95, No. 26, (December 1998), pp. 15688-15693, ISSN 0027-8424

Tollefsen, S., Tjelle, T. E., Schneider, J. Harboe, M., Wiker, H. G., Hewinson, G., Huygen, K. & Mathiesen, I. (2002). Improved cellular and humoral immune responses against *Mycobacterium tuberculosis* antigens after intramuscular DNA immunisation combined with muscle electroporation. *Vaccine*, Vol.20, No. 27-28, (September 2002), pp. 3370-3378, ISSN 0264-410X

Turner, J., Rhoades, E. R., Keen, M., Belisle, J. T., Frank, A. A. & Orme, I. M. (2000). Effective preexposure tuberuclosis vaccines fail to protect when they are given in an immunotherapeutic mode. *Infection and Immunity*, Vol. 68, No. 3, (March 2000), pp. 1706-1709, ISSN 0019-9567

van Pinxteren, L. A. H., Cassidy, J. P., Smedegaard, B. H. C., Agger, E. M. & Anersen, P. (2000). Control of latent *Mycobacterium tuberculosis* infection is dependent on CD8 T cells. *European Journal of Immunology*, Vol.30, No. 12, (December 2000), pp. 3689-3698, ISSN 0014-2980

Walzl, G., Ronacher, K., Hanekom, W., Scriba, T. J. & Zumla, A. (2011). Immunological biomarkers of tuberculosis. *Nature Reviews Immunology*, Vol.11, No. 5, (May 2011), pp. 343-354, ISSN 1474-1733

Wang, L. X., Nagata, T., Tsujimura, K., Uchijima, M., Seto, S. & Koide, Y. (2009). Identification of HLA-DR4-restricted T-cell epitope on MPT51 protein, a major secreted protein derived from *Mycobacterium tuberculosis* using MPT51 overlapping peptides screening. *Vaccine*, Vol.28, No. 8, (February 2009), pp. 2026-2031, ISSN 0264-410X

Wiker, H. G. & Harboe, M. (1992). The antigen 85 complex: a major secretion product of *Mycobacterium tuberculosis*. *Microbiological Reviews*, Vol.56, No. 4, (December 1992), pp. 648-661, ISSN 1092-2172

Winau, F., Weber, S., Sad, S., de Diego, J., Hoops, S. L., Breiden, B., Sandhoff, K., Brinkmann, V., Kaufmann, S. H. E. & Schaible, U. E. (2006). Apoptotic vesicles crossprime CD8 T cells and protect against tuberculosis. *Immunity*, Vol.24, No. 1, (January 2006), pp. 105-117, ISSN 1074-7613

World Health Organization. (2010). *WHO Report 2010 Global tuberculosis control*. Available from http://www.who.int/tb/publications/global_report/2010/pdf/full_report.pdf.

Yoshida, A., Nagata, T., Uchijima, M., Higashi, T. & Koide, Y. (2000). Advantage of gene gun-mediated over intramuscular inoculation of plasmid DNA vaccine in reproducible induction of specific immune responses. *Vaccine*, Vol.18, No. 17, (March 2000), pp. 1725-1729, ISSN 0264-410X

Yoshida, S., Tanaka, T., Kita, Y., Kuwayama, S., Kanamaru, N., Muraki, Y., Hashimoto, S., Inoue, Y., Sakatani, M., Kobayashi, E., Kaneda, Y. & Okada, M. (2006). DNA vaccine using hemagglutinating virus of Japan-liposome encapsulating combination encoding mycobacterial heat shock protein 65 and interleukin-12 confers protection against *Mycobacterium tuberculosis* by T cell activation. *Vaccine*, Vol.24, No. 8, (February 2006), pp. 1191-1204, ISSN 0264-410X

Zhang, X., Divangahi, M., Ngai, P., Santosuosso, M., Millar, J., Zganiacz, A., Wang, J., Bramson, J. & Xing, Z. (2007). Intramuscular immunization with a monogenic plasmid DNA tuberculosis vaccine: Enhanced immunogenicity by electroporation and co-expression of GM-CSF transgene. *Vaccine*, Vol.25, No. 7, (January 2007), pp. 1342-1352, ISSN 0264-410X

2

Vaccines Against *Mycobacterium tuberculosis*: An Overview from Preclinical Animal Studies to the Clinic

Rhea N. Coler, Susan L. Baldwin, and Steven G. Reed

Infectious Disease Research Institute (IDRI) Seattle,
USA

1. Introduction

More than a decade ago the World Health Organization (WHO) declared tuberculosis (TB) a global emergency and called on the biomedical community to strengthen its efforts to combat this scourge. The WHO predicts that by 2020 almost one billion people will be infected, with 35 million dying from the disease if research for new approaches to the management of this disease is unsuccessful (1). Designing a better TB vaccine is a high priority research goal. This chapter will review the various strategies currently being used to prevent and treat TB. In spite of the numerous new vaccine candidates in clinical trials, and several others in the preclinical pipeline, no clear TB vaccine development strategy has emerged.

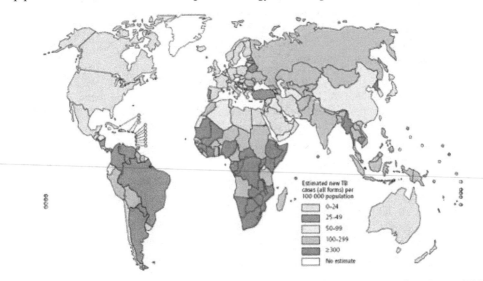

Fig. 1. Estimated TB incidence rates, by country, 2009 [http://para410.com/biophysical(2)].

Despite TB control programs, *Mycobacterium tuberculosis* (Mtb), a facultative bacterial pathogen, remains the most common cause of infectious disease-related mortality worldwide. Nearly 2 billion people are estimated to be infected with TB. Figure 1 shows the global distribution of TB incidence rates in 2009. Nearly 10 million individuals developed active TB globally (range, 8.9 million–9.9 million; equivalent to 137 cases per 100,000 population), and 1.7 million HIV-negative and HIV-positive people died of TB or related complications (3). TB has now become the leading cause of death in HIV-positive patients and is thought to accelerate the progression of HIV disease (4). Worldwide, 1 in every 3 people is infected with Mtb (5) and may harbor *Mycobacterium* bacilli in their lungs, thus serving as an important reservoir (6). Most of these TB cases occur in India, China, Africa and Indonesia, where 1 in every 8 deaths is a result of TB (7).

Resistance to single anti-mycobacterial agents has long been recognized. Fortunately, the standardized use of multiple agents to treat active disease and the common use of directly observed therapy (DOT), where a health care worker ensures chemotherapy regimens are taken by patients as recommended, have made a significant impact on mitigating treatment regimens and mortality. Unfortunately, the evolution of drug resistance has led to the emergence of TB strains resistant to multiple agents, including those medications used as standard first-line therapies. Fifty million of those infected have multi-drug resistant (MDR)-TB, a disease caused by Mtb strains that are resistant to both isoniazid and rifampicin with or without resistance to other first line drugs. The incidence of MDR-TB is rapidly growing, and the total number of estimated cases has steadily increased. The estimated global incidence of MDR-TB was 275,000 cases in 2000 and 440,000 cases in 2008 (8, 9). Nevertheless, the true prevalence of MDR-TB is likely under-recognized as many developing countries endemic for TB lack appropriate lab facilities, diagnostic resources and epidemiological capabilities (10). MDR strains do not appear to cause disease more readily than their drug sensitive counterparts, but HIV-positive individuals infected with MDR-TB have higher mortality rates, perhaps because HIV infection causes a malabsorption of TB drugs. This, and the fact that MDR-TB can require 24 months or more of drug therapy compared to 6-9 months for drug sensitive strains, can lead to acquired drug resistance and up to a 300-fold increase in drug costs (11).

Since the discovery of MDR-TB in the 1990s, the resistance pattern of TB has continued to evolve, and isolates resistant to both first- and second-line agents, termed extensively drug-resistant TB (XDR-TB), have been identified. Like MDR-TB, XDR-TB has been identified worldwide and now represents 2% of all cases of culture-positive TB (10).

Societal costs associated with MDR-TB are higher than for drug-susceptible TB due to longer hospitalization, longer treatment with more expensive and toxic medications, greater productivity losses, and higher rates of treatment failure and mortality. There have been recent reports of greater than 20% and 80% mortality attributable to MDR-TB and XDR-TB, respectively, with less than 60% of disease free MDR-TB patients after a mean drug treatment period of four years (12). In the U.S., where there are on average 300 newly reported cases of MDR-TB annually, this disease is very expensive to treat and current estimates suggest it is more than ten times as expensive as drug-sensitive infections (13-15).

2. BCG...then and now...

The bacille Calmette-Guérin (BCG) vaccine, derived from an attenuated strain of *Mycobacterium bovis*, has been used to vaccinate over 3 billion people throughout the world for more than 80 years since 1928. BCG lacks the genomic 'Region of Difference' (RD1) which encodes the ESX-1 secretion system, including the immunodominant 6-kDa Mtb antigen ESAT-6, included in the Hybrid 1 (ESAT-6/Ag85) vaccine (described in more detail in a later section of this chapter) and in IFN-γ release assays (IGRA's) used to diagnose Mtb (16, 17). The overriding dogma is that BCG protects against primary childhood TB, but its role in consistently protecting against adult pulmonary disease is minimal (18). Indeed, the efficacy of BCG in several field trials has been variable (19). The suggested reasons for the variability observed include differences in the BCG strains – resulting from inconsistent laboratory culture conditions which caused gene deletions or attenuated organisms (20), poor handling of the vaccine, doses and vaccination schedules in the various field trials (21), interference from environmental mycobacteria (22-24), and poor nutrition or genetic variability in the populations immunized (25, 26). Several analyses have identified genetic changes within some BCG substrains such as in the *phoP-phoR* system that has occurred along the way since BCG Pasteur was first derived.

Except in cases where infants are HIV-seropositive, BCG is considered safe. This has led to development of other vaccines that either enhance the immune responses resulting from BCG immunization, for example by insertion of specific genes present in virulent *M. tuberculosis* but which have been lost in the avirulent BCG vaccine - the recombinant forms of BCG (rBCG) - or, more broadly, are capable of boosting the effects of BCG. Recent studies have demonstrated that the new rBCG vaccines are more immunogenic, inducing effector and memory T cells, however one potential concern is that many of these rBCGs encode antigens such as Ag85A, CFP-10 etc. that are immunodominant. Recent data suggest that these antigens are highly conserved and are used by the bacteria as a ploy to cause damage in the lungs resulting in escape of the mycobacteria bacilli and increased transmission. It is important to demonstrate whether the new rBCGs can protect against clinical strains. Furthermore, because BCG is designed to be administered only once, none of the rBCG strategies are likely to yield a successful vaccine superior to what we have now.

Over the last 10 years more than 170 TB vaccine candidates have been tested in mouse, guinea pig or non human primate models of TB (27-31). These include: (i) subunit vaccines consisting of mycobacterial preparations (32-34), culture filtrates (CF) or secreted molecules (35-39), proteins (40-53), lipoglycoproteins (54), and glycolipids (55-57); (ii) DNA vaccines (58-72); (iii) live, attenuated, nonpathogenic/auxotrophic or recombinant bacteria (73-81); and (iv) attenuated, nonmycobacterial vectors such as *Salmonella* or *Vaccinia* virus (77, 82-87). In addition, attempts at improving BCG by administering lower doses (88-90), oral delivery (91), and prime/boost protocols are being explored (59, 85, 92-94). Currently, several candidate vaccines are being prepared for testing primarily as pre-exposure vaccines in humans (27, 95, 96).

Vaccine approaches currently in clinical trials also include altered forms of BCG to increase the effectiveness of the treatment. One of the vaccines, rBCG30, is an engineered form of BCG (rBCG) that over expresses Ag85B (97). It has shown much greater efficacy than the parental Tice BCG vaccine, perhaps due to loss of virulence in the current BCG vaccines, and was shown to increase Ag85B-specific T cell proliferation and IFN-γ responses in humans (97). Another rBCG in human clinical trials is a rBCG that is a urease-deficient mutant that expresses the lysteriolysin O gene from *Listeria monocytogenes* (98). Using this approach the vaccine increases phagosomal acidification in the absence of the ureC enzyme, while expressing the lysteriolysin protein, Hly, which requires an acidic pH within the phagosome in order to damage/perforate the phagosomal membrane. This process allows the release of antigen into the cytoplasm and induces macrophage apoptosis, leading to enhanced CD8[+] T cell presentation through a cross-priming strategy. Other whole virus vaccine approaches have seen some success against TB. One, based on a recombinant modified vaccinia virus Ankara (MVA) vaccine which expresses the Mtb protein Ag85A, is currently in clinical trials (99). However, the complex nature of TB infections may very well require multiple weapons in our armamentarium. These may include not only the use of multiple Mtb antigens but also vaccines based on other adjuvant and delivery platforms.

A post-exposure vaccine, to be used in healthy individuals infected with Mtb or those recently exposed to MDR-TB, could also reduce the probability of going on to develop TB disease. It could work by limiting bacteria that cause TB or MDR-TB, that are residing in a dormant state, by preventing reactivation and/or by reducing the chance of reinfection by exogenous Mtb. Finally, a therapeutic vaccine could function alone, or alongside antibiotic regimens, for individuals with active TB disease and could potentially shorten the treatment period.

3. Immune responses required for development of a successful TB vaccine...

Advances in our knowledge of resistance to Mtb have emerged since the pioneering work of Mackaness (1960's, 1070's) who demonstrated a dependence on cellular immunity against mycobacterial infection (100, 101). Another key advancement to the development of vaccines against Mtb was made by Orme and Collins (1980's), who were the first to show that transfer of immunity against Mtb could be achieved with antigen-specific CD4 and CD8 T cells, and that metabolically active mycobacteria secreted key immunologically relevant antigens (102-106). A major new idea in the mid-1980's, that has shaped the development of vaccines against many different pathogens, was that of Mosmann with the discovery that there were two types of helper CD4 T cells: Thelper 1 and Thelper 2 cells, that secrete either IFNγ or IL-4 respectively (among other cytokines) (107). More recently, Sallusto et al. have defined memory T cell subsets which can be functionally separated based on their surface receptors, which further advance testing the capability of vaccine induction of long-lived immune responses (108, 109). Although our understanding of an effective immune response against Mtb is far from complete, some fundamentals have been identified, resulting in a number of TB vaccines that are now being tested in humans. Several of these advances in our knowledge of the host's resistance to Mtb are discussed in the remainder of this chapter.

Mycobacteria bacilli usually enter the host through aerosol droplets of 1-3 μM inhaled to the lung alveoli. Some bacilli remain in the lungs and evade adaptive immunity to persist in the lungs, often for the lifetime of the host, and some are transported to draining lymph nodes where dendritic cells (DC) prime T lymphocytes. Mtb undergoes an initial period of uninhibited growth within non-activated host macrophages (110). Cell mediated immunity (CMI) characterized by the expansion of antigen-specific T-lymphocytes that attract monocytes/macrophages to inhibit bacillary growth through the production of cytokines, plays a key role in the control of TB. Persistence of Mtb inside of mononuclear phagocytes and DCs during all stages of infection can occur via many mechanisms including down-regulating major histocompatibility complex (MHC) class II expression or presentation

(111), neutralizing the phagosomal pH, interference with autophagy, and by inducing the production of immunosuppressive cytokines such as interleukin (IL)-10 and tumor growth factor beta (TGF-β)(112-115). Mtb can also inhibit apoptosis through prostaglandin production (116) and can invade the cytosolic compartment (117). Recent data also showed that of the large number of CD4+ effector T cells recruited to the lungs of infected mice, few are stimulated to produce IFN-γ (118).

The hallmark of CMI to Mtb infection is the formation of solid granulomas from aggregates of mononuclear phagocytes and polymorphonuclear granulocytes in the lung with a center of infected macrophages surrounded by a marginal zone of lymphocytes (119, 120). The protective role of granulomas is confinement of bacilli in a space that is lacking in vascularity and alveolar air, preventing both replication and dissemination to other sites. Granulomas also serve as sites for priming of CD4+ and CD8+ T cells as well as germinal center B cells. Primed T cells are reported to be polyfunctional, secreting IFN-γ, TNF and IL-2 cytokines, and of the central memory lineage (Tcm) (121) (Figure 2). Studies in gene-deficient/knock out (KO) mice and through neutralization with antibodies, have demonstrated the importance of IFN-γ (122-131), CD4+, and CD8+ (132-141) T cells in the acquired immune response to Mtb.

CD4+ T cells traffic to the lung within 7-14 days following infection and produce IFN-γ (142, 143). Depletion of CD4+ T cells prior to Mtb infection leads to increased bacterial burden and shortened survival (138) and depletion of this subset in latently infected animals leads to rapid reactivation (144). In sublethally-irradiated mice, passive transfer of CD4+ T cells mediates reduced susceptibility to Mtb infection (145). In contrast, CD4- and MHC Class II-deficient mice are extremely susceptible to Mtb. Finally, clinical conditions that impair CD4+ T cell immunity, such as HIV infection, dramatically increase the likelihood of developing active TB.

Mice deficient in IFN-γ, an effector cytokine which defines Th1-type CD4+ T cells, are highly susceptible to Mtb infection (127, 146). These mice fail to produce nitric oxide (NO) synthase (127) and develop a disseminated form of disease, characterized by irregular granulomas and necrotic areas. Patients in whom the gene for the IFN-γ receptor is mutated are prone to infection with atypical mycobacteria (147). Strong Th1-type, antigen-specific IFN-γ-secreting T cells are found in peripheral blood mononuclear cells (PBMC) from healthy individuals with latent TB infections (LTBI), but are diminished in individuals with pulmonary TB (148, 149). Recent results also indicate that CD4+ effector T cells are activated at suboptimal frequencies in tuberculosis, and that increasing effector T cell activation in the lungs by providing one or more epitope peptides may be a successful strategy for TB therapy (150).

The protective role of TNF in the immune response to Mtb was demonstrated in mice with defects in genes for TNF (151, 152). Its critical role for humans was also revealed by the occurrence of reactivation TB in rheumatoid arthritis patients who received long-term therapy with anti-TNF antibodies (153). Recently, both IL-23 and IL-17 were shown to be essential in the establishment of protective pulmonary CD4+ T cell responses, along with the concurrent expression of the chemokines CXCL9, CXCL10 and CXCL11 (154, 155).

Studies in mice and humans support an important role of CD8+ T cells in TB immunity, particularly during LTBI. Adoptive transfer or *in vivo* depletion of CD8+ cells demonstrated that CD8+ cells could confer protection against subsequent Mtb challenge, although the effects were less pronounced than those seen with CD4+ T cells (156-158). Mtb can egress into the cytosolic compartment of infected DCs resulting in direct loading of MHC class I (117). Cross-priming, which involves apoptosis of macrophages infected with Mtb, uptake of vesicles carrying Mtb antigens by nearby DC, and antigen presentation of the vesicular antigens by MHC I to CD8 is an additional mechanism by which CD8+ T cells are stimulated (159). Mice deficient in class I processing and presentation, including deficiencies in β2 microglobulin (160, 161), TAP1 (162), CD8 , or Class Ia ($K^{b-/-}/D^{b-/-}$)(163), are all more susceptible to Mtb infection than wild-type animals. In humans, Mtb-specific CD8+ T cells have been identified in Mtb-infected individuals and include CD8+ T cells that are classically (164-169), non-classically (170, 171), and CD1 restricted (172, 173).

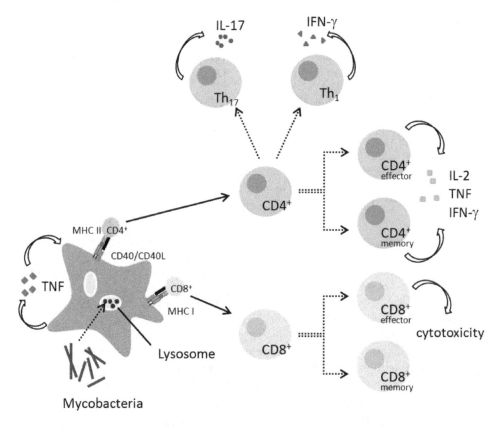

Fig. 2. The Cellular Host Response to TB. After infection of the host lung, macrophages and DCs infected with Mtb stimulate CD4+ and CD8+ T cells. CD4+ T cells are polarized into Th1 and Th17 effector cells or memory T cells secreting multiple cytokines including IFN-γ, TNF and IL-2. CD8+ memory T cells may be cytolytic and may secrete TNF and IFN-γ.

Infection with Mtb induces robust T cell responses yet adaptive immunity fails to eradicate *M. tuberculosis*. Mechanisms for the limited efficacy of the adaptive immune response in tuberculosis are hypothesized to fall into two categories: either the T cell effector functions are not effective because of failed or inappropriate responses induced by the infected cells; or the T cells recruited to the site of infection do not optimally perform the effector functions required for immune clearance. The ability of M. *tuberculosis* to resist and inhibit the TNF and IFN-γ-induced microbicidal responses of the phagocytic cells it infects is one immune evasion strategy in vivo. Another is that only a small fraction of the CD4 + effector T cells in the lungs is activated to synthesize IFN-γ. Identification of the elements of this host-pathogen interaction may lead to the development of therapies that target antigen gene suppression and inhibition of antigen presentation and provide a novel strategy for overcoming bacterial persistence in vivo, leading to better outcomes in Mtb infected individuals.

4. Designing a sub-unit vaccine from start to finish...

This section highlights the development of a new subunit vaccine, ID93/GLA-SE, and briefly discusses the other human TB vaccine candidates in the pipeline (see Table I).

Preclinical studies with a new TB subunit vaccine, ID93/GLA-SE, have been conducted and this vaccine is ready for testing in Phase I human clinical studies. This vaccine now joins 14 others, which are currently being tested in humans (Table I). The selection of the proteins for ID93 involved the generation of an Mtb protein library based on H37Rv proteins that were within the known immunogenic EsX and PE/PPE classes, between 6 and 70 kDa and with low homology with the human genome (less than 30%) (174). A comprehensive analysis was then performed on over 100 potential candidate antigens selected based on genome mining and expression as recombinant proteins. These candidate antigens were then down-selected based on IFN-γ production from human PBMCs in patients that were PPD(+) and which were non-responsive in PPD(-) patient samples. In combination with the TLR9 agonist, CpG ODN 1826, the vaccine candidates were then tested for efficacy in the C57BL/6 mouse aerosol model of Mtb infection. The ID93 fusion protein consists of four selected Mtb proteins: Rv3619, Rv1813, Rv3620, and Rv2608 (the cumulative molecular weights of each individual protein define the "93" in ID93). Three of the proteins are associated with Mtb virulence (Rv2608, Rv3619, and Rv3620) and one with latency (Rv1813). Rv2608 is a member of the PE/PPE family, Rv3619 and 3620 are in the EsX family of proteins and Rv1813 is expressed under hypoxic conditions (174). Similar to other fusion proteins, including Mtb72f, Ag85B-ESAT6, Ag85B-TB10 and H56, the fusion of more than one Mtb antigen leads to increased vaccine efficacy. Another similarity of these subunit vaccines is the need for an adjuvant to elicit maximum efficacy.

The adjuvant selected for use with the ID93 vaccine is a synthetic toll-like receptor (TLR4) agonist called glucopyranosyl lipid adjuvant (or GLA). This molecule has been extensively characterized in many biological systems, including mice, guinea pigs, ferrets (unpublished results), hamsters, non-human primates (NHPs) and humans (52, 175, 176). Early on, the Mtb72F subunit vaccine, in Phase II human clinical trials, included AS02A as its adjuvant. AS02A consists of a biological TLR4 agonist called monophosphoryl lipid A (MPL), derived from *Salmonella minnesota* mixed with QS21 and an oil-in-water formulation (177).

Other TB vaccine candidates currently in clinical trials include four different categories of vaccines: a) recombinant protein vaccines; b) recombinant live vaccines; c) viral vectored vaccines; and d) whole cell, inactivated or disrupted mycobacterial vaccines (Table 1). The recombinant subunit vaccines will be briefly described below.

	Protein/Vaccine	Adjuvant
Recombinant Proteins		
M72	fusion protein of Mtb32 and Mtb39 (72kDa)	AS02A: MPL and QS21
Hybrid 1	fusion protein of Ag85B and ESAT-6	IC31 (Intercell): ss oligodeoxynucleotide and peptide (KLKL5KLK)
Hybrid 1	fusion protein of Ag85B and ESAT-6	CAF01: cationic liposomes
HyVac4: AERAS-404	fusion protein of Ag85B and TB10.4	IC31 (Intercell): ss oligodeoxynucleotide and peptide (KLKL5KLK)
Recombinant Live Vaccines		
VPM1002: rBCG(delta)ureC:Hly	urease deficient; expresses listeriolysin (Hly) from *L. monocytogenes*	*NA*
rBCG30 (Tice strain): AERAS-422	rBCG30; overexpresses Ag85B	*NA*
rBCG (AFRO-1 strain): AERAS-422	rBCG30; overexpresses Ag85A, Ag85B and Rv3407 and expresses perfringolysin O	*NA*
Viral Vectored Vaccines		
MVA85A: AERAS-485	MVA (Modified vaccinia virus Ankara) expressing Ag85A	*NA*
Crucell Ad35: AERAS-402	Ad35 (non-replicating Adenovirus 35) expressing Ag85A, Ag85B and TB10.4	*NA*
Ad5Sg85A	Ad5 (non-replicating Adenovirus 5) expressing Ag85A	*NA*
Whole Cell Inactivated or Disrupted Vaccines		
M. vaccae	Inactivated whole cell mycobacteria	*NA*
Mw [*M. indicus pranii* (MIP)]	Whole cell saprophytic mycobacteria	*NA*
RUTI	Fragmented *M. tuberculosis* cells	*NA*
M. smegmatis	Whole cell extract	*NA*

Table 1. TB vaccines in human clinical trials (178), [TB vaccine candidates-2010; www.stoptb.org/wg/new_vaccines(2)].

The M72 (Mtb72F) + AS01 (or AS02A) vaccine was originally developed by Corixa and the Infectious Disease Research Institute (Seattle, WA) and clinical trials are currently being sponsored by GlaxoSmithKline (GSK) and Aeras. This vaccine is a fusion of tandomly linked proteins, Mtb32(C), Mtb39, and Mtb32(N) which showed efficacy in mice, guinea pigs, and NHPs (179-181) and is currently being evaluated in humans. This vaccine includes an AS01 adjuvant (GSK), which comprises the TLR4 agonist, monophosphoryl lipid A (MPL), QS21 and liposomes. In the first phase I clinical trial, Mtb72F combined with the AS02A adjuvant, which includes MPL, QS21, and an oil-in-water emulsion, the vaccine was locally reactogenic but the adverse events were mostly mild and transient and thus had an acceptable tolerability in humans (177). Immunologically, three doses of the Mtb72F/AS02A vaccine (given at 0, 1 and 2 months) induces both humoral and cellular responses in healthy PPD-negative adults (18-40 years of age); IL-2 and IFN-γ is elicited in PBMCs by ELISPOT and increased antigen-specific CD4+ T cells expressing CD40L, IL-2, TNF-α and IFN-γ by intracellular cytokine staining (ICS) are also induced.

The Hybrid-1 vaccine developed by the Statens Serum Institute, includes a fusion of the Mtb proteins antigen 85B and ESAT6. This vaccine, Hybrid 1, which is being evaluated in human clinical trials, is adjuvanted with either the Intercell adjuvant system, IC31 or with a liposomal adjuvant CAF01. CAF01 adjuvant is considered a cationic liposome, and is formulated with quaternary ammonium lipid N, N'-dimethyl-N,N'-dioctadecylammonium (DDA) plus a synthetic mycobacterial cord factor, α,α'-trehalose 6,6'-dibeheneate (TDB) (182-184). The IC31 adjuvant signals through TLR9, and contains the following KLK poly-peptide KLKL$_5$KLK-COOH and a non-CpG oligonucleotide ODN1a, consisting of a phosphodiester backbone ODN, 5'-ICI CIC ICI CIC ICI CIC ICI CIC IC-3' (185). Both adjuvant systems, CAF01 and IC31, elicit strong Th1 inducing activities and protection in animal models of tuberculosis when combined with the Ag85B-ESAT6 fusion (185-189).

Another subunit vaccine in development by the same group that developed the Hybrid-1 vaccine is the H56 vaccine which includes a fusion of Hybrid 1 and a latency-associated protein, Rv2660c, which is activated during hypoxic conditions (50). The H56 vaccine, formulated in CAF01, shows a 10-fold reduction in lung bacterial load in the mouse model in a head-to-head comparison with their precursor subunit vaccine, the Hybrid 1 vaccine, containing only Ag85B and ESAT6. In addition, the authors demonstrate that the H56 vaccine is capable of protecting against reactivation when tested after Mtb exposure in a modified Cornell mouse model. HyVac4/AERAS-404 combined with IC31 is also in clinical trials, and includes a fusion of the Mtb antigens Ag85B and TB10.4. Replacement of the ESAT-6 protein with TB10.4 in this vaccine, conserves the use of ESAT-6 for diagnostic purposes (16, 190). This vaccine induces polyfunctional CD4 T cells, which express IFN-γ, TNF-α and IL-2, correlating with protective efficacy in the mouse model against Mtb (191) and guinea pig model using a BCG prime/subunit boost strategy (192).

5. Conclusion

Today, an ambitious portfolio of novel vaccines, drug regimens, and diagnostic tools for TB is being supported by various research funding agencies. Mathematical modeling of TB to evaluate the potential benefits of novel interventions under development and those not yet in the portfolio suggest that: neonatal vaccination with an effective portfolio vaccine would decrease TB incidence by 39% to 52% by 2050, while drug regimens that shorten treatment duration and are efficacious against drug-resistant strains could reduce incidence by 10-27%. Clearly, TB elimination will require one or more effective vaccines. Importantly, new vaccines should have the potential to be effective against clinical strains representing all the major geographical regions.

6. References

[1] http://www.who.int/mediacentre/factsheets/fs104/en. WHO Fact Sheet No. 104, November 2010.

[2] http://www.stoptb.org/

[3] WHO. Global tuberculosis control. WHO Report 2010. Geneva, World Health Organization.

[4] Nunn P, Reid A, De Cock KM. Tuberculosis and HIV infection: the global setting. J Infect Dis. 2007;196 Suppl 1:S5-14.

[5] Sudre P, ten Dam G, Kochi A. Tuberculosis: a global overview of the situation today. BullWorld Health Organ. 1992;70(2):149-59.

[6] Kochi A. The global tuberculosis situation and the new control stratgey of the World Health Organization. 1082. Tubercle1991. p. 1-16.

[7] Cegielski JP, Chin DP, Espinal MA, Frieden TR, Rodriquez Cruz R, Talbot EA, et al. The global tuberculosis situation. Progress and problems in the 20th century, prospects for the 21st century. Infect Dis Clin North Am. 2002;16(1):1-58.

[8] Dye C, Espinal MA, Watt CJ, Mbiaga C, Williams BG. Worldwide incidence of multidrug-resistant tuberculosis. Journal of Infectious Diseases. 2002;185(8):1197-202.

[9] WHO. Multidrug and extensively drug-resistant TB (M/XDR-TB): 2010 global report on surveillance and response. Geneva; 2010 Contract No.: Document Number |.

[10] Zignol M, Wright A, Jaramillo E, Nunn P, Raviglione MC. Patients with previously treated tuberculosis no longer neglected. Clin Infect Dis. 2007;44(1):61-4.

[11] Bock NN, Jensen PA, Miller B, Nardell E. Tuberculosis infection control in resource-limited settings in the era of expanding HIV care and treatment. J Infect Dis. 2007;196 Suppl 1:S108-13.

[12] Goble M, Iseman MD, Madsen LA, Waite D, Ackerson L, Horsburgh CR, Jr. Treatment of 171 patients with pulmonary tuberculosis resistant to isoniazid and rifampin. New England Journal of Medicine. 1993;328(8):527-32.

[13] Burman WJ, Dalton CB, Cohn DL, Butler JR, Reves RR. A cost-effectiveness analysis of directly observed therapy vs self-administered therapy for treatment of tuberculosis. Chest. 1997;112(1):63-70.

[14] Wilton P, Smith RD, Coast J, Millar M, Karcher A. Directly observed treatment for multidrug-resistant tuberculosis: an economic evaluation in the United States of America and South Africa. Int J Tuberc Lung Dis. 2001;5(12):1137-42.

[15] Dye C. Doomsday postponed? Preventing and reversing epidemics of drug-resistant tuberculosis. Nature reviews. 2009;7(1):81-7.

[16] Lalvani A, Pathan AA, McShane H, Wilkinson RJ, Latif M, Conlon CP, et al. Rapid detection of Mycobacterium tuberculosis infection by enumeration of antigen-

specific T cells. American journal of respiratory and critical care medicine. 2001;163(4):824-8.

[17] Mori T, Sakatani M, Yamagishi F, Takashima T, Kawabe Y, Nagao K, et al. Specific detection of tuberculosis infection: an interferon-gamma-based assay using new antigens. American journal of respiratory and critical care medicine. 2004;170(1):59-64.

[18] Fine PE. Variation in protection by BCG: implications of and for heterologous immunity. Lancet. 1995;346(8986):1339-45.

[19] Colditz GA, Brewer TF, Berkey CS, Wilson ME, Burdick E, Fineberg HV, et al. Efficacy of GCG vaccine in the prevention of tuberculosis: meta-analysis of the published literature. 1088. JAMA. 1994;271:698-702.

[20] Behr MA. BCG--different strains, different vaccines? The Lancet infectious diseases. 2002;2(2):86-92.

[21] Behr MA, Wilson MA, Gill WP, Salamon H, Schoolnik GK, Rane S, et al. Comparative genomics of BCG vaccines by whole-genome DNA microarray [see comments] 7. Science. 1999;284(5419):1520-3.

[22] Brandt L, Feino CJ, Weinreich OA, Chilima B, Hirsch P, Appelberg R, et al. Failure of the Mycobacterium bovis BCG vaccine: some species of environmental mycobacteria block multiplication of BCG and induction of protective immunity to tuberculosis. Infection and Immunity. 2002;70(2):672-8.

[23] Palmer DR, Krzych U. Cellular and molecular requirements for the recall of IL-4-producing memory CD4(+)CD45RO(+)CD27(-) T cells during protection induced by attenuated Plasmodium falciparum sporozoites. EurJ Immunol. 2002;32(3):652-61.

[24] Rook GA, Bahr GM, Stanford JL. The effect of two distinct forms of cell-mediated response to mycobacteria on the protective efficacy of BCG 2084. Tubercle. 1981;62(1):63-8.

[25] Fine PE. BCG: the challenge continues. ScandJ InfectDis. 2001;33(4):243-5.

[26] Liu J, Tran V, Leung AS, Alexander DC, Zhu B. BCG vaccines: their mechanisms of attenuation and impact on safety and protective efficacy. Human vaccines. 2009;5(2):70-8.

[27] Ginsberg AM. What's new in tuberculosis vaccines? BullWorld Health Organ. 2002;80(6):483-8.

[28] Orme IM. Prospects for new vaccines against tuberculosis 207. Trends Microbiol. 1995;3(10):401-4.

[29] Orme IM. Progress in the development of new vaccines against tuberculosis 889. IntJTubercLung Dis. 1997;1(2):95-100.

[30] Orme IM. The search for new vaccines against tuberculosis. Journal of Leukocyte Biology. 2001;70(1):1-10.

[31] Orme IM, Belisle JT. TB vaccine development: after the flood 825. Trends Microbiol. 1999;7(10):394-5.

[32] Brehmer W, Anacker RL, Ribi E. Immunogenicity of cell walls from various mycobacteria against airborne tuberculosis in mice 772. Journal of Bacteriology. 1968;95(6):2000-4.

[33] Chugh IB, Kansal R, Vinayak VK, Khuller GK. Protective efficacy of different cell-wall fractions of Mycobacterium tuberculosis 329. Folia Microbiol(Praha). 1992;37(6):407-12.

[34] Pal DP, Shriniwas. Role of cellwall vaccine in prophylaxis of tuberculosis 564. Indian Journal of Medical Research. 1977;65(3):340-5.

[35] Andersen P. Effective vaccination of mice against Mycobacterium tuberculosis infection with a soluble mixture of secreted mycobacterial proteins. Infection and Immunity. 1994;62(6):2536-44.

[36] Boesen H, Jensen BN, Wilcke T, Andersen P. Human T-cell responses to secreted antigen fractions of Mycobacterium tuberculosis. Infection and Immunity. 1995;63(4):1491-7.

[37] Haslov K, Andersen A, Nagai S, Gottschau A, Sorensen T, Andersen P. Guinea pig cellular immune responses to proteins secreted by Mycobacterium tuberculosis 1286. Infection and Immunity. 1995;63(3):804-10.

[38] Horwitz MA, Lee BW, Dillon BJ, Harth G. Protective immunity against tuberculosis induced by vaccination with major extracellular proteins of Mycobacterium tuberculosis. ProcNatlAcadSciUSA. 1995;92(5):1530-4.

[39] Hubbard RD, Flory CM, Collins FM. Immunization of mice with mycobacterial culture filtrate proteins 1838. Clinical and Experimental Immunology. 1992;87(1):94-8.

[40] Alderson MR, Bement T, Day CH, Zhu L, Molesh D, Skeiky YA, et al. Expression cloning of an immunodominant family of Mycobacterium tuberculosis antigens using human CD4(+) T cells. J Exp Med. 2000;191(3):551-60.

[41] Andersen AB, Hansen EB. Structure and mapping of antigenic domains of protein antigen b, a 38,000-molecular-weight protein of Mycobacterium tuberculosis 2152. Infection and Immunity. 1989;57(8):2481-8.

[42] Brandt L, Elhay M, Rosenkrands I, Lindblad EB, Andersen P. ESAT-6 subunit vaccination against Mycobacterium tuberculosis 2383. Infection and Immunity. 2000;68(2):791-5.

[43] Coler RN, Campos-Neto A, Ovendale P, Day FH, Fling SP, Zhu L, et al. Vaccination with the T cell antigen Mtb 8.4 protects against challenge with Mycobacterium tuberculosis. J Immunol. 2001;166(10):6227-35.

[44] Collins HL, Kaufmann SH. Prospects for better tuberculosis vaccines. Lancet InfectDis. 2001;1(1):21-8.

[45] Dillon DC, Alderson MR, Day CH, Lewinsohn DM, Coler R, Bement T, et al. Molecular characterization and human T-cell responses to a member of a novel Mycobacterium tuberculosis mtb39 gene family. Infect Immun. 1999;67(6):2941-50.

[46] Skeiky YA, Lodes MJ, Guderian JA, Mohamath R, Bement T, Alderson MR, et al. Cloning, Expression, and Immunological Evaluation of Two Putative Secreted Serine Protease Antigens of Mycobacterium tuberculosis 1. Infection and Immunity. 1999;67(8):3998-4007.

[47] Skeiky YA, Ovendale PJ, Jen S, Alderson MR, Dillon DC, Smith S, et al. T cell expression cloning of a Mycobacterium tuberculosis gene encoding a protective antigen associated with the early control of infection. J Immunol. 2000;165(12):7140-9.

[48] Sorensen AL, Nagai S, Houen G, Andersen P, Andersen AB. Purification and characterization of a low-molecular-mass T-cell antigen secreted by Mycobacterium tuberculosis 1285. Infection and Immunity. 1995;63(5):1710-7.

[49] Weinrich OA, van Pinxteren LA, Meng OL, Birk RP, Andersen P. Protection of mice with a tuberculosis subunit vaccine based on a fusion protein of antigen 85b and esat-6. Infection and Immunity. 2001;69(5):2773-8.

[50] Aagaard C, Hoang T, Dietrich J, Cardona PJ, Izzo A, Dolganov G, et al. A multistage tuberculosis vaccine that confers efficient protection before and after exposure. Nat Med. 2011.

[51] Baldwin SL, Bertholet S, Kahn M, Zharkikh I, Ireton GC, Vedvick TS, et al. Intradermal immunization improves protective efficacy of a novel TB vaccine candidate. Vaccine. 2009;27(23):3063-71. PMCID: 2743149.

[52] Bertholet S, Ireton GC, Ordway DJ, Windish HP, Pine SO, Kahn M, et al. A defined tuberculosis vaccine candidate boosts BCG and protects against multidrug-resistant Mycobacterium tuberculosis. Sci Transl Med. 2010;2(53):53ra74.

[53] Aagaard C, Hoang T, Dietrich J, Cardona PJ, Izzo A, Dolganov G, et al. A multistage tuberculosis vaccine that confers efficient protection before and after exposure. Nature medicine. 2011;17(2):189-94.

[54] Vordermeier HM, Zhu X, Harris DP. Induction of CD8+ CTL recognizing mycobacterial peptides 138. Scandinavian Journal of Immunology. 1997;45(5):521-6.

[55] Anacker RL, Matsumoto J, Ribi E, Smith RF, Yamamoto K. Enhancement of resistance of mice to tuberculosis by purified components of mycobacterial lipid fractions. J InfectDis. 1973;127(4):357-64.

[56] Mara M, Galliova J, Sir Z, Mohelska H, Pruchova J, Julak J. Biochemistry of BCG lipids and their role in antituberculous immunity and hypersensitivity. J HygEpidemiolMicrobiolImmunol. 1975;19(4):444-52.

[57] Reggiardo Z, Shamsuddin AK. Granulomagenic activity of serologically active glycolipids from Mycobacterium bovis BCG 574. Infection and Immunity. 1976;14(6):1369-74.

[58] D'Souza S, Rosseels V, Denis O, Tanghe A, De Smet N, Jurion F, et al. Improved tuberculosis DNA vaccines by formulation in cationic lipids. Infection and Immunity. 2002;70(7):3681-8.

[59] Feng CG, Palendira U, Demangel C, Spratt JM, Malin AS, Britton WJ. Priming by DNA immunization augments protective efficacy of Mycobacterium bovis Bacille Calmette-Guerin against tuberculosis. Infection and Immunity. 2001;69(6):4174-6.

[60] Huygen K. DNA vaccines: application to tuberculosis 36. IntJTubercLung Dis. 1998;2(12):971-8.

[61] Huygen K, Content J, Denis O, Montgomery DL, Yawman AM, Deck RR, et al. Immunogenicity and protective efficacy of a tuberculosis DNA vaccine 2456. NatMed. 1996;2(8):893-8.

[62] Kamath AT, Feng CG, Macdonald M, Briscoe H, Britton WJ. Differential protective efficacy of DNA vaccines expressing secreted proteins of Mycobacterium tuberculosis 23. Infection and Immunity. 1999;67(4):1702-7.

[63] Kamath AT, Hanke T, Briscoe H, Britton WJ. Co-immunization with DNA vaccines expressing granulocyte-macrophage colony-stimulating factor and mycobacterial secreted proteins enhances T-cell immunity, but not protective efficacy against mycobacterium tuberculosis [In Process Citation] 11. Immunology. 1999;96(4):511-6.

[64] Lowrie DB, Silva CL, Colston MJ, Ragno S, Tascon RE. Protection against tuberculosis by a plasmid DNA vaccine. Vaccine. 1997;15(8):834-8.

[65] Lowrie DB, Silva CL, Tascon RE. DNA vaccines against tuberculosis. Immunology and Cell Biology. 1997;75(6):591-4.

[66] Lozes E, Huygen K, Content J, Denis O, Montgomery DL, Yawman AM, et al. Immunogenicity and efficacy of a tuberculosis DNA vaccine encoding the components of the secreted antigen 85 complex. Vaccine. 1997;15(8):830-3.

[67] Silva CL, Bonato VL, Lima VM. DNA encoding individual mycobacterial antigens protects mice against tuberculosis. BrazJ MedBiolRes. 1999;32(2):231-4.

[68] Tanghe A, Content J, Van Vooren JP, Portaels F, Huygen K. Protective efficacy of a DNA vaccine encoding antigen 85A from Mycobacterium bovis BCG against Buruli ulcer. Infection and Immunity. 2001;69(9):5403-11.

[69] Tascon RE, Colston MJ, Ragno S, Stavropoulos E, Gregory D, Lowrie DB. Vaccination against tuberculosis by DNA injection. NatMed. 1996;2(8):888-92.

[70] Ulmer JB, Liu MA, Montgomery DL, Yawman AM, Deck RR, DeWitt CM, et al. Expression and immunogenicity of Mycobacterium tuberculosis antigen 85 by DNA vaccination 130. Vaccine. 1997;15(8):792-4.

[71] Ulmer JB, Montgomery DL, Tang A, Zhu L, Deck RR, DeWitt C, et al. DNA vaccines against tuberculosis 30. NovartisFoundSymp. 1998;217:239-46.

[72] Velaz-Faircloth M, Cobb AJ, Horstman AL, Henry SC, Frothingham R. Protection against Mycobacterium avium by DNA vaccines expressing mycobacterial antigens as fusion proteins with green fluorescent protein 845. Infection and Immunity. 1999;67(8):4243-50.

[73] Bahr GM, Shaaban MA, Gabriel M, al Shimali B, Siddiqui Z, Chugh TD, et al. Improved immunotherapy for pulmonary tuberculosis with Mycobacterium vaccae. Tubercle. 1990;71(4):259-66.

[74] Chambers MA, Williams A, Gavier-Widen D, Whelan A, Hall G, Marsh PD, et al. Identification of a mycobacterium bovis BCG auxotrophic mutant that protects guinea pigs against M. bovis and hematogenous spread of mycobacterium tuberculosis without sensitization to tuberculin [In Process Citation] 2403. Infection and Immunity. 2000;68(12):7094-9.

[75] Collins DM, Wilson T, Campbell S, Buddle BM, Wards BJ, Hotter G, et al. Production of avirulent mutants of Mycobacterium bovis with vaccine properties by the use of illegitimate recombination and screening of stationary-phase cultures. Microbiology. 2002;148(Pt 10):3019-27.

[76] Dhar N, Rao V, Tyagi AK. Recombinant BCG approach for development of vaccines: cloning and expression of immunodominant antigens of M. tuberculosis [In Process Citation]. FEMS Microbiology Letters. 2000;190(2):309-16.

[77] Hess J, Kaufmann SH. Development of live recombinant vaccine candidates against tuberculosis. ScandJ InfectDis. 2001;33(10):723-4.

[78] Hondalus MK, Bardarov S, Russell R, Chan J, Jacobs WR, Jr., Bloom BR. Attenuation of and protection induced by a leucine auxotroph of Mycobacterium tuberculosis. Infection and Immunity. 2000;68(5):2888-98.

[79] Horwitz MA, Harth G, Dillon BJ, Maslesa-Galic S. Recombinant bacillus calmette-guerin (BCG) vaccines expressing the mycobacterium tuberculosis 30-kDa major secretory protein induce greater protective immunity against tuberculosis than conventional BCG vaccines in a highly susceptible animal model [In Process Citation]. ProcNatlAcadSciUSA. 2000;97(25):13853-8.

[80] Sambandamurthy VK, Wang X, Chen B, Russell RG, Derrick S, Collins FM, et al. A pantothenate auxotroph of Mycobacterium tuberculosis is highly attenuated and protects mice against tuberculosis. NatMed. 2002;8(10):1171-4.

[81] Waddell RD, Chintu C, Lein AD, Zumla A, Karagas MR, Baboo KS, et al. Safety and immunogenicity of a five-dose series of inactivated Mycobacterium vaccae vaccination for the prevention of HIV-associated tuberculosis. Clinical Infectious Diseases. 2000;30 Suppl 3:S309-15.:S309-S15.

[82] Feng CG, Blanchard TJ, Smith GL, Hill AV, Britton WJ. Induction of CD8+ T-lymphocyte responses to a secreted antigen of Mycobacterium tuberculosis by an attenuated vaccinia virus. Immunology and Cell Biology. 2001;79(6):569-75.

[83] Hess J, Grode L, Hellwig J, Conradt P, Gentschev I, Goebel W, et al. Protection against murine tuberculosis by an attenuated recombinant Salmonella typhimurium vaccine strain that secretes the 30-kDa antigen of Mycobacterium bovis BCG 2472. FEMS Immunology and Medical Microbiology. 2000;27(4):283-9.

[84] Malin AS, Huygen K, Content J, Mackett M, Brandt L, Andersen P, et al. Vaccinia expression of mycobacterium tuberculosis-secreted proteins: tissue plasminogen activator signal sequence enhances expression and immunogenicity of M. tuberculosis Ag85 [In Process Citation]. MicrobesInfect. 2000;2(14):1677-85.

[85] McShane H, Brookes R, Gilbert SC, Hill AV. Enhanced immunogenicity of CD4(+) t-cell responses and protective efficacy of a DNA-modified vaccinia virus Ankara prime-boost vaccination regimen for murine tuberculosis. Infection and Immunity. 2001;69(2):681-6.

[86] Mollenkopf HJ, Groine-Triebkorn D, Andersen P, Hess J, Kaufmann SH. Protective efficacy against tuberculosis of ESAT-6 secreted by a live Salmonella typhimurium vaccine carrier strain and expressed by naked DNA. Vaccine. 2001;19(28-29):4028-35.

[87] Zhu X, Venkataprasad N, Ivanyi J, Vordermeier HM. Vaccination with recombinant vaccinia viruses protects mice against Mycobacterium tuberculosis infection 114. Immunology. 1997;92(1):6-9.

[88] Bretscher P, Menon J, Power C, Uzonna J, Wei G. A case for a neonatal, low-dose BCG vaccination trial. ScandJ InfectDis. 2001;33(4):253-7.

[89] Bretscher PA. Prospects for low dose BCG vaccination against tuberculosis 248. Immunobiology. 1994;191(4-5):548-54.

[90] Power CA, Wei G, Bretscher PA. Mycobacterial dose defines the Th1/Th2 nature of the immune response independently of whether immunization is administered by the intravenous, subcutaneous, or intradermal route. Infection and Immunity. 1998;66(12):5743-50.

[91] Hoft DF, Brown RM, Belshe RB. Mucosal bacille calmette-Guerin vaccination of humans inhibits delayed-type hypersensitivity to purified protein derivative but induces mycobacteria-specific interferon-gamma responses. Clinical Infectious Diseases. 2000;30 Suppl 3:S217-22.:S217-S22.

[92] Brooks JV, Frank AA, Keen MA, Bellisle JT, Orme IM. Boosting vaccine for tuberculosis. Infection and Immunity. 2001;69(4):2714-7.

[93] Griffin JF, Chinn DN, Rodgers CR, Mackintosh CG. Optimal models to evaluate the protective efficacy of tuberculosis vaccines. Tuberculosis(Edinb). 2001;81(1-2):133-9.

[94] Griffin JF, Mackintosh CG, Slobbe L, Thomson AJ, Buchan GS. Vaccine protocols to optimise the protective efficacy of BCG. Tubercle and Lung Disease. 1999;79(3):135-43.

[95] McShane H, Behboudi S, Goonetilleke N, Brookes R, Hill AV. Protective immunity against Mycobacterium tuberculosis induced by dendritic cells pulsed with both CD8(+)- and CD4(+)-T-cell epitopes from antigen 85A. Infection and Immunity. 2002;70(3):1623-6.

[96] Reed SG, Alderson MR, Dalemans W, Lobet Y, Skeiky YAW. Prospects For a Better Vaccine Against Tuberculosis. Tuberculosis(Edinb). 2003;83(1-3):213-9.

[97] Hoft DF, Blazevic A, Abate G, Hanekom WA, Kaplan G, Soler JH, et al. A new recombinant bacille Calmette-Guerin vaccine safely induces significantly enhanced tuberculosis-specific immunity in human volunteers. The Journal of infectious diseases. 2008;198(10):1491-501. PMCID: 2670060.

[98] Grode L, Seiler P, Baumann S, Hess J, Brinkmann V, Nasser Eddine A, et al. Increased vaccine efficacy against tuberculosis of recombinant Mycobacterium bovis bacille Calmette-Guerin mutants that secrete listeriolysin. The Journal of clinical investigation. 2005;115(9):2472-9. PMCID: 1187936.

[99] McShane H. Tuberculosis vaccines: beyond bacille Calmette-Guerin. Philosophical transactions of the Royal Society of London Series B, Biological sciences. 2011;366(1579):2782-9. PMCID: 3146779.

[100] Mackaness GB. The Immunological Basis of Acquired Cellular Resistance. The Journal of experimental medicine. 1964;120:105-20. PMCID: 2137723.

[101] Mackaness GB. Resistance to intracellular infection. The Journal of infectious diseases. 1971;123(4):439-45.

[102] Orme IM. The kinetics of emergence and loss of mediator T lymphocytes acquired in response to infection with Mycobacterium tuberculosis. Journal of Immunology. 1987;138(1):293-8.

[103] Orme IM. Induction of nonspecific acquired resistance and delayed-type hypersensitivity, but not specific acquired resistance in mice inoculated with killed mycobacterial vaccines. Infection and Immunity. 1988;56(12):3310-2.

[104] Orme IM. Characteristics and specificity of acquired immunologic memory to Mycobacterium tuberculosis infection. Journal of Immunology. 1988;140(10):3589-93.

[105] Orme IM. Development of new vaccines and drugs for TB: limitations and potential strategic errors. Future microbiology. 2011;6(2):161-77. PMCID: 3122326.

[106] Orme IM, Collins FM. Protection against Mycobacterium tuberculosis infection by adoptive immunotherapy. Requirement for T cell-deficient recipients. Journal of Experimental Medicine. 1983;158(1):74-83.

[107] Mosmann TR, Cherwinski H, Bond MW, Giedlin MA, Coffman RL. Two types of murine helper T cell clone. I. Definition according to profiles of lymphokine activities and secreted proteins. Journal of immunology. 1986;136(7):2348-57.

[108] Sallusto F, Langenkamp A, Geginat J, Lanzavecchia A. Functional subsets of memory T cells identified by CCR7 expression. Current topics in microbiology and immunology. 2000;251:167-71.

[109] Sallusto F, Lenig D, Forster R, Lipp M, Lanzavecchia A. Two subsets of memory T lymphocytes with distinct homing potentials and effector functions. Nature. 1999;401(6754):708-12.

[110] Russell DG. Who puts the tubercle in tuberculosis? Nature reviews. 2007;5(1):39-47.

[111] Noss EH, Harding CV, Boom WH. Mycobacterium tuberculosis inhibits MHC class II antigen processing in murine bone marrow macrophages. Cell Immunol. 2000;201(1):63-74.

[112] Deretic V. Autophagy as an immune defense mechanism. Curr Opin Immunol. 2006;18(4):375-82.

[113] Hirsch CS, Johnson JL, Ellner JJ. Pulmonary tuberculosis. CurrOpinPulmMed. 1999;5(3):143-50.

[114] Rojas RE, Balaji KN, Subramanian A, Boom WH. Regulation of human CD4(+) alphabeta T-cell-receptor-positive (TCR(+)) and gammadelta TCR(+) T-cell responses to Mycobacterium tuberculosis by interleukin-10 and transforming growth factor beta. Infection and Immunity. 1999;67(12):6461-72.

[115] Turner J, Gonzalez-Juarrero M, Ellis DL, Basaraba RJ, Kipnis A, Orme IM, et al. In vivo IL-10 production reactivates chronic pulmonary tuberculosis in C57BL/6 mice. J Immunol. 2002;169(11):6343-51.

[116] Divangahi M, Desjardins D, Nunes-Alves C, Remold HG, Behar SM. Eicosanoid pathways regulate adaptive immunity to Mycobacterium tuberculosis. Nature immunology. 2010;11(8):751-8.

[117] van der Wel N, Hava D, Houben D, Fluitsma D, van Zon M, Pierson J, et al. M. tuberculosis and M. leprae translocate from the phagolysosome to the cytosol in myeloid cells. Cell. 2007;129(7):1287-98.

[118] Bold TD, Banaei N, Wolf AJ, Ernst JD. Suboptimal activation of antigen-specific CD4+ effector cells enables persistence of M. tuberculosis in vivo. PLoS pathogens. 2011;7(5):e1002063. PMCID: 3102708.

[119] Flynn JL. Lessons from experimental Mycobacterium tuberculosis infections. Microbes and infection / Institut Pasteur. 2006;8(4):1179-88.

[120] Ulrichs T, Kaufmann SH. New insights into the function of granulomas in human tuberculosis. J Pathol. 2006;208(2):261-9.

[121] Day TA, Koch M, Nouailles G, Jacobsen M, Kosmiadi GA, Miekley D, et al. Secondary lymphoid organs are dispensable for the development of T-cell-mediated immunity during tuberculosis. Eur J Immunol. 2010;40(6):1663-73.

[122] Appelberg R. Protective role of interferon gamma, tumor necrosis factor alpha and interleukin-6 in Mycobacterium tuberculosis and M. avium infections. Immunobiology. 1994;191(4-5):520-5.

[123] Appelberg R, Castro AG, Pedrosa J, Silva RA, Orme IM, Minoprio P. Role of gamma interferon and tumor necrosis factor alpha during T-cell-independent and -dependent phases of Mycobacterium avium infection. Infection and Immunity. 1994;62(9):3962-71.

[124] Chackerian AA, Perera TV, Behar SM. Gamma interferon-producing CD4+ T lymphocytes in the lung correlate with resistance to infection with Mycobacterium tuberculosis. Infection and Immunity. 2001;69(4):2666-74.

[125] Flesch I, Kaufmann SH. Mycobacterial growth inhibition by interferon-gamma-activated bone marrow macrophages and differential susceptibility among strains of Mycobacterium tuberculosis 1356. Journal of Immunology. 1987;138(12):4408-13.

[126] Flynn JL. Why is IFN-gamma insufficient to control tuberculosis? [letter] 2328. Trends Microbiol. 1999;7(12):477-8.

[127] Flynn JL, Chan J, Triebold KJ, Dalton DK, Stewart TA, Bloom BR. An essential role for interferon gamma in resistance to Mycobacterium tuberculosis infection 1422. Journal of Experimental Medicine. 1993;178(6):2249-54.

[128] Kaufmann SH. Role of T-cell subsets in bacterial infections 2500. Current Opinion In Immunology. 1991;3(4):465-70.

[129] Kawamura I, Tsukada H, Yoshikawa H, Fujita M, Nomoto K, Mitsuyama M. IFN-gamma-producing ability as a possible marker for the protective T cells against Mycobacterium bovis BCG in mice. J Immunol. 1992;148(9):2887-93.

[130] Sugawara I, Yamada H, Kazumi Y, Doi N, Otomo K, Aoki T, et al. Induction of granulomas in interferon-gamma gene-disrupted mice by avirulent but not by virulent strains of Mycobacterium tuberculosis. J MedMicrobiol. 1998;47(10):871-7.

[131] Cooper AM, Dalton DK, Stewart TA, Griffin JP, Russell DG, Orme IM. Disseminated tuberculosis in interferon gamma gene-disrupted mice. The Journal of experimental medicine. 1993;178(6):2243-7. PMCID: 2191280.

[132] Andersen P, Smedegaard B. CD4(+) T-cell subsets that mediate immunological memory to Mycobacterium tuberculosis infection in mice. Infect Immun. 2000;68(2):621-9. PMCID: 97184.

[133] Bloom BR, Flynn J, McDonough K, Kress Y, Chan J. Experimental approaches to mechanisms of protection and pathogenesis in M. tuberculosis infection. Immunobiology. 1994;191(4-5):526-36.

[134] Caruso AM, Serbina N, Klein E, Triebold K, Bloom BR, Flynn JL. Mice deficient in CD4 T cells have only transiently diminished levels of IFN-gamma, yet succumb to tuberculosis. Journal of Immunology. 1999;162(9):5407-16.

[135] Ladel CH, Blum C, Dreher A, Reifenberg K, Kaufmann SH. Protective role of gamma/delta T cells and alpha/beta T cells in tuberculosis [published erratum appears in Eur J Immunol 1995 Dec;25(12):3525]. European Journal of Immunology. 1995;25(10):2877-81.

[136] Ladel CH, Daugelat S, Kaufmann SH. Immune response to Mycobacterium bovis bacille Calmette Guerin infection in major histocompatibility complex cla. European Journal of Immunology. 1995;25(2):377-84.

[137] Ladel CH, Szalay G, Riedel D, Kaufmann SH. Interleukin-12 secretion by Mycobacterium tuberculosis-infected macrophages. Infection and Immunity. 1997;65(5):1936-8.

[138] Leveton C, Barnass S, Champion B, Lucas S, De Souza B, Nicol M, et al. T-cell-mediated protection of mice against virulent Mycobacterium tuberculosis. Infect Immun. 1989;57(2):390-5. PMCID: 313109.

[139] Munk ME, Gatrill AJ, Kaufmann SH. Target cell lysis and IL-2 secretion by gamma/delta T lymphocytes after activation with bacteria. Journal of Immunology. 1990;145(8):2434-9.

[140] Stenger S, Mazzaccaro RJ, Uyemura K, Cho S, Barnes PF, Rosat JP, et al. Differential effects of cytolytic T cell subsets on intracellular infection. Science. 1997;276(5319):1684-7.

[141] Tascon RE, Stavropoulos E, Lukacs KV, Colston MJ. Protection against Mycobacterium tuberculosis infection by CD8+ T cells requires the production of gamma interferon. Infection and Immunity. 1998;66(2):830-4.

[142] Caruso AM, Serbina N, Klein E, Triebold K, Bloom BR, Flynn JL. Mice deficient in CD4 T cells have only transiently diminished levels of IFN-gamma, yet succumb to tuberculosis 14. Journal of Immunology. 1999;162(9):5407-16.

[143] Serbina NV, Flynn JL. Early emergence of CD8(+) T cells primed for production of type 1 cytokines in the lungs of Mycobacterium tuberculosis-infected mice 1413. Infection and Immunity. 1999;67(8):3980-8.

[144] Scanga CA, Mohan VP, Yu K, Joseph H, Tanaka K, Chan J, et al. Depletion of CD4(+) T cells causes reactivation of murine persistent tuberculosis despite continued expression of interferon gamma and nitric oxide synthase 2. Journal of Experimental Medicine. 2000;192(3):347-58.

[145] Orme IM. Characteristics and specificity of acquired immunologic memory to Mycobacterium tuberculosis infection 406. Journal of Immunology. 1988;140(10):3589-93.

[146] Cooper AM, Dalton DK, Stewart TA, Griffin JP, Russell DG, Orme IM. Disseminated tuberculosis in interferon gamma gene-disrupted mice 1389. Journal of Experimental Medicine. 1993;178(6):2243-7.

[147] Newport MJ, Huxley CM, Huston S, Hawrylowicz CM, Oostra BA, Williamson R, et al. A mutation in the interferon-gamma-receptor gene and susceptibility to mycobacterial infection 1537. New England Journal of Medicine. 1996;335(26):1941-9.

[148] Hirsch CS, Toossi Z, Othieno C, Johnson JL, Schwander SK, Robertson S, et al. Depressed T-cell interferon-gamma responses in pulmonary tuberculosis: analysis of underlying mechanisms and modulation with therapy. Journal of Infectious Diseases. 1999;180(6):2069-73.

[149] Zhang M, Lin Y, Iyer DV, Gong J, Abrams JS, Barnes PF. T-cell cytokine responses in human infection with Mycobacterium tuberculosis 1481. Infection and Immunity. 1995;63(8):3231-4.

[150] Bold TD, Banaei N, Wolf AJ, Ernst JD. Suboptimal activation of antigen-specific CD4+ effector cells enables persistence of M. tuberculosis in vivo. PLoS pathogens. 2011;7(5):e1002063. PMCID: 3102708.

[151] Bean AG, Roach DR, Briscoe H, France MP, Korner H, Sedgwick JD, et al. Structural deficiencies in granuloma formation in TNF gene-targeted mice underlie the heightened susceptibility to aerosol Mycobacterium tuberculosis infection, which is not compensated for by lymphotoxin. J Immunol. 1999;162(6):3504-11.

[152] Flynn JL, Goldstein MM, Chan J, Triebold KJ, Pfeffer K, Lowenstein CJ, et al. Tumor necrosis factor-alpha is required in the protective immune response against Mycobacterium tuberculosis in mice 221. Immunity. 1995;2(6):561-72.

[153] Keane J, Gershon S, Wise RP, Mirabile-Levens E, Kasznica J, Schwieterman WD, et al. Tuberculosis associated with infliximab, a tumor necrosis factor alpha-neutralizing agent. New England Journal of Medicine. 2001;345(15):1098-104.

[154] Khader SA, Bell GK, Pearl JE, Fountain JJ, Rangel-Moreno J, Cilley GE, et al. IL-23 and IL-17 in the establishment of protective pulmonary CD4+ T cell responses after vaccination and during Mycobacterium tuberculosis challenge. Nature immunology. 2007;8(4):369-77.

[155] Khader SA, Pearl JE, Sakamoto K, Gilmartin L, Bell GK, Jelley-Gibbs DM, et al. IL-23 compensates for the absence of IL-12p70 and is essential for the IL-17 response during tuberculosis but is dispensable for protection and antigen-specific IFN-gamma responses if IL-12p70 is available. J Immunol. 2005;175(2):788-95.

[156] Muller I, Cobbold SP, Waldmann H, Kaufmann SH. Impaired resistance to Mycobacterium tuberculosis infection after selective in vivo depletion of L3T4+ and Lyt-2+ T cells 1355. Infection and Immunity. 1987;55(9):2037-41.

[157] Orme IM. The kinetics of emergence and loss of mediator T lymphocytes acquired in response to infection with Mycobacterium tuberculosis. J Immunol. 1987;138(1):293-8.

[158] Silva CL, Silva MF, Pietro RC, Lowrie DB. Protection against tuberculosis by passive transfer with T-cell clones recognizing mycobacterial heat-shock protein 65 1628. Immunology. 1994;83(3):341-6.

[159] Winau F, Hegasy G, Kaufmann SH, Schaible UE. No life without death--apoptosis as prerequisite for T cell activation. Apoptosis. 2005;10(4):707-15.

[160] Flynn JL, Goldstein MM, Triebold KJ, Koller B, Bloom BR. Major histocompatibility complex class I-restricted T cells are required for resistance to Mycobacterium tuberculosis infection 302. ProcNatlAcadSciUSA. 1992;89(24):12013-7.

[161] Ladel CH, Daugelat S, Kaufmann SH. Immune response to Mycobacterium bovis bacille Calmette Guerin infection in major histocompatibility complex class I- and II-deficient knock-out mice: contribution of CD4 and CD8 T cells to acquired resistance. EurJ Immunol. 1995;25(2):377-84.

[162] Behar SM, Dascher CC, Grusby MJ, Wang CR, Brenner MB. Susceptibility of mice deficient in CD1D or TAP1 to infection with Mycobacterium tuberculosis 1000. Journal of Experimental Medicine. 1999;189(12):1973-80.

[163] Rolph MS, Raupach B, Kobernick HH, Collins HL, Perarnau B, Lemonnier FA, et al. MHC class Ia-restricted T cells partially account for beta2-microglobulin-dependent resistance to Mycobacterium tuberculosis. EurJ Immunol. 2001;31(6):1944-9.

[164] Lalvani A, Brookes R, Wilkinson RJ, Malin AS, Pathan AA, Andersen P, et al. Human cytolytic and interferon gamma-secreting CD8+ T lymphocytes specific for Mycobacterium tuberculosis 1052. ProcNatlAcadSciUSA. 1998;95(1):270-5.

[165] Lewinsohn DM, Briden AL, Reed SG, Grabstein KH, Alderson MR. Mycobacterium tuberculosis-reactive CD8+ T lymphocytes: the relative contribution of classical versus nonclassical HLA restriction 2419. Journal of Immunology. 2000;165(2):925-30.

[166] Lewinsohn DM, Zhu L, Madison VJ, Dillon DC, Fling SP, Reed SG, et al. Classically restricted human CD8(+) T lymphocytes derived from mycobacterium tuberculosis-infected cells: definition of antigenic specificity [In Process Citation] 2420. Journal of Immunology. 2001;166(1):439-46.

[167] Mohagheghpour N, Gammon D, Kawamura LM, van Vollenhoven A, Benike CJ, Engleman EG. CTL response to Mycobacterium tuberculosis: identification of an

immunogenic epitope in the 19-kDa lipoprotein 61. Journal of Immunology. 1998;161(5):2400-6.

[168] Tan JS, Canaday DH, Boom WH, Balaji KN, Schwander SK, Rich EA. Human alveolar T lymphocyte responses to Mycobacterium tuberculosis antigens: role for CD4+ and CD8+ cytotoxic T cells and relative resistance of alveolar macrophages to lysis 1604. Journal of Immunology. 1997;159(1):290-7.

[169] Turner J, Dockrell HM. Stimulation of human peripheral blood mononuclear cells with live Mycobacterium bovis BCG activates cytolytic CD8+ T cells in vitro 184. Immunology. 1996;87(3):339-42.

[170] Heinzel AS, Grotzke JE, Lines RA, Lewinsohn DA, McNabb AL, Streblow DN, et al. HLA-E-dependent presentation of Mtb-derived antigen to human CD8+ T cells. Journal of Experimental Medicine. 2002;196(11):1473-81.

[171] Lewinsohn DM, Alderson MR, Briden AL, Riddell SR, Reed SG, Grabstein KH. Characterization of human CD8+ T cells reactive with Mycobacterium tuberculosis-infected antigen-presenting cells 1781. Journal of Experimental Medicine. 1998;187(10):1633-40.

[172] Moody DB, Reinhold BB, Reinhold VN, Besra GS, Porcelli SA. Uptake and processing of glycosylated mycolates for presentation to CD1b-restricted T cells 1772. Immunology Letters. 1999;65(1-2):85-91.

[173] Rosat JP, Grant EP, Beckman EM, Dascher CC, Sieling PA, Frederique D, et al. CD1-restricted microbial lipid antigen-specific recognition found in the CD8+ alpha beta T cell pool 1725. Journal of Immunology. 1999;162(1):366-71.

[174] Bertholet S, Ireton GC, Kahn M, Guderian J, Mohamath R, Stride N, et al. Identification of human T cell antigens for the development of vaccines against Mycobacterium tuberculosis. J Immunol. 2008;181(11):7948-57. PMCID: 2586986.

[175] Coler RN, Baldwin SL, Shaverdian N, Bertholet S, Reed SJ, Raman VS, et al. A synthetic adjuvant to enhance and expand immune responses to influenza vaccines. PloS one. 2010;5(10):e13677. PMCID: 2965144.

[176] Coler RN, Bertholet S, Moutaftsi M, Guderian JA, Windish HP, Baldwin SL, et al. Development of Glucopyranosyl Lipid A, a Synthetic TLR4 Agonist, as a Vaccine Adjuvant. PloS one. 2011;6(1):e16333.

[177] Von Eschen K, Morrison R, Braun M, Ofori-Anyinam O, De Kock E, Pavithran P, et al. The candidate tuberculosis vaccine Mtb72F/AS02A: Tolerability and immunogenicity in humans. Human vaccines. 2009;5(7):475-82.

[178] Rowland R, McShane H. Tuberculosis vaccines in clinical trials. Expert review of vaccines. 2011;10(5):645-58.

[179] Brandt L, Skeiky YA, Alderson MR, Lobet Y, Dalemans W, Turner OC, et al. The protective effect of the Mycobacterium bovis BCG vaccine is increased by coadministration with the Mycobacterium tuberculosis 72-kilodalton fusion polyprotein Mtb72F in M. tuberculosis-infected guinea pigs. Infect Immun. 2004;72(11):6622-32.

[180] Reed SG, Coler RN, Dalemans W, Tan EV, DeLa Cruz EC, Basaraba RJ, et al. Defined tuberculosis vaccine, Mtb72F/AS02A, evidence of protection in cynomolgus monkeys. Proceedings of the National Academy of Sciences of the United States of America. 2009;106(7):2301-6. PMCID: 2650151.

[181] Skeiky YA, Alderson MR, Ovendale PJ, Guderian JA, Brandt L, Dillon DC, et al. Differential immune responses and protective efficacy induced by components of a tuberculosis polyprotein vaccine, Mtb72F, delivered as naked DNA or recombinant protein. J Immunol. 2004;172(12):7618-28.

[182] Agger EM, Rosenkrands I, Hansen J, Brahimi K, Vandahl BS, Aagaard C, et al. Cationic liposomes formulated with synthetic mycobacterial cordfactor (CAF01): a versatile adjuvant for vaccines with different immunological requirements. PloS one. 2008;3(9):e3116. PMCID: 2525815.

[183] Davidsen J, Rosenkrands I, Christensen D, Vangala A, Kirby D, Perrie Y, et al. Characterization of cationic liposomes based on dimethyldioctadecylammonium and synthetic cord factor from M. tuberculosis (trehalose 6,6'-dibehenate)-a novel adjuvant inducing both strong CMI and antibody responses. Biochim Biophys Acta. 2005;1718(1-2):22-31.

[184] Holten-Andersen L, Doherty TM, Korsholm KS, Andersen P. Combination of the cationic surfactant dimethyl dioctadecyl ammonium bromide and synthetic mycobacterial cord factor as an efficient adjuvant for tuberculosis subunit vaccines. Infect Immun. 2004;72(3):1608-17. PMCID: 356055.

[185] Agger EM, Rosenkrands I, Olsen AW, Hatch G, Williams A, Kritsch C, et al. Protective immunity to tuberculosis with Ag85B-ESAT-6 in a synthetic cationic adjuvant system IC31. Vaccine. 2006;24(26):5452-60.

[186] Kamath AT, Rochat AF, Christensen D, Agger EM, Andersen P, Lambert PH, et al. A liposome-based mycobacterial vaccine induces potent adult and neonatal multifunctional T cells through the exquisite targeting of dendritic cells. PloS one. 2009;4(6):e5771. PMCID: 2685976.

[187] Kamath AT, Rochat AF, Valenti MP, Agger EM, Lingnau K, Andersen P, et al. Adult-like anti-mycobacterial T cell and in vivo dendritic cell responses following neonatal immunization with Ag85B-ESAT-6 in the IC31 adjuvant. PloS one. 2008;3(11):e3683. PMCID: 2577009.

[188] Langermans JA, Doherty TM, Vervenne RA, van der Laan T, Lyashchenko K, Greenwald R, et al. Protection of macaques against Mycobacterium tuberculosis infection by a subunit vaccine based on a fusion protein of antigen 85B and ESAT-6. Vaccine. 2005;23(21):2740-50.

[189] Olsen AW, Williams A, Okkels LM, Hatch G, Andersen P. Protective effect of a tuberculosis subunit vaccine based on a fusion of antigen 85B and ESAT-6 in the aerosol guinea pig model. Infect Immun. 2004;72(10):6148-50. PMCID: 517547.

[190] Brock I, Weldingh K, Leyten EM, Arend SM, Ravn P, Andersen P. Specific T-cell epitopes for immunoassay-based diagnosis of Mycobacterium tuberculosis infection. J Clin Microbiol. 2004;42(6):2379-87. PMCID: 427833.

[191] Aagaard C, Hoang TT, Izzo A, Billeskov R, Troudt J, Arnett K, et al. Protection and polyfunctional T cells induced by Ag85B-TB10.4/IC31 against Mycobacterium tuberculosis is highly dependent on the antigen dose. PloS one. 2009;4(6):e5930. PMCID: 2691953.

[192] Skeiky YA, Dietrich J, Lasco TM, Stagliano K, Dheenadhayalan V, Goetz MA, et al. Non-clinical efficacy and safety of HyVac4:IC31 vaccine administered in a BCG prime-boost regimen. Vaccine. 2010;28(4):1084-93.

3

Identification of CD8+ T Cell Epitopes Against *Mycobacterium tuberculosis*

Fei Chen, Yanfeng Gao and Yuanming Qi

Department of Bioengineering, Zhengzhou University, Zhengzhou
China

1. Introduction

Although the effective immune response against *Mycobacterium tuberculosis* (*M. tuberculosis*, Mtb) is primarily due to cell-mediated immunity, the mechanisms by which T cells participate in the control of infection are still not completely understood. The importance of CD8+ T cells in the immune response to tuberculosis has been recognized by many researchers [1]. Experimental evidence from the murine model indicated that CD8+ T cells could be important to the control of *Mycobacterium tuberculosis* infection *in vivo* [2-5]. The isolation of *M. tuberculosis*-specific CD8+ T cells from infected mice and human clearly showed that this subset could be induced during infection [6-8]. Reports on epitope-specific *M. tuberculosis* reactive CD8+ T cells, which are present at very high frequencies in the peripheral blood of PPD positive individuals and patients with active tuberculosis, support the importance of CD8+ T cells to the immunity of *M. tuberculosis* and emphasize that the CD8+ T cell subset should be considered to the design of new anti-tuberculosis vaccines [9, 10]. CD8+ T cells may contribute to the control of *M. tuberculosis* infection through four mechanisms: (1) Cytokine release, such as IFN-γ and TNF-α; (2) Cytotoxicity via granule-dependent exocytosis pathway; (3) Cytotoxicity mediated through Fas/Fas ligand interaction; (4) Direct microbicidal activity.

The pathogen's antigens are processed by antigen presenting cells (APCs) and digested into short peptides. Consequently, these non-self peptides are presented to the surface of the infected cells or APCs through the loading of the major histocompatibility complex (MHC) or called human leukocyte antigen (HLA) in human. These peptide/MHC complexes are recognized by specific T-cells that perform immune responses, such as cytotoxicity (in the case of class I MHC). These peptides which act as the markers of the pathogens are called T cell epitopes [11]. The identification of novel cytotoxic T lymphocyte (CTL) epitopes is important to the analysis of the involvement of CD8+ T cells in *M. tuberculosis* infection as well as the anti-Mtb vaccine development. However, only a small number of MHC-I-restricted CTL epitopes have been identified within a few of *M. tuberculosis* proteins. The step to develop epitope-based vaccines include: (1) antigen selection; (2) epitope prediction; (3) epitope identification; (4) vaccine prototype engineering; (5) immunization and challenge studies. In this chapter we mainly focused on the strategy to identify CD8+ T cell epitopes against *Mycobacterium tuberculosis*. It includes: selection of the antigens; Prediction the CD8+ T cell epitopes; Synthesis and modification of the epitopes; Identification of epitopes by *in vitro* and *in vivo* assays; Development of CD8+ T cell epitope-based vaccines.

2. Selection of antigens from *Mycobacterium tuberculosis*

An essential step towards the development of novel vaccines against Mtb is gaining more information on the antigenic architecture of *Mycobacterium tuberculosis* to identify T-cell epitopes responsible for eliciting protective immune responses. Determination of the complete genome sequence of *Mycobacterium tuberculosis* facilitated this step considerably. The H37Rv strain of *Mycobacterium tuberculosis* has been found extensive, worldwide application in biomedical research because it has retained full virulence in animal models. Cole et al reported the complete genome sequence of H37Rv in 1998 [12]. This progress in genomics makes it possible that we can find corresponding protein sequences through submitting to publicly accessible sequence databases such as GenBank and TB database [13].

The Mtb genome contains about 4,203 open reading frames, nearly half of which are categorized as 'hypothetical proteins' with unknown function. Although secreted proteins are generally associated with protective immune responses, no proteins or protein families have yet been shown to fully protect against the active Mtb infection. Screening each protein from these 4,023 open reading frames by using human serum and gel electrophoresis would be time-consuming and costly method of identifying new vaccine candidates. Bioinformatics tools provide more practical means to rapidly identify potential epitopes and antigens for Mtb vaccines development. A range of approaches have been utilized to select proteins for analysis prior to epitope mapping. For example, whole genome analysis can be performed in order to identify candidate vaccine components, or alternatively, bioinformatics tools that select proteins according to their secretion characteristics can be used to narrow the number of proteins evaluated in the next step [14-16]. Frieder et al used pepmixes created by Micro-Scale SPOT™ to map T cell epitopes in 389 proteins of *Mycobacterium tuberculosis* [17]. These proteins are sorted by their known or likely known function such as PPE/PE, cell wall, cell processes, virulence, detoxification, and adaptation. Some CD8+ T cell epitopes identified by researchers were listed in **Table 1.**

So far, antigens in *Mycobacterium tuberculosis* from which CD8+ T cell epitopes were identified are mainly focused on secretory proteins, lipoproteins, such as Ag85-complex, ESAT-6, CFP10, 16kDa protein, 19kDa lipoprotein and so on. But there are few studies focused on the membrane proteins like the drug efflux pumps which play important role in the drug-resistant of *Mycobacterium tuberculosis*. Researchers in our lab tried to identify novel CD8+ T cell epitopes from these antigens and found several novel CD8+ T cell epitopes which could elicit potent immune responses both *in vitro* and *in vivo* [32].

3. Prediction of the CD8+ T cell epitopes

The lack of simple methods to identify relevant T-cell epitopes, the high mutation rate of many pathogens, and restriction of T-cell response to epitopes due to human lymphocyte

Protein name	Gene description	Amino acid position	HLA allele	Frequency	References
Ag85A	mycolyltransferases	48-56	HLA-A2	1/20,693PBMCs (Elispot)	[18]
		242-250	HLA-A2	1/3,300 PBMCs (tetramer) 1/23,779 PBMCs (Elispot) 1/3,750 PBMCs (tetramer)	
Ag85B	mycolyltransferases	143–152 199–207 264–272	HLA-A2 HLA-A2 HLA-B35	ND Undetectable (tetramer) ND	[19, 20]
Ag85C	mycolyltransferases	204–212	HLA-B35	1/13,700–1/22,200 PBMCs	[20]
ESAT-6	Early secretory antigen target	69–76 82–90 21–29	HLA-B53 HLA-A2 HLA-A6802	1/700 CD8+ 1/2,500 PBMCs 1/2,100 CD8+	[21, 22]
CFP10	10kDa culture filtrate antigen	2–9 2–12 3–11 75–83 2–11 49–58 85–94 71–79 76–85	HLA-B4501 HLA-B4501 HLA-B0801 HLA-B1502 HLA-B44 HLA-B44 HLA-B3514 HLA-B14 HLA-B3514	1/101 CD8+ 1/125 CD8+ 1/645 CD8+ 1/145 CD8+ 1/700 CD8+ 1/7,000 CD8+ 1/2,100 CD8+ 1/438–1/1,602 PBMCs 1/437–1/2,427 PBMCs	[11, 23, 24]
CFP21	cutinase precursor	134-142	HLA-A2	3/5000-1/10000 PBMCs ((Elispot))	[25]

Protein name	Gene description	Amino acid position	HLA allele	Frequency	References
Mtb8.4	low molecular weight T-cell antigen	5–15 32–40	HLA-B1501 HLA-B3514	1/10,416 CD8+ 1/1,190 CD8+	[23]
Mtb9.8	Hypothetical protein	3–11 53–61	HLA-A0201 HLA-B0801	<1/25,000 CD8+ 1/2,840 CD8+	[23]
Mtb39	PPE family protein	144–153 346–355	HLA-B44 HLA-B44	ND ND	[26]
16kDa protein	heat shock protein	21–29 120–128	HLA-A2 HLA-A2	1/1,000 CD8+ 1/800 CD8+	[19]
19kDa lipoprotein	19 kDa lipoprotein antigen precursor	88–97	HLA-A2	ND	[27]
38kDa protein	periplasmic phosphate-binding lipoprotein	8–17	HLA-A0201	1/331 CD8+	[28]
Hsp65	chaperonin	369–377	HLA-A2	ND	[29]
Rv0341	isoniazid inductible gene protein	33–42 33–44 33–45	HLA-A2 HLA-A2 HLA-A2	ND ND ND	[30]
Rv2903c	signal peptidase	201–209	HLA-B35	Undetectable	[31]
Rv1410c	aminoglycosides/tetracycline -transport integral membrane protein	510-518	HLA-A0201	3/2500 PBMCs	[32]
GlnA1	glutamine synthetase	308–316	HLA-A2	ND	[33]
SodA	superoxide dismutase	160–168	HLA-A2	ND	[32]
AlaDH	delta-aminolevulinic acid dehydratase	160–169	HLA-A2	ND	[32]
Hemolysin	cytotoxin/hemolysin	73–82	HLA-A0201	1/353 CD8+	[28]

Table 1. CD8+ T cell epitopes identified in *Mycobacterium tuberculosis*

antigen (HLA) polymorphism have significantly hindered the development of cytotoxic T-lymphocyte (CTL) epitope-based or epitope-driven vaccines. As the development of bioinformatics, computer-driven algorithms methods for predicting CD8+ T cell epitopes are used as important tools to the vaccine design. These tools offer a significant advantage over other methods of epitope selection because high-throughput screening can be performed in silico, followed by consequent immunological experiments *in vitro* and *in vivo* [34]. Traditionally, the identification of T cell epitopes required the synthesis of overlapping peptides that spanned the entire length of a protein, followed by experimental assays for each peptide, such as *in vitro* intracellular cytokine staining, to determine the T cell activation. This method is economically viable only for single protein or pathogen that consists of fewer proteins. As a result, alternative computational approaches have been developed for the prediction of T cell epitopes, which have significantly decreased the experimental burden that is associated with epitope identification. Computer-driven algorithms are now routinely employed to sort through protein sequences for linear strings of amino acids that confirm to previously established patterns known to be associated with the binding to antigen presenting molecules (such as MHC) and stimulation of T cells. These peptide strings, once proven to stimulate T cells *in vitro* or *in vivo*, are considered as T cell epitopes.

A lot of computational algorithms have been developed to predict CTL epitopes in pathogen protein sequences (some of these are listed in **Table 2**). In reality, using only one computational algorithm to predict CTL epitopes may lead to large number of false positives and false negatives. Later and more comprehensive validations using data from several different prediction softwares are accurate and of high value in reducing the cost for epitope identification. Researchers in our lab used several prediction servers and identified novel CTL epitopes successfully [25, 32].

4. Synthesis and modification of the epitopes

Solid phase peptide synthesis (SPPS) offers important advantages over the synthesis in solution, in which coupling reactions can be carried out more rapidly and nearly to completion using an excess of the activated amino acid derivative, which can be removed at the end of the reaction by simple washing operations. The introduction of Fmoc protecting group into SPPS by Carpino in 1970 allowed the entire process of SPPS to be carried out under milder reactive conditions [35]. As a result of this chemical progress, nowadays the synthesis of many peptides can be smoothly accomplished by manual or automate-assisted SPPS and even longer proteins can be synthesized by coupling protected segments or more efficiently by chemical ligation with unprotected peptide segments [36].

The immunogenicity of the native epitope is often weak. Substitutions at main anchor positions to increase the complementarity between the peptide and HLA binding cleft constitute a common procedure to improve the binding capacity and immunogenicity of the native epitope. In 1993, Ruppert et al determined that the 'canonical' HLA-A2.1 motif could be defined as leucine (L) or methione (M) at position 2 (P2) and leucine (L), valine (V), or isoleucine (I) at position 9 (P9) [37]. In 2000, Tourdot et al demonstrated that residue tyrosine (Y) at position 1 (P1) could enhance the affinity of epitope to HLA-I molecule [38]. These results suggested that an altered peptide ligand (APL) might be used to exploit a latent capacity of the T cell repertoire to respond more effectively to the native epitope. We also used this strategy to modify the related positions and found the binding capacity and immunogenicity of some epitopes improved [25, 32]. The second strategy is to modify the amino acids with a side chain protruding out of the peptide binding cleft of the HLA molecule, because these amino acids may participate in T cell receptor (TCR) recognition. If they are substituted by amino acids with other properties, a mutated epitope may bind more efficiently to TCR or elicit a more diverse TCR reservoir [39, 40].

ID	server	Abbreviation	Prediction algorithm
1	BIMAS	BIMAS	Matrix[a]
2	HLA Ligand	HLA_LI	Matrix[a]
3	IEDB (ANN)	IEDB_ANN	ANN[b]
4	IEDB (ARB)	IEDB_ARB	Matrix[a]
5	IEDB (SMM)	IEDB_SMM	Matrix[a]
6	MAPPP (Bimas)	MAPPP_B	Matrix[a]
7	MAPPP(SYFPEITHI)	MAPPP_S	Matrix[a]
8	MHC Binder Prediction	MHC_BP	Matrix[a]
9	MHC-BPS	MHC-BPS	SVM[c]
10	MHC-I (Multiple matrix)	MHCI_MM	Structure-based model
11	MHC-I (Single matrix)	MHCI_SM	Structure-based model
12	MHCPred (Interactions)	MHCP_I	Partial least square
13	MHCPred (Amino Acids)	MHCP_AA	Partial least square
14	MULTIPRED (ANN)	MULTI_ANN	ANN[b]
15	MULTIPRED (HMM)	MULTI_HMM	HMM[d]
16	MULTIPRED (SVM)	MULTI_SVM	SVM[c]
17	NetMHC (ANN)	NETM_ANN	ANN[b]
18	NetMHC (Weight Matrix)	NETM_WM	Matrix[a]
19	nHLAPred (ANNPred)	NHP_ANN	ANN[b]
20	nHLAPred (ComPred)	NHP_CP	ANN[b] and Matrix[a]
21	PepDist	PEPDIST	distance function
22	PeptideCheck (Matrix)	PEPC_M	Matrix[a]
23	Predep	PREDEP	Structure-based model
24	ProPred1	PROPRED	Matrix[a]
25	Rankpep	RANKPEP	Matrix[a]
26	SMM	SMM	Matrix[a]
27	SVMHC (MHCPEP)	SVMHC_M	SVM[c]
28	SVMHC (SYFPEITHI)	SVMHC_S	SVM[c]
29	SVRMHC	SVRMHC	SVM[c]
30	SYFPEITHI	SYFPEITHI	Matrix[a]

a: binding matrices
b: artificial neural networks
c: support vector machines
d: hidden Markov models

Table 2. Some epitope prediction servers

5. Identification of epitopes by *in vitro* and *in vivo* assays

The immunogenicity of epitopes predicted through appropriate prediction softwares should be identified by a series of *in vitro* and *in vivo* assays. Only epitopes which are proven to stimulate T cells *in vitro* or *in vivo* can be used as potential subunit components for the design of vaccines against tuberculosis. Because there are various techniques to identify specific T-cell epitopes, the question arises about how to select and combine these techniques to screen peptides more efficiently and rapidly.

According to the processing and presenting progress of T cell epitopes and their ability to specifically stimulate T cells in an MHC allele-restricted manner. The pathway of MHC-I eptiope presentation has been exhibited and the process comprise three main steps: firstly, endogenous proteins are digested into short peptides by proteasomes; secondly, special epitopes are selected to load onto MHC-I molecule within the endoplasmic reticulum; finally, the peptide/MHC complexes are transferred to cell surface and to stimulate specific T-cell receptors on T cells. Therefore, there are three essential elements for a random peptide to be considered as MHC-I restricted T cell epitope. First, the peptide must be naturally processed into an optimal length via a proteasome dependent pathway. Second, the peptide should have the affinity to bind to the corresponding MHC-I molecule. Finally, and perhaps the most important, the peptide must have the ability to induce a T-cell-specific response after its presentation on an MHC-I molecule [11]. Thus, the techniques to evaluate the three features of a given peptide can be classified into three corresponding types: MHC-binding assay; T cell specific antigenicity assay; Verification of the natural processing of the peptide.

5.1 MHC binding assay

Various methods have been developed to evaluate the binding affinity of peptides to MHC-I molecule. Standard peptide binding inhibition assay is a common method used to quantitatively measure the binding affinity of the target peptides [41]. The MHC-I transfected cell line binding assay was utilized in many labs for its simplicity, repeatability and quantifiability for determining peptide and MHC-binding affinities [25, 32].

5.2 T cell specific antigenicity assay

Peptides with atypical anchoring residues for a related MHC-I allele always display very low binding affinity for MHC-I molecule tested *in vitro*. However, some of these peptides may possess potent antigenicity to induce robust and specific T cell responses. Therefore, it is commonly considered that the most definitive means of defining an epitope is to test peptide-specific T cell responses. Numerous techniques are currently utilized in peptide specific T cell determination, including MHC tetramer staining, enzyme-linked immunospot (ELISPOT) assay, intracellular cytokine staining (ICS), cytotoxicity assay (such as lactate dehydrogenase release assay and ^{51}Cr release assay) and T-cell proliferation assay [18-33].

5.3 Verification of the natural processing of the peptide

Some artificially synthesized peptides have the potent immunogenicity to trigger specific T cell responses and binding affinity to the related MHC molecules *in vitro*. However, these peptides cannot be generated through natural processing and presenting steps [42]. Therefore, demonstrating that a given peptide is processed naturally is a prerequisite to epitope identification. There are two conventional techniques by using reversed phase high-performance liquid chromatography (RP-HPLC) and mass spectrometry (MS) to analyze if a peptide is naturally processed. One method is to manipulate the peptide through the following procedures: (1) Target cells are transfected with specific MHC-I allele; (2) The cells are harvested, and the MHC molecules expressed on the surface of the cells are purified; (3) The peptides bound to the MHC molecules are acid-eluted, purified and finally analyzed by MS [43]. The other technique is to cleave the longer peptides which include the potential epitopes with purified proteasome complexes *in vitro*. Then, production of peptides by the digestion is analyzed by RP-HPLC and MS [44]. However, the results of this method must be analyzed carefully, because proteasome digestion can only generate the proper C terminus of the MHC-loaded peptides [11].

6. Development of CD8$^+$ T cell epitope-based vaccines

One of the approaches to find effective and safe vaccines is epitope-based DNA vaccination that enables focusing of the immune response on important and highly conserved epitopes [45]. This provides the opportunity to use specific epitopes to shift the immune system toward a Th1 or a Th2-mediated immune response and eliminate the unwanted responses. Besides that, CTL epitope-based immunization has the advantage of eliciting immune response only against the protective epitope and avoidance of epitope drift in *Mycobacterium tuberculosis* infection [46].

In many cases, a single CTL epitope-based DNA vaccine could not be fully protective against the Mtb infection. Development of epitope-based vaccines has been hampered for its relatively low antigenicity. Thus, different vaccine patterns and delivery methodologies have been developed, which include synthetic multivalent peptide vaccine, recombinant protein vaccine, DNA vaccine, viral vector, protein carrier, and adjuvant, to solve the problem. Studies of Mtb in human indicate that the induction of broad T-cell mediated immunity to Mtb and Type 1 cytokines including interleukin-2 (IL-2), interferon-γ (IFN-γ), and tumor necrosis factor α (TNF-α) are essential for Mtb vaccine design [47]. Vaccines based on CTL epitopes represent a logical approach to generate effective cellular immunity in both the prophylactic and therapeutic settings because multiple epitopes can be incorporated into the vaccine design with the goal of inducing broadly reactive responses composed of multiple CTL clones directed against different epitopes. DNA vaccines derived from multiple epitopes have been reported to induce broad CTL responses against HIV, HBV, and SARS-CoV [48-50]. Although epitope-based vaccines are often thought to be limited with respect to HLA polymorphism and population coverage, the use of supertype-restricted epitopes, those capable of binding with significant affinity to multiple related HLA alleles, provides a means to address this problem [51]. There are several problems which need to be solved in the future studies of epitope-based Mtb vaccines, such as the safety of the DNA vaccine, the development of better adjuvants, the difference and mutation among the Mtb strains, complete clearance of the Mtb, the results from challenge models in rats or guinea pigs inconsistent with that of clinical trials.

7. References

[1] Lazarevic, V. and Flynn J. (2002). CD8+ T cells in tuberculosis. Am J Respir Crit Care Med 166(8): 1116-1121.

[2] Flynn, J. L. and Chan J. (2001). Immunology of tuberculosis. Annu Rev Immunol 19: 93-129.

[3] Flynn, J. L., Goldstein, M. M. et al. (1992). Major histocompatibility complex class I-restricted T cells are required for resistance to Mycobacterium tuberculosis infection. Proc Natl Acad Sci U S A 89(24): 12013-12017.

[4] Sousa, A. O., Mazzaccaro, R. J. et al. (2000). Relative contributions of distinct MHC class I-dependent cell populations in protection to tuberculosis infection in mice. Proc Natl Acad Sci U S A 97(8): 4204-4208.

[5] D'Souza, C. D., Cooper, A. M. et al. (2000). A novel nonclassic beta2-microglobulin-restricted mechanism influencing early lymphocyte accumulation and subsequent resistance to tuberculosis in the lung. Am J Respir Cell Mol Biol 23(2): 188-193.

[6] Serbina, N. V. and Flynn J. L. (1999). Early emergence of CD8(+) T cells primed for production of type 1 cytokines in the lungs of Mycobacterium tuberculosis-infected mice. Infect Immun 67(8): 3980-3988.

[7] Stenger, S., Mazzaccaro, R. J. et al. (1997). Differential effects of cytolytic T cell subsets on intracellular infection. Science 276(5319): 1684-1687.

[8] Rosat, J. P., Grant, et al. E. P. (1999). CD1-restricted microbial lipid antigen-specific recognition found in the CD8+ alpha beta T cell pool. J Immunol 162(1): 366-371.

[9] Lewinsohn, D. M., Briden, A. L. et al. (2000). Mycobacterium tuberculosis-reactive CD8+ T lymphocytes: the relative contribution of classical versus nonclassical HLA restriction. J Immunol 165(2): 925-930.

[10] Lewinsohn, D. M., Zhu, L. et al. (2001). Classically restricted human CD8+ T lymphocytes derived from Mycobacterium tuberculosis-infected cells: definition of antigenic specificity. J Immunol 166(1): 439-446.

[11] Liu, J., Zhang, S. et al. (2011). Revival of the identification of cytotoxic T-lymphocyte epitopes for immunological diagnosis, therapy and vaccine development. Exp Biol Med (Maywood) 236(3): 253-267.

[12] Cole, S. T., Brosch, R. et al. (1998). Deciphering the biology of Mycobacterium tuberculosis from the complete genome sequence. Nature 393(6685): 537-544.

[13] Galagan, J. E., Sisk, P. et al. (2010). TB database 2010: overview and update. Tuberculosis (Edinb) 90(4): 225-235.

[14] Sbai, H., Mehta, A. et al. (2001). Use of T cell epitopes for vaccine development. Curr Drug Targets Infect Disord 1(3): 303-313.

[15] Gomez, M., Johnson, S. et al. (2000). Identification of secreted proteins of Mycobacterium tuberculosis by a bioinformatic approach. Infect Immun 68(4): 2323-2327.

[16] McMurry, J., Sbai, H. et al. (2005). Analyzing Mycobacterium tuberculosis proteomes for candidate vaccine epitopes. Tuberculosis (Edinb) 85(1-2): 95-105.

[17] Frieder M., Lewinsohn D. M. (2009). T-cell epitope mapping in Mycobacterium tuberculosis using pepmixes created by micro-scale SPOT- synthesis. Methods Mol Biol 524:369-382.

[18] Smith, S. M., Brookes, R. et al. (2000). Human CD8+ CTL specific for the mycobacterial major secreted antigen 85A. J Immunol 165(12): 7088-7095.

[19] Geluk, A., van Meijgaarden, K. E. et al. (2000). Identification of major epitopes of Mycobacterium tuberculosis AG85B that are recognized by HLA-A*0201-restricted CD8+ T cells in HLA-transgenic mice and humans. J Immunol 165(11): 6463-6471.

[20] Klein, M. R., Smith, S. M. et al. (2001). HLA-B*35-restricted CD8 T cell epitopes in the antigen 85 complex of Mycobacterium tuberculosis. J Infect Dis 183(6): 928-934.

[21] Lalvani, A., Brookes, R. et al. (1998). Human cytolytic and interferon gamma-secreting CD8+ T lymphocytes specific for Mycobacterium tuberculosis. Proc Natl Acad Sci U S A 95(1): 270-275.

[22] Pathan, A. A., Wilkinson, K. A. et al. (2000). High frequencies of circulating IFN-gamma-secreting CD8 cytotoxic T cells specific for a novel MHC class I-restricted Mycobacterium tuberculosis epitope in M. tuberculosis-infected subjects without disease. Eur J Immunol 30(9): 2713-2721.

[23] Lewinsohn, D. A., Winata, E. et al. (2007). Immunodominant tuberculosis CD8 antigens preferentially restricted by HLA-B. PLoS Pathog 3(9): 1240-1249.

[24] Shams, H., Klucar, P. et al. (2004). Characterization of a Mycobacterium tuberculosis peptide that is recognized by human CD4+ and CD8+ T cells in the context of multiple HLA alleles. J Immunol 173(3): 1966-1977.

[25] Lv, H., Gao, Y. et al. (2010). Identification of a novel cytotoxic T lymphocyte epitope from CFP21, a secreted protein of Mycobacterium tuberculosis. Immunol Lett 133(2): 94-98.

[26] Lewinsohn, D. A., Lines, R. A. et al. (2002). Human dendritic cells presenting adenovirally expressed antigen elicit Mycobacterium tuberculosis--specific CD8+ T cells. Am J Respir Crit Care Med 166(6): 843-848.

[27] Mohagheghpour, N., Gammon, D. et al. (1998). CTL response to Mycobacterium tuberculosis: identification of an immunogenic epitope in the 19-kDa lipoprotein. J Immunol 161(5): 2400-2406.

[28] Shams, H., Barnes, P. F. et al. (2003). Human CD8+ T cells recognize epitopes of the 28-kDa hemolysin and the 38-kDa antigen of Mycobacterium tuberculosis. J Leukoc Biol 74(6): 1008-1014.

[29] Charo, J., Geluk, A. et al. (2001). The identification of a common pathogen-specific HLA class I A*0201-restricted cytotoxic T cell epitope encoded within the heat shock protein 65. Eur J Immunol 31(12): 3602-3611.

[30] Flyer, D. C., Ramakrishna, V. et al. (2002). Identification by mass spectrometry of CD8(+)-T-cell Mycobacterium tuberculosis epitopes within the Rv0341 gene product. Infect Immun 70(6): 2926-2932.

[31] Klein, M. R., Hammond, A. S. et al. (2002). HLA-B*35-restricted CD8(+)-T-cell epitope in Mycobacterium tuberculosis Rv2903c. Infect Immun 70(2): 981-984.

[32] Zhu, Y. H., Gao, Y. F. et al. (2011). Identification of novel T cell epitopes from efflux pumps of Mycobacterium tuberculosis. Immunol Lett. 140(1-2):68-73

[33] Dong, Y., Demaria, S. et al. (2004). HLA-A2-restricted CD8+-cytotoxic-T-cell responses to novel epitopes in Mycobacterium tuberculosis superoxide dismutase, alanine dehydrogenase, and glutamine synthetase. Infect Immun 72(4): 2412-2415.

[34] Martin, W., Sbai, H. et al. (2003). Bioinformatics tools for identifying class I-restricted epitopes. Methods 29(3): 289-298

[35] Carpino, L.A. (1970) 9-Fluorenylmethoxycarbonyl function, a new base-sensitive amino-protecting group. J. Am. Chem. Soc 92:5748 .

[36] Coin, I., Beyermann, M. et al. (2007). Solid-phase peptide synthesis: from standard procedures to the synthesis of difficult sequences. Nat Protoc 2(12): 3247-3256.

[37] Ruppert, J., Sidney, J. et al. (1993). Prominent role of secondary anchor residues in peptide binding to HLA-A2.1 molecules. Cell 74(5): 929-937.

[38] Tourdot, S., Scardino, A. et al. (2000). A general strategy to enhance immunogenicity of low-affinity HLA-A2.1-associated peptides: implication in the identification of cryptic tumor epitopes. Eur J Immunol 30(12): 3411-3421.

[39] Slansky, J. E., Rattis, F. M. et al. (2000). Enhanced antigen-specific antitumor immunity with altered peptide ligands that stabilize the MHC-peptide-TCR complex. Immunity 13(4): 529-538.

[40] Windhagen, A., Scholz, C. et al. (1995). Modulation of cytokine patterns of human autoreactive T cell clones by a single amino acid substitution of their peptide ligand. Immunity 2(4): 373-380.

[41] Altfeld, M. A., Livingston, B. et al. (2001). Identification of novel HLA-A2-restricted human immunodeficiency virus type 1-specific cytotoxic T-lymphocyte epitopes predicted by the HLA-A2 supertype peptide-binding motif. J Virol 75(3): 1301-1311.

[42] Toma, A., Laika, T. et al. (2009). Recognition of human proinsulin leader sequence by class I-restricted T-cells in HLA-A*0201 transgenic mice and in human type 1 diabetes. Diabetes 58(2): 394-402.

[43] Oelke, M., Maus, M. V. et al. (2003). Ex vivo induction and expansion of antigen-specific cytotoxic T cells by HLA-Ig-coated artificial antigen-presenting cells. Nat Med 9(5): 619-624.

[44] Pinkse, G. G., Tysma, O. H. et al. (2005). Autoreactive CD8 T cells associated with beta cell destruction in type 1 diabetes. Proc Natl Acad Sci U S A 102(51): 18425-18430.

[45] Wilson, C. C., McKinney, D. et al. (2003). Development of a DNA vaccine designed to induce cytotoxic T lymphocyte responses to multiple conserved epitopes in HIV-1. J Immunol 171(10): 5611-5623.

[46] Pouriayevali, M. H., Bamdad, T. et al. (2011). Full length antigen priming enhances the CTL epitope-based DNA vaccine efficacy. Cell Immunol 268(1): 4-8.

[47] Kaufmann, S. H. and Hess J. (1999). Impact of intracellular location of and antigen display by intracellular bacteria: implications for vaccine development. Immunol Lett 65(1-2): 81-84.

[48] Thomson, S. A., Sherritt, M. A. et al. (1998). Delivery of multiple CD8 cytotoxic T cell epitopes by DNA vaccination. J Immunol 160(4): 1717-1723.

[49] An, L. L., Rodriguez, F. et al. (2000). Quantitative and qualitative analyses of the immune responses induced by a multivalent minigene DNA vaccine. Vaccine 18(20): 2132-2141.

[50] Alexander, J., Oseroff, C. et al. (1997). Derivation of HLA-A11/Kb transgenic mice: functional CTL repertoire and recognition of human A11-restricted CTL epitopes. J Immunol 159(10): 4753-4761.

[51] Sette, A. and Sidney J. (1999). Nine major HLA class I supertypes account for the vast preponderance of HLA-A and -B polymorphism. Immunogenetics 50(3-4): 201-212.

4

Towards a New Challenge in TB Control: Development of Antibody-Based Protection

Armando Acosta[1]*, Yamile Lopez[1],
Norazmi Mohd Nor[2], Rogelio Hernández Pando[3],
Nadine Alvarez[1] and Maria Elena Sarmiento[1]
[1]Instituto Finlay, La Habana,
[2]School of Health Sciences, Universiti Sains Malaysia, Kelantan,
[3]Experimental Pathology Section, National Institute of Medical Sciences and Nutrition,
Mexico City,
[1]Cuba
[2]Malaysia
[3]Mexico

1. Introduction

Throughout history tuberculosis (TB) has been a health problem for humanity. In the beginning of civilization when human population densities were sparse, this disease may have been fairly harmless. However, with the increase in population densities, probably from the 17th to 19th centuries, TB took epidemic proportions [1].

Bacille Calmette Guérin (BCG), the only licensed vaccine against TB, has been shown to be effective in preventing meningeal and miliary TB in children. However, the efficacy of this vaccine in preventing adult pulmonary TB is questionable. Despite widespread vaccination with BCG, nearly 2 million people die each year from TB. Furthermore, the World Health Organization no longer recommends BCG vaccination of children with HIV or HIV-positive mothers due to safety concerns, leaving many infants without any protection against this disease. While drug therapies exist to combat TB infection, the implentation of suitable treatment is often difficult in the countries hardest hit by the disease and a fact complicated by the limited effectiveness of the current therapeutic schemes at treating drug resistant strains of TB [2-4].

Nowadays there is an increasing realization of the need of new animal models to test vaccine efficacy in more realistic scenarios overcoming the limitations of the current models in use. In addition, the elucidation of the significance of humoral defense against intracellular pathogens, in particular against *Mycobacterium tuberculosis*, constitutes an exciting new approach to improve the rational design of new vaccines, therapies and diagnostics.

---

* Corresponding Author

2. Reshaping the classical paradigm

In order to develop improved vaccines and new methods for the control of TB, an important element is the discovery of markers to measure the effector mechanisms of the protective immune response against *M. tuberculosis*. For many years Cellular Mediated Immunity (CMI) was attributed as the exclusive defence mechanism against intracellular pathogens. The Th1/Th2 classical paradigm prevailed for a long time and directed the development of vaccines according to this theory [5].

Based on this point of view, only intracellular pathogens could be effectively controlled by granulomatous inflammation induced by a Th1 response whereas a Th2 response induces antibody production that control extracellular pathogens and parasites. However, the question arises of what really constitutes the true demarcation between "extracellular and intracellular"? In the infectious cycle of several intracellular pathogens, they could be found in the extracellular space and *vice versa*. In the specific case of *M. tuberculosis*, it can be localized extracellularly at the beginning of the infection in the upper respiratory tract as well as in advanced stages of the disease after the rupture of granulomatous lesions [6]. In the case of *Erhlichia* spp specific antibodies could mediate protection against [7], possibly by blocking cellular entry or promoting the expression of proinflammatory cytokines [8;9]. It has been demonstrated that this obligate intracellular pathogen has also an extracellular phase that may include replication which could be targeted by specific antibodies [10].

For certain viral pathogens, the induction of Antibody Mediated-Immunity is sufficient to prevent infection, as has been clearly demonstrated by the almost complete eradication of smallpox with the use of vaccines that elicited antibody-mediated immunity [11]. There are several prokaryotic and eukaryotic intracellular pathogens for which antibody have been shown to modify the course of infection by different mechanisms, as reviewed extensively by Casadevall and colleagues [12-14]. Nowadays, it is well established that an efficient combination of both humoral and cellular immune mechanisms could be the best choice to control certain diseases produced by intracellular pathogens [15;16].

In 2005, de Valiere and colleagues reported for the first time that human antimycobacterial antibodies stimulates the Th1 response instead of diminishing it, as was thought previously [17].

3. Protective role of antibodies: Epidemiological evidence

There is accummulated evidence in the last few decades on the influence of antibodies in the development of pulmonary or disseminated TB. Children with low serum IgG against sonicated mycobacterial antigens and LAM, or those who cannot mount antibody responses to these antigens, were predisposed to dissemination of the bacteria [18]. In another report, Kamble and colleagues reported that *M. leprae* reactive salivary IgA antibodies could be quite important in a mucosal protective immunity [19]. In one study carried out on the Mexican Totonaca Indian population, the presence of high antibody titers to Ag85 complex antigens were observed in patients with non-cavitary TB and in patients who were cured with anti-TB chemotherapy. In contrast, patients without such antibodies had a poor outcome of the disease [20].

4. Experimental studies

4.1 Animal models for the evaluation of the role of antibodies in TB infection

One important criterion for the evaluation of the role of specific antibodies in the protection against TB is the use of animal models. Currently, there is no optimal model to reproduce the infection as it occurs in humans [21]. Several animal models have been used to evaluate different aspects. One crucial aspect is the delivery of inoculums, where several routes of inoculation have been employed as intravenous, intraperitoneal, intranasal, aerosol and intratracheal [22]. The geographical location, genetic factors of the host, the presence of environmental mycobacteria and other concomitant infections like helminthiasis, are factors that have to be considered when designing animal experiments [23].

The study of the distribution of monoclonal and polyclonal antibody formulations in different organs and tissues of mice after administration by different routes, including the use of backpack models have been reported [24-26]. Each model has its advantages and drawbacks. For example, the backpack model is very useful for the evaluation of the protective role of IgA, but poses ethical problems in long term experiments due to the increase in tumour size over time produced by the inoculated hybridoma [27].

In prophylactic and therapeutic models, antibody formulations have been administered via the intranasal, intravenous and intraperitoneal routes and combined with cytokines and antibiotics [28,29] before and/or after the infectious challenge.

The administration of *M. tuberculosis* pre-coated with antibodies [30,31] in different models of infection have also contributed to understanding the interactions between host and microbe.

Another approach has been the use of knockout mice models for IgA, polymeric immunoglobulin receptor (pIgR) and B cells, as will be discussed later.

4.2 Experimental studies with antibodies

A great number of studies involving antibodies as inoculum have been conducted as far back as the end of the 19th century. These experiments can be grouped in several categories: serum therapies, mouse polyclonal antibodies, human polyclonal antibodies including commercial human gamma globulins, secretory human IgA (hsIgA) and studies with monoclonal antibodies.

4.2.1 Serum therapies

Serum therapy experiments were conducted from the second half of the 19th century. Immune sera was generated by immunizing animals with different microbial fractions and administered either to animals or humans. The results obtained were either variable, inconclusive or contradictory, due to differences in the methods of serum preparation or its administration, and the lack of appropriate experimental controls [32]. These controversial results led to the perceived minor role of antibodies in the defence against intracellular pathogens.

Why these results were considered "controversial"? Immune serum is a polyclonal preparation that includes antibodies to multiple specificities and isotypes; consequently, polyclonal sera may contain blocking antibodies [33] and antibodies of different functional categories that can affect the outcome of infection. For example, IgG3 murine monoclonal antibodies protects against *Streptococcus pneumoniae* and *M. tuberculosis* but fails to protect against *C. neoformans* [34]. Moreover, results from animal studies are not always reflective of the Ig isotype function in humans. Besides intrinsic factors associated to the antibody structure, other parameters such as the genetic background of the microbe and the immunocompetence of the host could alter the outcome of antibody protection experiments. For some microorganisms (*Legionella pneumophila* and *C. neoformans*), passive antibody therapy efficacy depends on the mouse strain used [35]. In the same way, some microbial strains are more susceptible to the effects of antibodies. The animal model used is another important parameter that varies between different experiments cited in the literature. Timing, the route of infection, the magnitude of the infecting inoculum and the variables to measure efficacy are some of the critical parameters in antibody protection studies [36].

Despite its controversial nature, the results obtained with serum therapy were valuable, demonstrating some beneficial effect of serum on the course of TB in humans, mainly in cases of early or localized TB [37]. Moreover, it was demonstrated that long periods of treatment were necessary to achieve a sustained effect [38].

4.2.2 Polyclonal mouse antibodies

A recent study re-examined the usefulness of immune serum in the context of a therapeutic vaccine against TB [39]. This vaccine, called RUTI, is generated from detoxified *M. tuberculosis* cell fragments that facilitate a balanced T helper response to a wide range of antigens along with intense antibody production. Local accumulation of specific CD8+ T cells and a strong humoral response after immunization are characteristic features of RUTI, features that contribute to its protective properties. In this study, immune serum was generated by immunizing mice with RUTI. Severe Combined Immunodeficiency (SCID) mice were infected with *M. tuberculosis* and treated with chemotherapy for 3–8 weeks. After chemotherapy they were treated for up to 10 weeks with intraperitoneal injections of immune serum. Mice treated with immune serum from RUTI vaccinated animals showed significant decreases in lung CFU as well as reduction in the extent of granulomatous response and abscess formation in comparisson with controls. These results suggest that protective serum antibodies can be elicited by vaccination, and that antibodies may be usefully combined with chemotherapy [29,40].

4.2.3 Human gammaglobulins

4.2.3.1 Human polyclonal antibodies

The first evidence of the stimulatory role upon cellular immunity of specific antibodies in experimental mycobacterial infections was reported by Valiere and colleagues in 2005. In this study, serum samples containing specific antimycobacterial antibodies were obtained from volunteers vaccinated twice with BCG by the intradermal route. Significant titres of IgG antibodies against lipoarabinomannan (LAM) were detected in the volunteers. Moreover, BCG internalization into phagocytic cells was significantly increased in the presence of BCG induced antibodies as were the inhibitory effects of neutrophils and macrophages on mycobacterial growth. Furthermore, these antibodies induced significant production of IFN-γ by CD4+ and CD8+ T cells [17].

4.2.3.2 IgG formulations

Roy and colleagues demonstrated that the treatment of *M. tuberculosis*-infected mice with a single cycle of human intravenous Ig resulted in substantially reduced bacterial loads in the spleen and lungs when administered either at early or at late stage of infection [41].

The effect of the administration of a commercial preparation of human gammaglobulins in a mouse model of intranasal infection with BCG was evaluated by our group. We demonstrated the passage of specific antibodies to saliva and lung lavage following the intranasal or intraperitoneal administration of human gammaglobulins to mice. This treatment inhibited BCG colonization of the lungs of treated mice. A similar inhibitory effect was observed after infection of mice with gammaglobulin-opsonized BCG [42]. The same formulation was evaluated also in a mouse model of intratracheal infection with *M. tuberculosis*. Animals receiving human gammaglobulins intranasally 2h before intratracheal challenge showed a significant decrease in lung bacilli load compared to non-treated animals. When *M. tuberculosis* was pre-incubated with the gammaglobulin before challenge the same effect was observed. The protective effect of the gammaglobulin formulation was abolished after pre-incubation with *M. tuberculosis* [30]. These results suggest a potential role of specific human antibodies in the defence against mycobacterial infections.

Taken together these studies provide consistent support for the potential use of gammaglobulins and their beneficial immunomodulatory effects in tuberculosis. The results of certain knockout mouse studies and the gammaglobulin experiments indicate that B cells and their products mediate protection against *M. tuberculosis* [43-45]. However, the important question that remains is whether B-cell responses can be augmented to improve immunity against *M. tuberculosis* through immunotherapy or vaccination.

4.2.3.3 Purified human secretory IgA

Human secretory IgA (hsIgA) is the major class of antibody associated with immune protection of the mucosal surfaces [46]. Colostrum volume is above 100 mL in humans during the first three days after delivery [47]. The high percentage of (hsIgA) in human colostrum [48] strongly suggests its important role in passive immune protection against gastrointestinal and respiratory infections [49]. In one study performed by our group, hsIgA from human colostrum was obtained by anion exchange and gel filtration chromatographic methods, using DEAE Sepharose FF and Superose 6 preparative grade, respectively [50]. HsIgA was administered intranasally to BALB/c mice, and the level of this immunoglobulin in several biological fluids was determined by ELISA. The results showed the presence of this antibody in the saliva of animals that received the hsIgA, at all time intervals studied. In tracheobronchial lavage, hsIgA was detected at 2 and 3 hours after inoculation in animals that received the hsIgA [51]. Similar studies were performed by Falero and colleagues with monoclonal antibodies of IgA and IgG class [52]. Following demostration that hsIgA could be detected in several biological secretions after intranasal administration, the protective effect of this formulation against *M. tuberculosis* challenge was evaluated. Mice challenged with *M. tuberculosis* preincubated with hsIgA showed a statistically significant decrease in the mean number of viable bacteria recovered from the lungs compared to control mice and to the group that received the hsIgA before challenge with *M. tuberculosis*. Moreover, an increased level of iNOS production was also reported (Alvarez et al., mannuscript in preparation). Consistently with this result, a better organization of granulomatous areas with foci of lymphocytes and abundant activated macrophages were observed in the lungs of mice of the group that received *M. tuberculosis* pre-incubated with hsIgA sacrificed at 2 months post-challenge. Untreated animals, however, showed an increased area of bronchiectasis and atelectasis as well as fibrin deposits, accumulation of activated macrophages and lymphocytes. The pneumonic areas were more prominent in the untreated animals than in the groups treated with hsIgA and *M. tuberculosis* pre-incubated with hsIgA (Alvarez et al., mannuscript in preparation)

4.2.4 Studies performed with monoclonal antibodies

Since the first report on the use of the monoclonal antibody Mab 9d8 against *M. tuberculosis*, many similar studies have been reported [53;54]. This IgG3 monoclonal antibody (Mab) generated against arabinomannan (AM) capsular polysaccharide, increased thesurvival of intratracheally infected mice when the *M. tuberculosis* Erdman strain was pre-coated with it. In this study, a longer survival associated with an enhanced granulomatous response in the lungs was found as compared to controls receiving an isotype-specific non-related Mab [31].

Another Mab, SMITB14, directed against the AM portion of LAM prolonged the survival of intravenously infected mice associated with reduced lung CFU and prevention of weight loss. In this study, the authors demonstrated that protection was independent of the antibody Fc portion, because the F(ab')2 fragment also conferred a similar protective effect [55].

In another study, mice receiving the Mab 5c11 (an IgM antibody that recognizes other mycobacterial arabinose-containing carbohydrates in addition to AM) intravenously prior to Mannosylated lipoarabinomannan (ManLAM) administration, showed a significant clearance of ManLAM and redirection of this product to the hepatobiliary system. This study strongly supports an indirect effect of certain antibodies on the course of mycobacterial infection, altering problably the pharmacokinetics of mycobacterial components and contributing to protection against TB [56].

Heparin Binding Hemagglutinin Adhesin (HBHA) is a surface-exposed glycoprotein involved in the mycobacterial binding to epithelial cells and in mycobacterial dissemination [57]. Monoclonal antibodies 3921E4 (IgG2a) and 4057D2 (IgG3) directed against HBHA were used to coat mycobacteria before administration to mice. In this study, spleen CFUs were reduced while lung CFUs did not [58]. These results suggest that binding of these antibodies to HBHA impede mycobacterial dissemination.

The protective efficacy of a monoclonal antibody, TBA61, IgA anti-Acr administered intranasally before and after the intranasal or aerosol challenge with *M. tuberculosis* was demonstrated in a previous work [59]. In another series of experiments carried out by López and colleagues, the protective effect of this Mab administered intratracheally before an intratracheal challenge with virulent mycobacteria was evaluated. At 21 days post-infection, pre-treatment of mice with TBA61 caused a significant decrease in viable bacteria in the lungs compared to control mice or those treated with the Mab against the 38-kDa protein (TBA84). Consistent with the reduction of viable bacteria following treatment with TBA61, the area of peribronchial inflammation was also statistically smaller in this group compared to the control group [60].

When the lungs of mice were histologically examined, granulomas were better organized in the infected animals that had received TBA61 than in controls or mice treated with TBA84. The reduction of CFU in lungs of the treated group was associated with milder histopathological changes, as indicated by the organization of the granulomas and less pneumonic area. The fact that this Mab promotes granuloma formation in mice infected intratracheally with *M. tuberculosis* strongly suggests the close interaction between antibody-mediated immunity and cell-mediated immunity to induce protection against intracellular pathogens (61). Some of the results obtained in the evaluation of TBA61 monoclonal antibody under different conditions are listed in the Table 1.

MAb, delivery route and inoculation regime	Challenge	Days selected for Organ Harvesting	Parameter measured		References
			CFU reduction	Histopathology	
TBA61 i.n (-3h, +3h, 6h) TBA61 i.n (-3h) TBA61 i.n (+3h) TBA61 i.n (-3h, +3h)	H37Rv i.n, aerosol	9 days	Significant reduction of CFU post-challenge	nd	59
TBA61 i.n + IFN-γ i.n (-3h, -2h, +2h, +7h)	H37Rv i.n, aerosol	9, 21 and 28 days	Significant reduction of CFU post-challenge	Significant reduction of the granulomatous area in the lungs of treated as, compared to untreated mice	28
TBA61 i.t (-3h)	H37Rv i.t	24h, 72h, 21 days	Significant reduction at 21 days post-challenge	Less interstitial and peribronchial inflammation. Well-organized granuloma	60

Table 1. Results from different experimental approaches involving a monoclonal antibody against *M. tuberculosis* 16 kDa protein (TBA61). Note: i.n: intranasal; i.t: intratracheal

The 16 kDa protein (Acr antigen) has been defined as a major membrane protein peripherally associated with the membrane [62] carrying epitopes restricted to tubercle bacilli on the basis of B-cell recognition [63,64]. The Acr antigen is present on the surface of tubercle bacilli and is highly expressed in organisms growing within infected macrophages, allowing it to be potentially targeted by specific antibodies either inside infected cells as well as extracellulary.

A novel immunotherapy, combining treatment with anti-IL-4 antibodies, IgA antibody against 16 kDa protein and IFN-γ, showed the potential for passive immunoprophylaxis against TB. In genetically deficient IL-4-/- BALB/c mice, infection in both lungs and spleen was substantially reduced for up to 8 weeks. Reconstitution of IL-4-/- mice with rIL-4 increased bacterial counts to wild-type levels and making mice refractory to protection by IgA/IFN-γ [65].

More recently, Balu and colleagues reported a novel human IgA1 Mab, constructed using a single-chain variable fragment clone selected from an Ab phage library. The purified Mab monomer revealed high binding affinities for the mycobacterial α-crystallin Ag and for the human FcαRI (CD89) IgA receptor. Intranasal inoculations with the monoclonal antibody and recombinant mouse IFN-γ significantly inhibited pulmonary H37Rv infection in mice transgenic for human CD89 but not in CD89-negative littermate controls, suggesting that binding to CD89 was necessary for the IgA-imparted passive protection. The Mab added to human whole-blood or monocyte cultures inhibited luciferase-tagged H37Rv infection although not for all tested blood donors. Inhibition of the infection by the antibody was synergistic with human rIFN-γ in cultures of purified human monocytes but not in whole-blood cultures. The demonstration of the mandatory role of FcαRI (CD89) for human IgA-mediated protection is important for understanding the mechanisms involved and also for translating this approach towards the development of passive immunotherapy for TB [66].

In all the studies analyzed, it is possible to assert that different mechanisms of action of monoclonal and polyclonal antibodies are involved in the protection against TB. Some of these mechanisms will be discussed later in this chapter.

4.2.5 Studies performed in transgenic mice

Mouse models with deficiency in antibody production can be useful in understanding certain roles of the antibodies in protection against mycobacterial infections. However, knockout mouse studies can lead to premature conclusions regarding the role of a particular component of immunity, if not interpreted carefully. Additionally, experimental conditions can have marked effects on the results.

Rodríguez and colleagues reported that IgA deficient (IgA-/-) mice and wild type non-targeted littermate (IgA+/+) were immunized by intranasal route with the mycobacterium surface antigen PstS-1. These authors showed that IgA-/- mice were more susceptible to BCG infection compared to IgA+/+ mice, as revealed by the higher bacterial loads in the lungs and bronchoalveolar lavage (BAL). More importantly, analysis of the cytokine responses revealed a reduction in the IFN-γ and TNF-α production in the lungs of IgA-/- compared to IgA+/+ mice, suggesting that IgA may play a role in protection against mycobacterial infections in the respiratory tract. Furthermore, these authors demonstrated that immunized pIgR-/- mice were more susceptible to BCG infection than immunized wild-type mice [67].

In the attempt to elucidate whether humoral immunity has a special role in the defence against TB, different experiments with B cell knockout mice were performed by several authors. In 1996, Vordermeier and colleagues developed an infection model of TB in μ chain knockout Ig- mice. Organs from *M. tuberculosis* infected IgG- mice had three to eight fold elevated counts of viable bacilli compared with those from normal mice. This result suggested that B cells play a role in the containment of murine tuberculous infection [68]. In another study, B cell gene disrupted mice (B cell KO) and controls were infected by aerosol with *M. tuberculosis* to allow the latter group to generate an antibody response in the upper respiratory tract. They were subsequetly given chemotherapy to destroy remaining bacilli and then re-challenged by aerosol exposure. The results of this study, however, revealed no differences in the ability of animals to control this second infection, indicating that, in this low dose pulmonary infection model at least, any local production of antibodies neither impeded nor enhanced the expression of specific acquired resistance [69].

In another series of experiments the role of B cells during early immune responses to infection with a clinical isolate of *M. tuberculosis* (CDC 1551) was evaluated. In this study, despite comparable bacterial loads in the lungs, less severe pulmonary granuloma formation and delayed dissemination of bacteria from lungs to peripheral organs were observed in BKO mice. Additional analysis of lung cell populations revealed greater numbers of lymphocytes, especially CD8+ T cells, macrophages, and neutrophils in wild-type and reconstituted mice than in BKO mice. Thus, less severe lesion formation and delayed dissemination of bacteria found in BKO mice were dependent on B cells, (not antibodies, at least in this study) and were associated with altered cellular infiltrate to the lungs [70].

This latter result differs to the study carried out by Maglione and colleagues in which B cell-/- mice had exacerbated immunopathology corresponding with elevated pulmonary recruitment of neutrophils upon aerosol challenge with *M. tuberculosis* Erdman strain. Infected B cell-/- mice showed increased production of IL-10 in the lungs, whereas IFN-γ, TNF-α, and IL-10R remain unchanged from wild type. B cell-/- mice had enhanced susceptibility to infection when aerogenically challenged with 300 CFU of *M. tuberculosis* corresponding with elevated bacterial burden in the lungs but not in the spleen or liver [43].

Together these studies reveal that B cells may have a greater role in the host defence against *M. tuberculosis* than previously thought.

5. Possible mechanisms of action

Secretions found on mucosal surfaces contain significant levels of Igs, particularly, IgA. This immunoglobin has direct and indirect functional roles to combat infectious agents such as viruses and bacteria that cross the mucosal barrier. Moreover, experimental evidences suggest that the IgA associated with the pIgR may neutralize pathogens and antigens intracellularly during their transport from the basolateral to the apical zone of epithelial cells [71,72]. In addition, as demonstrated previously, IgA may interact with Gal-3 (an intracellular binding β-galactosidase lectin), and interfere with the interaction of mycobacteria with the phagosomal membrane, resulting in the decrease of bacterial survival and replication in the phagosome [73].

As reported by several authors, antibodies may be critical, at least during the extracellular phases of intracellular facultative pathogens. Antibodies may act by interfering with adhesion, neutralizing toxins and activating complement. Moreover, antibodies may be able to penetrate recently infected cells and bind to the internalised pathogen, increasing the antigen processing (74). It is well accepted that antibodies play a crucial role in modulating the immune response by activating faster secretion of selected cytokines that in turn, contribute to more efficient and rapid Th1 response [74,75], increasing the efficacy of co-stimulatory signals, enhancing Antibody Dependent Cellular Cytotoxicity responses (ADCC) and the homing of immune cells to the lungs after the respiratory infection [13,76-81].

Examples of relevant action mechanisms of antibodies have been discussed by Glatman-Freedman [82].

6. Potential applications

Future applications of antibody formulations for the control of TB may include treatment of patients infected with Multidrug Resistant (MDR) strains, combination with the standard treatment in order to achieve faster therapeutic effects, and administration to recent contacts of TB patients with special attention to risk groups [85].

On the other hand, the induction of specific antibody responses by vaccination in addition to the stimulation of cell mediated immunity could be a novel strategy for the development of new generation prophylactic and therapeutic vaccines against TB.

The prevailing dogma about the uncertain role of antibodies in the protection against TB has somewhat limited the study of B cell immunodominant epitopes which have been mainly related with the development of serodiagnosis assays [86]. Consequently, little information is available on B cell epitopes that could potentially contribute to protection or therapy. With the development of bioinformatics tools for bacterial genome analysis, it has been possible to predict *in silico* microbial regions that trigger immune responses relevant for protection and vaccine development.

Our group is currently developing a candidate experimental vaccine based on proteoliposomes from *M. smegmatis*. In one study, bibliographic search was used to identify highly expressed proteins in active, latent and reactivation phases of TB [87]. The subcellular localization of the selected proteins was defined according to the report on the identification and localization of 1044 *M. tuberculosis* proteins using two-dimensional, capillary high-performance liquid chromatography coupled with mass spectrometry (2DLC/MS) method [88] and using prediction algorithms.

Taking into consideration the cell fractions potentially included in the proteoliposome, from the previously identified proteins, the ones located in the cell membrane and cell wall, as well as those which are secreted and homologous to those of *M. smegmatis* were selected. The regions of the selected proteins containing promiscuous B and T cell epitopes were determined [87]. Thus the *M. smegmatis* proteolipomes were predicted to contain multiple B and T epitopes which are potentially cross reactive with those of *M. tuberculosis*. It is important to note that there could be conformational B epitopes and additional epitopes related with lipids and carbohydrates included in the proteoliposomes that could reinforce the humoral cross reactivity.

Considering the results of the *in silico* analysis, proteoliposomes of *M. smegmatis* were obtained and their immunogenicity was studied in mice [89]. In addition to cellular immune effectors recognizing antigens from *M. tuberculosis*, cross reactive humoral immune responses of several IgG subclasses corresponding with a combined Th1 and Th2 pattern against antigenic components of *M. tuberculosis* were elicited. These findings were in concordance with the *in silico* predictions [87,89]. It is interesting to note that differences in the pattern of humoral recognition of lipidic components was dependent on the characteristics of the adjuvant used, which could have relevance for the development of vaccines which includes lipidic components [89]. Currently studies are underway to evaluate the protective capacity of *M. smegmatis* proteoliposomes in challenge models with *M. tuberculosis* in mice.

Bioinformatics tools for prediction of T and B epitopes were also employed for the design of multiepitopic constructions, which were used to obtain recombinant BCG strains. Based on this prediction, B cell epitopes from ESAT-6, CFP-10, Ag85B and MTP40 proteins were selected and combined with T cell epitopes of the 85B protein and fused to 8.4 protein [90]. A significant IgG antibody response against specific B cell epitopes of ESAT-6 and CFP-10 was obtained in mice immunized with the recombinant strain. After studying the specific response of spleen cells by lymphoproliferation assay and detection of intracellular cytokines in CD4 + and CD8 + subpopulations, the recognition of T epitopes was also observed. The response showed a Th1 pattern after immunization with this recombinant strain (Mohamud, R, et al. manuscript in preparation). In another series of experiments, recombinant BCG strains expressing several combinations of multiepitopic constructions were used to immunize BALB/c mice subcutaneously and challenged intratracheally with the *M. tuberculosis* H37Rv strain. Recombinant BCG strains expressing T epitopes from 85BAg fused to Mtb8.4 protein and BCG expressing a HSP60 T cell epitope plus different combinations of B cell epitopes from 85BAg, Mce1A, L7/L12, 16 kDa, HBHA, ESAT6, CFP10 and MTP40 and combinations of B cell epitopes alone produced significant reductions in lung CFU compared with BCG (Norazmi MN, manuscript in preparation).

The cumulative works reviewed above related with the use of antibody formulations and vaccines suggest that antibodies if present at the right moment at the site of infection can provide protection against *M. tuberculosis*. This concept opens the way to the development of a new generation of vaccines that elicit specific IgA and/or IgG antibodies able to protect at the port of entry against the infection and directed to bacteria in the infected tissues.

An antibody-based vaccine could be implemented against TB. Such antibodies should recognize the pathogen immediately after its entry into the host, mainly at the mucosal surfaces, where these antibodies must be strategically induced [91]. This vaccine has to induce IgA and IgG antibodies that can inactivate bacterial components essential for the microbial survival in the host, activate complement for direct lysis of the cells, opsonize bacteria to promote their capture by phagocytic cells and induce stimulation of specific cellular immune responses.

Although no serological tests for diagnosis of TB are recommended [92], due to the generation of false results as well as incorrect treatments, for many other pathogens, the availability of serological diagnostic tests has been of great value, in particular in poor countries. In some cases, it constitutes the best protection correlate [93].

In the specific case of TB, several studies of the antibody response have been developed [94]. A number of factors have been described to contribute to the variation of antibody response during the disease. Some of these factors are associated to the pathogen (strain variation, micro-environment and growth state of bacteria). Not less important are the factors related to the host, mainly the previous exposure to antigen and host genetics [95].

On the other hand, only a small fraction of the genomic regions of *M. tuberculosis* encoding proteins has been explored. Currently, novel immunoassay platforms are being used to dissect the entire proteome of *M. tuberculosis*, including reacting protein microarrays with sera from TB patients and controls [96,97]. These studies could lead to the discovery of new antigens that may constitute a suitable diagnostic marker as well as to the identification of correlates of protection.

The study of the role of specific antibodies in the defense against tuberculosis is opening new possibilities for the future development of new vaccines, diagnostics and therapies against the disease. It is envisaged that new discoveries will arise from the ongoing studies in this area that will expedite the introduction of new strategies in the fight against tuberculosis.

7. Acknowledgements

The authors' work was partly supported by the Ministry of Science, Technology & Innovation, Malaysia [Grant No. 304.PPSK.6150079.N106 & 10-01-05-MEB002] and USM Research University Grant [1001.PPSK.812005] and CONACyT (contract 84456)

8. References

[1] Jacob JT, Mehta AK, Leonard MK. Acute forms of tuberculosis in adults. Am J Med 2009;122(1):12-7.

[2] Chung KT, Biggers CJ. Albert Leon Charles Calmette (1863-1933) and the antituberculous BCG vaccination. Perspect Biol Med 2001;44(3):379-89.

[3] Davies PD. Medical classics. La Boheme and tuberculosis. BMJ 2008;337:a2587.

[4] Gradmann C. Robert Koch and tuberculosis: the beginning of medical bacteriology. Pneumologie 2009 Dec;63(12):702-8.

[5] Gor DO, Rose NR, Greenspan NS. TH1-TH2: a procrustean paradigm. Nat Immunol 2003 Jun;4(6):503-5.

[6] Grosset J. *Mycobacterium tuberculosis* in the extracellular compartment: an underestimated adversary. Antimicrob Agents Chemother 2003;47(3):833-6.

[7] Kaylor PS, Crawford TB, McElwain TF, Palmer GH. Passive transfer of antibody to *Ehrlichia risticii* protects mice from ehrlichiosis. Infect Immun 1991 Jun;59(6):2058-62.

[8] Lee EH, Rikihisa Y. Anti-*Ehrlichia chaffeensis* antibody complexed with *E. chaffeensis* induces potent proinflammatory cytokine mRNA expression in human monocytes through sustained reduction of IkappaB-alpha and activation of NF-kappaB. Infect Immun 1997;65(7):2890-7.

[9] Messick JB, Rikihisa Y. Inhibition of binding, entry, or intracellular proliferation of *Ehrlichia risticii* in P388D1 cells by anti-*E. risticii* serum, immunoglobulin G, or Fab fragment. Infect Immun 1994;62(8):3156-61.

[10] Li JS, Winslow GM. Survival, replication, and antibody susceptibility of *Ehrlichia chaffeensis* outside of host cells. Infect Immun 2003;71(8):4229-37.

[11] Fooks AR, Schadeck E, Liebert UG, et al. High-level expression of the measles virus nucleocapsid protein by using a replication-deficient adenovirus vector: induction of an MHC-1-restricted CTL response and protection in a murine model. Virology 1995;210(2):456-65.

[12] Casadevall A. Antibody-based therapies for emerging infectious diseases. Emerg Infect Dis 1996;2(3):200-8.

[13] Casadevall A, Pirofski LA. Antibody-mediated regulation of cellular immunity and the inflammatory response. Trends Immunol 2003;24(9):474-8.

[14] Casadevall A, Pirofski LA. A reappraisal of humoral immunity based on mechanisms of antibody-mediated protection against intracellular pathogens. Adv Immunol 2006;91:1-44.

[15] Macedo GC, Bozzi A, Weinreich HR, Bafica A, Teixeira HC, Oliveira SC. Human T cell and antibody-mediated responses to the *Mycobacterium tuberculosis* recombinant 85A, 85B, and ESAT-6 antigens. Clin Dev Immunol 2011;2011:351573.

[16] Kidd P. Th1/Th2 balance: the hypothesis, its limitations, and implications for health and disease. Altern Med Rev 2003;8(3):223-46.

[17] de Valiere S, Abate G, Blazevic A, Heuertz RM, Hoft DF. Enhancement of innate and cell-mediated immunity by antimycobacterial antibodies. Infect Immun 2005;73(10):6711-20.

[18] Costello AM, Kumar A, Narayan V, et al. Does antibody to mycobacterial antigens, including lipoarabinomannan, limit dissemination in childhood tuberculosis? Trans R Soc Trop Med Hyg 1992;86(6):686-92.

[19] Kamble RR, Shinde VS, Madhale SP, Jadhav RS. Study of cross-reactivity of *Mycobacterium leprae* reactive salivary IgA with other environmental mycobacteria. Indian J Lepr 2009;81(2):63-8.

[20] Sánchez-Rodríguez C, Estrada-Chávez C, García-Vigil J, et al. An IgG antibody response to the antigen 85 complex is associated with good outcome in Mexican Totonaca Indians with pulmonary tuberculosis. Int J Tuberc Lung Dis 2002;6(8):706-12.

[21] Ordway DJ and Orme IM. Animal models of Mycobacteria infection. Curr Protoc Immunol, 2011; Chapter 19: Unit 19.5.

[22] Dannenberg AM Jr. Perspectives on clinical and preclinical testing of new tuberculosis vaccines. Clin Microbiol Rev. 2010;23(4):781-94.

[23] Rook GA, Hernández-Pando R, Zumla A. Tuberculosis due to high-dose challenge in partially immune individuals: a problem for vaccination? J Infect Dis. 2009;199(5):613-8.

[24] Acosta A, Sarmiento ME, Gonzalez A, et al. Histopathologic and humoral study of Balb/c mice inoculated with BCG by different routes. Arch Med Res 1994;25(2):159-63.

[25] León A, Acosta A, Sarmiento ME, Estévez P, Martínez M, Pérez ME, Falero G, Infante JF, Fariñas M, Sierra G. Desarrollo de Biomodelos para la evaluación de la inmunidad de mucosa contra M. *tuberculosis*. Vaccimonitor, 2000;3:6-10.

[26] Acosta A, Olivares N, León A, López Y, Sarmiento ME, Cádiz A, Moya A, Falero G, Infante JF, Martínez M, Sierra G. A new approach to understand the defence mechanism against tuberculosis: role of specific antibodies. Biotecnología Aplicada 2003;20:130-133.

[27] Winner L 3rd, Mack J, Weltzin R, Mekalanos JJ, Kraehenbuhl JP, Neutra MR. New model for analysis of mucosal immunity: intestinal secretion of specific monoclonal immunoglobulin A from hybridoma tumors protects against Vibrio cholerae infection. Infect Immun. 1991 Mar;59(3):977-82.

[28] Reljic R. IFN-gamma therapy of tuberculosis and related infections. J Interferon Cytokine Res 2007;27(5):353-64.

[29] Guirado E, Amat I, Gil O, et al. Passive serum therapy with polyclonal antibodies against *Mycobacterium tuberculosis* protects against post-chemotherapy relapse of tuberculosis infection in SCID mice. Microbes Infect 2006;8(5):1252-9.

[30] Olivares N, Puig A, Aguilar D, et al. Prophylactic effect of administration of human gammaglobulins in a mouse model of tuberculosis. Tuberculosis (Edinb) 2009 May;89(3):218-20.

[31] Teitelbaum R, Glatman-Freedman A, Chen B, et al. A mAb recognizing a surface antigen of *Mycobacterium tuberculosis* enhances host survival. Proc Natl Acad Sci U S A 1998;95(26):15688-93.

[32] Casadevall A, Scharff MD. Return to the past: the case for antibody-based therapies in infectious diseases. Clin Infect Dis 1995;21(1):150-61.

[33] Joiner KA, Scales R, Warren KA, Frank MM, Rice PA. Mechanism of action of blocking immunoglobulin G for *Neisseria gonorrhoeae*. J Clin Invest 1985;76(5):1765-72.

[34] Yuan R, Casadevall A, Spira G, Scharff MD. Isotype switching from IgG3 to IgG1 converts a nonprotective murine antibody to *Cryptococcus neoformans* into a protective antibody. J Immunol 1995;154(4):1810-6.

[35] Eisenstein TK, Killar LM, Sultzer BM. Immunity to infection with *Salmonella typhimurium*: mouse-strain differences in vaccine- and serum-mediated protection. J Infect Dis 1984;150(3):425-35.

[36] Casadevall A. Antibody-mediated immunity against intracellular pathogens: two-dimensional thinking comes full circle. Infect Immun 2003;71(8):4225-8.

[37] Imaz MS, Zerbini E. Antibody response to culture filtrate antigens of *Mycobacterium tuberculosis* during and after treatment of tuberculosis patients. Int J Tuberc Lung Dis 2000;4(6):562-9.

[38] Glatman-Freedman A, Casadevall A. Serum therapy for tuberculosis revisited: reappraisal of the role of antibody-mediated immunity against *Mycobacterium tuberculosis*. Clin Microbiol Rev 1998;11(3):514-32.

[39] Guirado E, Gil O, Caceres N, Singh M, Vilaplana C, Cardona PJ. Induction of a specific strong polyantigenic cellular immune response after short-term chemotherapy controls bacillary reactivation in murine and guinea pig experimental models of tuberculosis. Clin Vaccine Immunol 2008;15(8):1229-37.

[40] Domingo M, Gil O, Serrano E, et al. Effectiveness and safety of a treatment regimen based on isoniazid plus vaccination with *Mycobacterium tuberculosis* cells' fragments: field-study with naturally *Mycobacterium caprae*-infected goats. Scand J Immunol 2009;69(6):500-7.

[41] Roy E, Stavropoulos E, Brennan J, et al. Therapeutic efficacy of high-dose intravenous immunoglobulin in *Mycobacterium tuberculosis* infection in mice. Infect Immun 2005;73(9):6101-9.

[42] Olivares N, León A, López Y, et al. The effect of the administration of human gamma globulins in a model of BCG infection in mice. Tuberculosis (Edinb) 2006;86(3-4):268-72.

[43] Maglione PJ, Xu J, Chan J. B cells moderate inflammatory progression and enhance bacterial containment upon pulmonary challenge with Mycobacterium tuberculosis. J Immunol 2007 Jun 1;178(11):7222-34.

[44] Maglione PJ, Xu J, Casadevall A, Chan J. Fc gamma receptors regulate immune activation and susceptibility during Mycobacterium tuberculosis infection. J Immunol 2008;180(5):3329-38.

[45] Maglione PJ, Chan J. How B cells shape the immune response against Mycobacterium tuberculosis. Eur J Immunol 2009;39(3):676-86.

[46] Woof JM, Kerr MA. The function of immunoglobulin A in immunity. J Pathol 2006;208(2):270-82.

[47] Sagodira S, Buzoni-Gatel D, Iochmann S, Naciri M, Bout D. Protection of kids against Cryptosporidium parvum infection after immunization of dams with CP15-DNA. Vaccine 1999;17(19):2346-55.

[48] Lawrence RM, Lawrence RA. Breast milk and infection. Clin Perinatol 2004;31(3):501-28.

[49] Reljic R, Williams A, Ivanyi J. Mucosal immunotherapy of tuberculosis: is there a value in passive IgA? Tuberculosis (Edinb) 2006;86(3-4):179-90.

[50] Alvarez N, Otero O, Falero-Diaz G, Cádiz A, Marcet R, Carbonell AE, Sarmiento ME, Mohd-Nor N, Acosta A. Purificacion de inmunoglobulina A secretora a partir de calostro humano. Vaccimonitor 2010; 19(3): 26-29.

[51] Alvarez N, Camacho F, Otero O, Borrero R, Acevedo R, Valdés Y, Díaz D, Fariñas M, Izquierdo L, Sarmiento ME, Norazmi Mohd, Acosta A. Biodistribution of secretory IgA purified from human colostrum in biological fluids of Balb/c mice. Vaccimonitor (In press)

[52] Falero-Diaz G, Challacombe S, Rahman D, et al. Transmission of IgA and IgG monoclonal antibodies to mucosal fluids following intranasal or parenteral delivery. Int Arch Allergy Immunol 2000;122(2):143-50.

[53] Glatman-Freedman A. The role of antibody-mediated immunity in defense against Mycobacterium tuberculosis: advances toward a novel vaccine strategy. Tuberculosis (Edinb) 2006;86(3-4):191-7.

[54] Ben mM, Gherissi D, Mouthon L, Salmon-Ceron D. Tuberculosis risk among patients with systemic diseases. Presse Med 2009;38(2):274-90.

[55] Hamasur B, Haile M, Pawlowski A, et al. Mycobacterium tuberculosis arabinomannan-protein conjugates protect against tuberculosis. Vaccine 2003;21(25-26):4081-93.

[56] Glatman-Freedman A, Mednick AJ, Lendvai N, Casadevall A. Clearance and organ distribution of Mycobacterium tuberculosis lipoarabinomannan (LAM) in the presence and absence of LAM-binding immunoglobulin M. Infect Immun 2000;68(1):335-41.

[57] Pethe K, Puech V, Daffe M, et al. Mycobacterium smegmatis laminin-binding glycoprotein shares epitopes with Mycobacterium tuberculosis heparin-binding haemagglutinin. Mol Microbiol 2001;39(1):89-99.

[58] Pethe K, Bifani P, Drobecq H, et al. Mycobacterial heparin-binding hemagglutinin and laminin-binding protein share antigenic methyllysines that confer resistance to proteolysis. Proc Natl Acad Sci U S A 2002;99(16):10759-64.

[59] Williams A, Reljic R, Naylor I, et al. Passive protection with immunoglobulin A antibodies against tuberculous early infection of the lungs. Immunology 2004;111(3):328-33.

[60] López Y, Yero D, Falero-Díaz G, et al. Induction of a protective response with an IgA monoclonal antibody against *Mycobacterium tuberculosis* 16kDa protein in a model of progressive pulmonary infection. Int J Med Microbiol 2009;299(6):447-52.

[61] López Y, Falero G, Yero D, Solís R, Sarmiento ME, Acosta A. Antibodies in the protection against mycobacterial infections: what have we learned? Procedia in Vaccinology 2010, 2:172-7.

[62] Lee BY, Hefta SA, Brennan PJ. Characterization of the major membrane protein of virulent *Mycobacterium tuberculosis*. Infect Immun 1992;60(5):2066-74.

[63] Coates AR, Hewitt J, Allen BW, Ivanyi J, Mitchison DA. Antigenic diversity of *Mycobacterium tuberculosis* and *Mycobacterium bovis* detected by means of monoclonal antibodies. Lancet 1981;2(8239):167-9.

[64] Sun R, Skeiky YA, Izzo A, et al. Novel recombinant BCG expressing perfringolysin O and the over-expression of key immunodominant antigens; pre-clinical characterization, safety and protection against challenge with *Mycobacterium tuberculosis*. Vaccine 2009;27(33):4412-23.

[65] Buccheri S, Reljic R, Caccamo N, et al. IL-4 depletion enhances host resistance and passive IgA protection against tuberculosis infection in BALB/c mice. Eur J Immunol 2007;37(3):729-37.

[66] Balu S, Reljic R, Lewis MJ, et al. A novel human IgA monoclonal antibody protects against tuberculosis. J Immunol 2011;186(5):3113-9.

[67] Rodríguez A, Tjarnlund A, Ivanji J, et al. Role of IgA in the defense against respiratory infections IgA deficient mice exhibited increased susceptibility to intranasal infection with *Mycobacterium bovis* BCG. Vaccine 2005;23(20):2565-72.

[68] Vordermeier HM, Venkataprasad N, Harris DP, Ivanyi J. Increase of tuberculous infection in the organs of B cell-deficient mice. Clin Exp Immunol, 1996;106:312-16

[69] Johnson CM, Cooper AM, Frank AA, Bonorino CBC, Wysoki LJ. *Mycobacterium tuberculosis* aerogenic rechallenge infections in B cell.deficient mice. Tubercle and Lung Disease (1997) 78(5&6), 257-261.

[70] Bosio CM, Gardner D, Elkins KL. Infection of B cell-deficient mice with CDC 1551, a clinical isolate of Mycobacterium tuberculosis: delay in dissemination and development of lung pathology. J Immunol. 2000;164(12):6417-25.

[71] Delbridge LM, O'Riordan MX. Innate recognition of intracellular bacteria. Curr Opin Immunol 2007;19(1):10-6.

[72] Phalipon A, Corthesy B. Novel functions of the polymeric Ig receptor: well beyond transport of immunoglobulins. Trends Immunol 2003;24(2):55-8.

[73] Reljic R, Ivanyi J. A case for passive immunoprophylaxis against tuberculosis. Lancet Infect Dis 2006;6(12):813-8.

[74] Igietseme JU, Eko FO, He Q, Black CM. Antibody regulation of Tcell immunity: implications for vaccine strategies against intracellular pathogens. Expert Rev Vaccines 2004;3(1):23-34.

[75] Moore AC, Hutchings CL. Combination vaccines: synergistic simultaneous induction of antibody and T-cell immunity. Expert Rev Vaccines 2007;6(1):111-21.

[76] Reynolds HY. Identification and role of immunoglobulins in respiratory secretions. Eur J Respir Dis Suppl 1987;153:103-16.

[77] Regnault A, Lankar D, Lacabanne V, et al. Fcgamma receptor-mediated induction of dendritic cell maturation and major histocompatibility complex class I-restricted antigen presentation after immune complex internalization. J Exp Med 1999;189(2):371-80.

[78] Ravetch JV, Bolland S. IgG Fc receptors. Annu Rev Immunol 2001;19:275-90.

[79] Robinson S, Charini WA, Newberg MH, Kuroda MJ, Lord CI, Letvin NL. A commonly recognized simian immunodeficiency virus Nef epitope presented to cytotoxic T lymphocytes of Indian-origin rhesus monkeys by the prevalent major histocompatibility complex class I allele Mamu-A*02. J Virol 2001;75(21):10179-86.

[80] Monteiro RC, Leroy V, Launay P, et al. Pathogenesis of Berger's disease: recent advances on the involvement of immunoglobulin A and their receptors. Med Sci (Paris) 2003;19(12):1233-41.

[81] Iankov ID, Petrov DP, Mladenov IV, et al. Protective efficacy of IgA monoclonal antibodies to O and H antigens in a mouse model of intranasal challenge with *Salmonella enterica* serotype Enteritidis. Microbes Infect 2004;6(10):901-10.

[82] Glatman-Freedman. The role of antibodies against tuberculosis. In: Norazmi MN, Acosta A, Sarmiento ME, eds. The Art&Science of tuberculosis vaccine development. 1st ed. Malaysia. Oxford University Press;, 2010. p.186-208.

[83] Chambers MA, Gavier-Widén D, Hewinson RG. Antibody bound to the surface antigen MPB85 of *Mycobacterium bovis* enhances survival against high dose and low dose challenge. Immunol Med Microbiol;41:93-100.

[84] Schlesinger LS and Horwitz MA. A role for natural antibody in the pathogenesis of leprosy: antibody in nonimmune serum mediates C3 fixation to the *Mycobacterium leprae* surface and hence phagocytosis by human mononuclear phagocytes. Infect Immun, 1994, 62(1): 280-289.

[85] Norazmi MN, Sarmiento ME, Acosta A. Recent advances in tuberculosis vaccine development. Curr Resp Med Rev, 2005;1(12):109-16.

[86] De Groot AS, McMurry J, Marcon L, et al. Developing an epitope-driven tuberculosis (TB) vaccine. Vaccine 2005;23(17-18):2121-31.

[87] Le Thuy Nguyen Thi, Reinier Borrero Maura, Sonsire Férnandez, Giselle Reyes, José Luis Perez, Fátima Reyes, María de los Angeles García, Midrey Fariñas, Juan Francisco Infante, Yanely Tirado, Alina Puig, Gustavo Sierra, Nadine Álvarez, Juan Carlos Ramírez, María Elena Sarmiento, Mohd-Nor Norazmi, Armando Acosta. Evaluation of the potential of *Mycobacterium smegmatis* as vaccine Candidate against tuberculosis by *in silico* and *in vivo* studies. VacciMonitor 2010;19 (1):20-6

[88] Mawuenyega KG, Forst CV, Dobos KM, et al. *Mycobacterium tuberculosis* functional network analysis by global subcellular protein profiling. Mol Biol Cell 2005;16(1):396-404.

[89] Rodríguez L, Tirado Y, Reyes F, et al. Proteoliposomes from *Mycobacterium smegmatis* induce immune cross-reactivity against *Mycobacterium tuberculosis* antigens in mice. Vaccine 2011; 29(37):6236-41.

[90] Acosta A, Norazmi MN, Sarmiento ME. Antibody mediated immunity- a missed opportunity in the fight against tuberculosis?Malaysian J Med Sci.2010;17(2):66-7.

[91] Kaufmann SH, Meinke AL, von GA. Novel vaccination concepts on the basis of modern insights into immunology. Bundesgesundheitsblatt Gesundheitsforschung Gesundheitsschutz 2009 Oct 18.

[92] Morris K. WHO recommends against inaccurate tuberculosis tests. The Lancet, 2011;377(9760): 113-4.

[93] Edwards KM. Development, Acceptance, and Use of Immunologic Correlates of Protection in Monitoring the Effectiveness of Combination Vaccines *Clin Infect Dis.* 2001; 33 (4): S274-S277.

[94] Velayudhan SK and Gennaro ML. Antibody responses in tuberculosis. In: Norazmi MN, Acosta A, Sarmiento ME, eds. The Art&Science of tuberculosis vaccine development. 1st ed. Malaysia. Oxford University Press;, 2010. p.186-208.

[95] Pottumarthy S, Wells VC and Morris AJ. A Comparison of Seven Tests for Serological Diagnosis of Tuberculosis. J Clin Microbiol. 2000; 38(6): 2227–2231.

[96] Michaud GA, Salcius M, Zhou F, Bangham R, Bonnin J, Guo H, et al. Analysing antibody specificity with whole proteome microarrays. Nat Biotechnol, 2003;21(12): 1509-12.

[97] Khan IH, Ravindran R, Yee J, Ziman M, Lewinsohn DM, Gennaro ML et al. Profiling antibodies to Mycobacterium tuberculosis by multiplex microbead suspension arrays for serodiagnosis of tuberculosis. Clin Vaccine Immunol, 2008;8(4):433-8.

5

Immunotherapy of Tuberculosis with IgA and Cytokines

Rajko Reljic[1] and Juraj Ivanyi[2]
[1]Clinical Sciences Division, St George's, University of London,
[2]Clinical and Diagnostic Sciences Department, Kings College London,
Guy's Campus of Kings College London
GB

1. Introduction

Immunotherapy of tuberculosis (TB) has long been considered to be a potential adjunct to chemotherapy, by targeting 'persister' organisms which are generated during chemotherapy. In this chapter, we briefly review the current immunotherapeutic approaches in TB and then focus in more detail on a novel form of combined immunotherapy (CIT), comprising an IgA monoclonal antibody (mAb) against the α-crystallin (Acr) antigen, IFN-γ and anti-IL-4 antibodies. CIT treatment significantly reduced new pulmonary infection and also the post-chemotherapy relapse in *Mycobacterium tuberculosis* infected BALB/c mice. Translation of this approach toward application in humans has been advanced by the development and characterization of a novel human IgA1 mAb which was generated by co-transfecting the V domains of the Acr-binding 2E9 scFv clone and IgA1 constant region domains into CHO-K1 cells. The monomeric 2E9IgA1 has strong binding affinities for Acr and for the human FcαRI/CD89 receptor. Intranasal inoculation of affinity purified 2E9IgA, and mouse IFN-γ inhibited *M. tuberculosis* pulmonary infection and granuloma formation in the lungs of CD89 transgenic, but not in littermate control mice. 2E9IgA1 also inhibited infection of human whole blood and monocyte cultures. Demonstration of the mandatory role of the FcαRI/CD89 receptor for passive protection is novel and important for the elucidation of mechanisms of IgA action. Further development of the described new human mAb is required for the translation of immunotherapy for the control of TB in humans.

2. Immunotherapy of TB

TB is a major killer, causing 1.5 million deaths annually, with the majority occurring in developing countries, also bearing the brunt of the rampant HIV epidemic. Although TB chemotherapy is highly effective, it is very protracted, lasting for six months or longer. This impacts negatively on completion rates, and defaulting leads to the emergence and spread of multi-drug resistant (MDR) strains of tubercle bacilli. Although new drugs have been proposed for treatment [1], the need for new therapies is of major concern in the fight against the MDR-TB. Arresting the global TB epidemic and also reducing the incidence of

MDR-TB could be achieved by shortening the duration of the treatment. Since combined drug and immunotherapy treatments probably carry the greatest potential, several immunotherapeutic approaches have been considered, with the three described below receiving most attention.

2.1 Immunotherapeutic vaccines

One of the first immunotherapeutic applications of vaccines to show some promise in a clinical trial was the heat-killed *Mycobacterium vaccae* [2]. Its mode of action has been proposed to be an enhancement of Th1 and down-regulation of Th2 cytokine expression. Multiple doses of vaccine are required to achieve faster bacteriological conversion, improved radiological picture and recovery of body weight. However, subsequent clinical trials with *M. vaccae* produced inconclusive (reviewed in [3]), or negative results [4, 5]. Plasmid DNA expressing mycobacterial antigens have also been evaluated for their therapeutic capacity. Thus, Hsp65-based DNA vaccine prevented the post-chemotherapy relapse in mice [6], while an Ag85-expressing DNA vaccine was effective in one [7], but not in another [8] study. A detoxified extract of *M. tuberculosis* in liposome form (termed RUTI), prevented post-chemotherapy relapse in the 'Cornell model', and was proposed for the immunoprophylactic treatment of latent tuberculous infection [9]; this vaccine has recently undergone a phase 1 clinical trial in Spain (Cardona-PJ, personal communication).

2.2 Cytokine therapy

Cytokines are highly pleiotropic proteins that can promote host immune defence mechanisms. For effective treatment of mycobacterial infections, the administered cytokines must first reach their target cells, bind to the specific receptors and finally, activate an intact signal transduction pathway to elicit a cellular response. Due to their pleiotropic activities, the dose and route of administration must be carefully considered, in order to avoid the risk of toxicity and other unwanted pharmacological effects. Several cytokines have been considered for treatment of mycobacterial infections, including IFN-γ, Il-2, IL-12, GM-CSF (granulocyte-macrophage colony-stimulating factor) and G-CSF (granulocyte colony-stimulating factor). In TB patients, Th1 cytokines are produced at high levels at the site of infection, but the systemic response is characterised by high levels of Th2 and reduced levels of Th1 cytokines [10, 11]. Given the established protective role of Th1 immunity to intracellular pathogens, this provides a strong rationale for using these cytokines as immunotherapeutic adjunct treatment for TB. Two small clinical trials utilising recombinant IL-2 reported a definitive benefit in TB patients [12, 13]. However, a subsequent large-scale randomized IL-2 trial of HIV-negative TB patients yielded disappointingly negative results. Paradoxically, it even appeared that IL-2 had a detrimental effect on bacillary clearance, probably due to IL-2-mediated induction of CD25 + regulatory T cells [14]. These studies show that although the cytokines carry a significant therapeutic potential, their application for treatment of TB is yet to be fully explored.

2.3 Monoclonal antibodies

Historically, the view that protective immunity against TB is imparted exclusively by T cells, but not by antibodies has been influenced by the assumption that antibodies cannot reach the bacilli which shelter within the phagosomes of infected macrophages. However, a review of the early literature on passive 'serum therapy' indicates both positive and negative results[15], with the one consistent theme being that such treatments appeared more effective in patients with early and localised TB rather than long-standing, chronic cases. With the development of modern approaches and tools, most notably the monoclonal antibody technology, it became possible to address the role of antibodies in intracellular infections in a far more controlled, reproducible fashion. Thus, significant new evidence emerged that antibodies can play a role in suppressing intracellular infections, including those caused by *Cryptococcus neoformans* [16], *Listeria monocytgenes* [17] and *Erlichia chaffensis* [18]. This led to a reappraisal of the role of antibodies in TB, which has recently been reviewed by us [19] and others [15, 20]. However, this approach still remains contentious, and further work is clearly needed to address the role of antibodies and their potential therapeutic application in TB and other intracellular infections.

3. Evidence for a therapeutic potential of antibodies in TB

The possible protective role of antibodies in *M. tuberculosis* infection has been indicated by clinical studies, showing that antibody titres to LAM [21] or Ag85 antigens [22] were higher in patients with milder forms of active TB. Support for a protective role comes also from animal experiments showing higher level of infection in mice genetically depleted of B cells (μ-chain knock-out)[23] or defective for IgA production [24].

Recently, a significant 100-fold reduction of the postchemotherapy relapse of pulmonary infection in SCID mice was reported following intraperitoneal inoculation of mouse antisera containing predominantly IgG antibodies [25]. These antibodies were stimulated by *M. tuberculosis* infection, chemotherapy and immunization of DBA/2 mice with a detoxified *M. tuberculosis* extract. In addition, intraperitoneal administration of a standard preparation of human gamma globulin from normal donors, reduced bacterial loads in the spleen and lungs of intravenously infected mice [26]. Antibodies could have played a role, since normal human sera contain high antibody titres for LAM and mycobacterial heat shock proteins [27].

Passive inoculation of mouse monoclonal antibodies (mAb) against a number of antigens was reported to be protective in mouse models of TB infection, but the mechanisms involved differed. Thus, pre-opsonization of intratracheally administered tubercle bacilli with IgG3 against LAM antigen [28] enhanced the granulomatous infiltration and prolonged the survival of mice, without affecting the bacterial load in the lungs, while an intravenously administered IgG1 against the same antigen decreased the bacterial load, and also prolonged survival [29]. The authors of both these studies suggested that antibody action involved blocking of the LAM-mediated uptake of bacilli by macrophages.

Another study, utilising an antibody against heparin-binding hemagglutinin (HBHA) glycoprotein, showed impaired bacterial dissemination from the lungs, due to the antibody inhibiting HBHA interaction with epithelial cells [30]. In addition to the above quoted passive protection studies, *in vitro* coating of *M. tuberculosis* bacilli with monoclonal anti-lipomannan IgG3 [28] or anti-MPB83 surface glycoprotein IgG1 [31] prolonged the survival (but not the infection of lungs) of infected mice.

Taken together, these studies have clearly demonstrated that antibodies can influence *M. tuberculosis* infection, despite the intracellular location, by probably interacting with the bacilli during the extracellular phase following the initial inhalation, or the release from apoptotic macrophages. No clinical trials have been conducted as yet, but they seem justified, subject to development and evaluation of 'humanised' mAbs.

4. Immunotherapy of TB with mouse IgA mAb TBA61

IgA is the most abundant antibody class in mucosal fluids, where it plays important anti-microbial roles involving several different mechanisms of action. The majority of the IgA found in mucosal fluids is secretory IgA (sIgA), which is formed when polymeric IgA binds to the poly-immunoglobulin receptor (PIGR), expressed on the basolateral side of epithelial membranes. While retaining a portion of PIGR, the antibody is then translocated into the mucosal lumen, where it can bind to invading pathogens, leading to their neutralisation or 'exclusion' of infection. sIgA can also intercept viruses infecting epithelial cells, during the process of antibody transcytosis [32]. These important functions of sIgA, coupled with its increased stability in harsh mucosal environment, make this form of IgA antibody particularly suitable for therapeutic purposes. Unfortunately, sIgA is difficult to make in recombinant form, though advances in expression technology have been made [33]. Therefore, most of the passive protection studies have been conducted with the serum forms of monomeric IgA.

IgA can bind to a number of different cellular receptors. In addition to the already mentioned PIGR on epithelial cells, the main Fc receptor of mononuclear cells for human IgA is CD89, though its mouse equivalent has not been identified. Other known IgA receptors include the asialoglycoprotein receptor, which plays a role in IgA catabolism by hepatocytes [34], the transferrin receptor, which binds IgA1 but not IgA2 [35] and the IgA/IgM receptor (Fcα/μR), which is expressed on B cells and monocytes [36].

IgA was reported to be protective against pathogenic bacteria in a number of studies, although the mechanisms of action appear different. For example, immune exclusion was reported as the key protective mechanism against *Salmonella typhimurium* [37] and *Vibrio cholera* [38], while agglutination was shown to play a role in inhibition of *Chlamydia trachomatis* genital infection [39]. In addition, binding to a defined virulence factor and neutralisation, were the mechanisms of inhibition of *Helicobacter felis* gastric infection [40], while multiple mechanisms were suggested for IgA-mediated inhibition of *Shigella flexneri* infection [41].

Transmission of mAbs against mycobacterial antigens into the lungs following intranasal (i.n.) or parenteral administration [42] was more efficient for IgA, than for IgG mAbs. When comparing these mAbs for their protective capacity in BALB/c mouse model of *M. tuberculosis* infection, the IgA mAb TBA61, which is specific for the α-crystallin (Acr, 16 kDa) antigen, was superior to both an IgG1 of the same antigen and epitope specificity, and also to another IgA mAb, specific for the PstS1 (38 kDa) antigen [43]. Both monomeric and polymeric form of IgA were found to be protective, inducing an approximately 10-fold reduction of the bacterial load in infected animals. Interestingly, both pre- and post-challenge mAb inoculations were required for optimal protection and the Acr antigen specificity and IgA isotype were both important for the observed inhibitory effect [43].

Acr is a small heat shock protein of *M. tuberculosis* which is expressed at particularly high levels during conditions of anoxia and stress during growth in macrophages [44, 45]. Although the protein is largely expressed in the cytosol, an increased association with the bacterial cell wall is observed under the conditions of stress and low oxygen concentration [46]. These conditions are present during the stationary phase of growth *in vitro* and also during the intracellular phase of infection. The recent evidence suggests that *M. tuberculosis* clinical strains recovered from the sputum of TB patients have a changed phenotype consistent with stationary, rather than actively dividing organisms [47], lending further support to the importance of the Acr antigens as the antibody target. Evidence from the guinea pig model of *M. tuberculosis* infection indicates that the majority of residual 'persister' bacilli following short-term drug treatment are extracellular [48]. Most likely, such non-dividing organisms would express high levels of cell wall associated Acr, making them a suitable target for anti-Acr IgA mAbs.

The IgA-mediated inhibition of the early *M. tuberculosis* infection in mice was transient, and therefore we explored the possibilities for extending and further enhancing the observed therapeutic effect. Cytokines play crucial roles in modulating immune responses to infection, and therefore, could be harnessed to aid therapeutic treatments. We considered the immune-stimulating cytokine IFN-γ, and the suppression/removal of Th2 cytokine IL-4, that can undermine protective immunity in TB. The rationale for inclusion of IFN-γ and also the neutralising anti-IL-4 antibodies, as well as the effect of combined immunotherapy is described in the following section.

5. Combined immunotherapy for TB with IgA, IFN-γ and anti-IL-4

5.1 Rationale for IFN-γ

IFN-γ has many important activities, such as activation of phagocytes, stimulation of antigen presentation, induction of cell proliferation and cell adhesion, and regulation of apoptosis. These important roles of IFN-γ for the immune responses to pathogens are best described in the context of the so-called Th1/Th2 paradigm. IL-12, another important cytokine, directly induces IFN-γ gene transcription and secretion in antigen-stimulated naive CD4+ cells [49], while in turn, IFN-γ induces IL-12 expression in macrophages and monocytes [50], thus creating a positive feedback loop. This leads against a Th1 type immune response to an intracellular infection. In contrast, Th2 cytokines IL-4, IL-13 and IL-10 suppress production of IL-12 by monocytes, and consequently also inhibit effector functions of IFN-γ, notably, the expression of inducible nitric oxide synthase [51, 52] and the respiratory burst [53].

The critical role of IFN-γ in the immunity to mycobacterial infections was confirmed in IFN-γ deficient mice, when two groups showed independently [54, 55] that mice with a disrupted IFN-γ gene were unable to control *M. tuberculosis* infection. The lack of protective immunity in IFN-γ deficient mice could be attributed exclusively to their inability to activate macrophages, since these mice otherwise developed antigen specific T cell responses, albeit more rapidly than the control mice [56]. Humans with a mutation in the IFN-γ receptor show enhanced susceptibility to TB [57] and the results of a first small scale clinical trial for treatment of MDR-TB with aerosolised IFN-γ [58] indicated a short-term treatment benefit. Therefore, IFN-γ may have a therapeutic potential for treatment of TB, although additional components may be required to achieve a more robust therapeutic effect [59].

5.2 Rationale for Th2-suppressing agents

The regulatory and potentially detrimental role of Th2 cytokines in TB has recently attracted considerable research interest, in relation to studies of both immunopathogenesis of TB and vaccine development. TB develops only in a small proportion (5-10%) of the exposed immunocompetent individuals. It is tempting to speculate that these individuals could have the normally protective innate and acquired immunity 'dis-regulated' by Th2 cell mediated inhibitory immune mechanisms. It has been proposed that IL-4 in particular, could downregulate the protective Th1 cytokine IFN-γ and lead to mediated toxicity and fibrosis [60].

However, the exact mechanism of the negative IL-4 effect on the course of mycobacterial infection is not fully understood. One possibility is that IL-4 inhibits the expression of nitric oxide synthase [61, 62] and since nitric oxide is a mandatory mediator of macrophage activation mediated killing of tubercle bacilli, its decreased levels could delay the clearance of mycobacterial infection [52].

Additional circumstantial evidence from experimental studies also points to a possible negative role of IL-4 in TB. Thus, β-glucan mediated inhibition of TGF-β, resulted in upregulated expression of IFN-γ and IL-2 and downregulated production of IL-4, leading to a significant reduction in bacterial counts in the absence of chemotherapy [63]. This was unfortunately associated with an increased risk of inflammation in the lungs, which required anti-inflammatory treatment for optimal anti-tuberculous effect.

Similarly, immunisation of M. tuberculosis infected mice with heat-killed M. vaccae resulted in decrease of bacterial burden in the lungs, which was correlated by decrease in IL-4 expression [64]. Two other immunotherapeutic vaccines have been proposed (though not tested in clinical trials), both interfering with Th2 cytokine expression levels. A DNA vaccine incorporating mycobacterial heat shock protein 65 (HSP65) was shown to be protective in mice [6] and the protection was clearly correlated with down-regulation of IL-4 production. More recently, a fragmented and detoxified M. tuberculosis based vaccine termed RUTI, was shown to be protective when given to chemotherapy-treated mice [9], and this effect was at least in part mediated by suppression of Th2 cytokine activity. Therefore, therapeutic approaches targeting Th2 cytokines could potentially be utilised for adjunctive treatment of TB.

6. Development and testing of CIT

IgA-mediated protection against early M. tuberculosis in mice could be further extended by co-inoculation with IFN-γ [65, 66]. IFN-γ was inoculated to mice i.n., 3 days before aerosol M. tuberculosis challenge, and then again together with IgA mAb, on the day of the infection and 2 days later. Co-administration of IgA and IFN-γ synergistically prolonged and enhanced the CFU-inhibitory effect of IgA alone and also reduced lung pathology [65].

IL-4 depleted or genetically deficient IL-4$^{-/-}$ mice are more resistant to M. tuberculosis infection; this could be reversed by reconstitution of mice with recombinant IL-4 [67, 68]. Combined treatment of mice with a neutralizing anti-IL-4 antibody, anti-α-crystallin IgA mAb and IFN-γ reduced lung infection with M. tuberculosis profoundly more than individual treatment regimens. Most importantly, however, this combined triple treatment with anti-IL-4 mAb, IgA and IFN-γ, prevented post-chemotherapy relapse of the infection in three different strains of mice [69], suggesting that CIT has the therapeutic potential for adjunctive application with standard TB treatment.

Multiple mechanisms are likely to be involved in protection against *M. tuberculosis* conferred by CIT. Some of them may operate on a cellular level (for example, stimulation of phagocytosis by IgA and IFN-γ), while others may involve more complex interactions within the immune system, resulting in modulation of the early response to *M. tuberculosis* infection. A schematic representation of some of the potential mechanisms of CIT action is depicted in Fig.1.

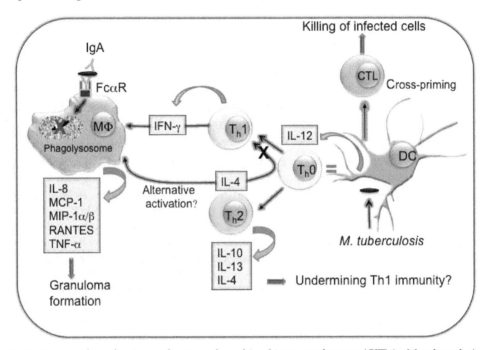

Fig. 1. Proposed mechanisms of action of combined immunotherapy (CIT) in *M. tuberculosis* infected hosts. Antibody could target extracellular bacteria and following their phagocytosis *via* IgA-receptor (indicated is human FcαR, though the mouse equivalent is not known), the bacilli are destroyed in phagolysosome. IFN-γ activates non-infected monocytes/macrophages, thus enhancing their bactericidal activity towards incipient infection. IL-4 could induce alternative activation of macrophages that does not lead to killing of intracellular organisms; in addition, it could also negatively modulate the early immune response to *M. tuberculosis*, by undermining the Th1 type response. Other, unknown mechanisms might also be involved, possibly including cytotoxicity of lymphocytes and granuloma formation.

7. Translational studies with human IgA

In order to further develop the combined TB immunotherapy for potential application in humans, a human IgA antibody specific for Acr antigen has been generated. As mentioned earlier, the human and mouse IgA systems differ significantly, both in terms of IgA structure and also the availability of IgA Fc receptors. Thus, IgA exists in two forms in humans, IgA1 and IgA2, while the mouse IgA exists in a single form, corresponding to IgA1. The most significant difference, however, is that there is a well characterised IgA-Fc receptor on human myeloid cells, CD89, which is responsible for much of the IgA-mediated anti-microbial activity [70-72], while an equivalent receptor in mice has not be identified. Therefore, it is an important consideration that therapeutic recombinant IgA antibodies should bind efficiently not only to the target antigen, but also to CD89 on monocytes/macrophages, the target cell population for immunotherapy.

A single chain Fv fragment (scFv) specific for Acr was generated using a human phage library and then expressed in CHO cells as a human IgA1 molecule with 'grafted' scFv epitope binding site [73]. The expressed 170 kDa recombinant IgA was purified by affinity chromatography and found to be glycosylated, with both N- and O-linked sugars present. The purified human antibody, termed 2E9IgA1, bound to both Acr (7.0 x 10^{-8}) and CD89 (2.9 x 10^{-6}), with both the affinity constants being well within the range for antibody-antigen and antibody-receptor type interactions, respectively.

The effect of 2E9IgA1 on *M. tuberculosis* infection was tested in mice transgenic for the human IgA receptor. Antibody was administered at the time of infection and again, at either 1 or 21 day after infection. Separate groups of mice were inoculated with IFN-γ or with both IFN-γ and IgA. The bacterial load in the lungs and spleen, as well as the immunopathology of the lungs were analysed four weeks later. Both 2E9IgA1 and IFN-γ caused partial reduction in bacterial load, but the greatest therapeutic effect was observed when the two were co-administered together, with the difference between treated and untreated animals being statistically highly significant [73]. Early and late treatment applications following challenge of mice with *M. tuberculosis* produced a similar therapeutic effect. Importantly though, the treatment had no significant effect on the infection in non-transgenic littermate controls, suggesting a mandatory role for CD89 in the observed reduction of infection. In agreement with decreased bacterial load in the lungs, the treated animals showed also reduced granulomatous infiltration of their lungs.

Studies on whole human blood cultures infected with *M. tuberculosis* showed that 2E9IgA1 reduced the infection at least in some donors. This effect required a relatively high concentration of the antibody (100 μg/ml) and the inhibition was apparent only when the ratio of bacteria:cell was 10 or less [73]. Interestingly, IFN-γ did not enhance the bactericidal effect of 2E9IgA in whole blood cultures although it did do so in purified human monocytes infected with *M. tuberculosis*. The outcome of the *in vitro* studies is generally consistent with the finding using mouse IgA, that the therapeutic effect *in vivo* was greater than the inhibition of infection *in vitro*, hence suggesting the involvement of complex *in vivo* mechanisms of antibody action.

These studies showed that the therapeutic potentials of 2E9IgA1 human mAb for tuberculosis deserve further evaluation in the form of CIT for treatment. The history of the past advances using IgA based CIT are summarised in Table 1.

Year	Stage of development	Reference
2000	TBA61 anti-Acr mAb generated and shown to be superior to IgG for transmission to lungs	[42]
2004	TBA61 IgA induced a 10-fold inhibition of early *M. tuberculosis* infection in BALB/c mice; however, inhibition was transient	[43]
2006	Co-administration of IgA and IFN-γ extended the duration of inhibition compared to IgA alone	[65]
2007	Addition of anti-IL-4 antibody profoundly enhanced the therapeutic effect of IgA and IFN-γ	[67]
2009	CIT (IgA, IFN-γ and anti-IL4) reduced significantly postchemotherapy relapse of *M. tuberculosis* infection in mice	[69]
2011	Human 2E9IgA1 anti-Acr mAb generated and shown to be protective, when co-administered with IFN-γ, in human IgA-receptor transgenic mice	[73]
Future research	Testing of 2E9IgA1-based CIT in non-human primates and subsequently, phase I human clinical trials	-

Table 1. Key stages of development of CIT based on IgA, IFN-γ and anti-IL-4

8. Targets for future research, development and clinical evaluation

There is scope for future research on the following different aspects of the combined immunotherapy:

1. *Mechanisms of IgA action.* We proposed previously that binding of mouse IgA to the intracellular lectin galectin 3 [74], which accumulates in phagosomes [75], could 'unblock' the *M. tuberculosis* induced inhibition of phagosome maturation [19]. In principle, galectin 3 could act as a mediator of the intracellular actions of IgA, considering that it has structural homology with TRIM21, which mediates the virus neutralizing activity of IgG antibodies [76].

2. *Studies in CD89 transgenic mice.* There is a need to demonstrate: i) if there is synergy between the actions of the 2E9IgA human antibody and anti-IL-4 antibodies or IL-4 antagonists; ii) if 2E9IgA based CIT can reduce the relapse of infection following short-term chemotherapy to an extent, which had been reported for the mouse TBA61-based CIT; iii) if CIT can reduce the MDR-TB infection.

3. *Development of 2E9IgA production.* It is necessary to modify the plastic adherent CHO-K1 transfectant cell line into a suspension growing variant [77], in order to increase the yield of IgA production. This is a prerequisite for producing the GMP-grade antibody in quantities required for evaluation in clinical trials.

4. *Evaluation of 2E9IgA based CIT in non-human monkey models of TB.* Macaques are eminently suitable, since they express the IgA/CD89 receptor [78] that can bind human IgA [79]. A suitable technique for aerosol delivery of IgA would need to be developed

using the approaches for the inhaled therapy with various agents [80]. Demonstrating protection against aerosol *M. tuberculosis* infection and pathology in the macaque model of infection would justify further evaluation in human clinical trials.

5. *Evaluation in HIV-positive, low CD4+cell patients.* They develop active TB at a high rate and need an alternative to the current combined chemotherapy for HIV and TB [81], because it associates with drug-drug interactions and toxicity.

6. *Evaluation in patients with drug-susceptible TB, as an adjunct to chemotherapy.* The potential benefit to the widest range of patients would be to shorten the duration of treatment. This would in turn lead to higher completion rates, reduced risk of relapse and MDR-TB. The rationale of this approach has recently been strengthened by the finding, that chemotherapy generated 'persister' bacilli are extracellular [48]; this makes them a suitable target for IgA-based CIT.

7. *Evaluation in MDR-TB and XDR-TB patients.* Existing difficulties in developing effective new drugs justify evaluation of CIT as a possible alternative approach.

9. References

[1] Andries K, Verhasselt P, Guillemont J, et al. A diarylquinoline drug active on the ATP synthase of Mycobacterium tuberculosis. Science 2005;307:223-7.

[2] Onyebujoh PC, Abdulmumini T, Robinson S, Rook GAW, Stanford JL. Immunotherapy with Mycobacterium-Vaccae As An Addition to Chemotherapy for the Treatment of Pulmonary Tuberculosis Under Difficult Conditions in Africa. Respiratory Medicine 1995;89:199-207.

[3] Stanford J, Stanford C, Grange J. Immunotherapy with Mycobacterium vaccae in the treatment of tuberculosis. Frontiers in Bioscience 2004;9:1701-19.

[4] Mwinga A, Nunn A, Ngwira B, et al. Mycobacterium vaccae (SRL172) immunotherapy as an adjunct to standard antituberculosis treatment in HIV-infected adults with pulmonary tuberculosis: a randomised placebo-controlled trial. Lancet 2002;360:1050-5.

[5] Johnson JL, Nunn AJ, Fourie PB, et al. Effect of Mycobacterium vaccae (SRL172) immunotherapy on radiographic healing in tuberculosis. International Journal of Tuberculosis and Lung Disease 2004;8:1348-54.

[6] Lowrie DB, Tascon RE, Bonato VLD, et al. Therapy of tuberculosis in mice by DNA vaccination. Nature 1999;400:269-71.

[7] Ha SJ, Jeon BY, Kim SC, et al. Therapeutic effect of DNA vaccines combined with chemotherapy in a latent infection model after aerosol infection of mice with Mycobacterium tuberculosis. Gene Therapy 2003;10:1592-9.

[8] Turner J, Rhoades ER, Keen M, Belisle JT, Frank AA, Orme IM. Effective preexposure tuberculosis vaccines fail to protect when they are given in an immunotherapeutic mode. Infection and Immunity 2000;68:1706-9.

[9] Cardona PJ, Arnat I, Gordillo S, et al. Immunotherapy with fragmented Mycobacterium tuberculosis cells increases the effectiveness of chemotherapy against a chronical infection in a murine model of tuberculosis. Vaccine 2005;23:1393-8.

[10] Toossi Z, Ellner JJ. Interaction of Leu-11 Reactive Lymphocytes and Adherent Cells in Suppression of Ppd-Induced Il-2 Production in Tuberculosis. Clinical Research 1986;34:A535.

[11] Vankayalapati R, Wizel B, Weis SE, et al. Serum cytokine concentrations do not parallel Mycobacterium tuberculosis - Induced cytokine production in patients with tuberculosis. Clinical Infectious Diseases 2003;36:24-8.

[12] Johnson BJ, Bekker LG, Rickman R, et al. rhuIL-2 adjunctive therapy in multidrug resistant tuberculosis: a comparison of two treatment regimens and placebo. Tubercle and Lung Disease 1997;78:195-203.

[13] Johnson BJ, Ress SR, Willcox P, et al. Clinical and Immune-Responses of Tuberculosis Patients Treated with Low-Dose Il-2 and Multidrug Therapy. Cytokines and Molecular Therapy 1995;1:185-96.

[14] Barnes PF. Immunotherapy for tuberculosis - Wave of the future or tilting at windmills? American Journal of Respiratory and Critical Care Medicine 2003;168:142-3.

[15] Glatman-Freedman A. Advances in antibody-mediated immunity against Mycobacterium tuberculosis: implications for a novel vaccine strategy. Fems Immunology and Medical Microbiology 2003;39:9-16.

[16] Mukherjee J, Scharff MD, Casadevall A. Protective Murine Monoclonal-Antibodies to Cryptococcus-Neoformans. Infection and Immunity 1992;60:4534-41.

[17] Edelson BT, Unanue ER. Intracellular antibody neutralizes Listeria growth. Immunity 2001;14:503-12.

[18] Li JSY, Yager E, Reilly M, et al. Outer membrane protein-specific monoclonal antibodies protect SCID mice from fatal infection by the obligate intracellular bacterial pathogen Ehrlichia chaffeensis. Journal of Immunology 2001;166:1855-62.

[19] Reljic R, Williams A, Ivanyi J. Mucosal immunotherapy of tuberculosis: Is there value in passive IgA? Tuberculosis 2006;86:179-90.

[20] Casadevall A. Antibody-mediated immunity against intracellular pathogens: Two-dimensional thinking comes full circle. Infection and Immunity 2003;71:4225-8.

[21] Costello AMD, Kumar A, Narayan V, et al. Does Antibody to Mycobacterial Antigens, Including Lipoarabinomannan, Limit Dissemination in Childhood Tuberculosis. Transactions of the Royal Society of Tropical Medicine and Hygiene 1992;86:686-92.

[22] Sanchez-Rodriguez C, Estrada-Chavez C, Garcia-Vigil J, et al. An IgG antibody response to the antigen 85 complex is associated with good outcome in Mexican Totonaca Indians with pulmonary tuberculosis. International Journal of Tuberculosis and Lung Disease 2002;6:706-12.

[23] Vordermeier HM, Venkatprasad N, Harris DP, Ivanyi J. Increase of tuberculous infection in the organs of B cell-deficient mice. Clinical and Experimental Immunology 1996;106:312-6.

[24] Rodriguez A, Tjarnlund A, Ivanji J, et al. Role of IgA in the defense against respiratory infections IgA deficient mice exhibited increased susceptibility to intranasal infection with Mycobacterium bovis BCG. Vaccine 2005;23:2565-72.

[25] Guirado E, Amat I, Gil O, et al. Passive serum therapy with polyclonal antibodies against Mycobacterium tuberculosis protects against post-chemotherapy relapse of tuberculosis infection in SCID mice. Microbes and Infection 2006;8:1252-9.

[26] Roy E, Stavropoulos E, Brennan J, et al. Therapeutic efficacy of high-dose intravenous immunoglobulin in Mycobacterium tuberculosis infection in mice. Infection and Immunity 2005;73:6101-9.

[27] Jackett PS, Bothamley GH, Batra HV, Mistry A, Young DB, Ivanyi J. Specificity of Antibodies to Immunodominant Mycobacterial Antigens in Pulmonary Tuberculosis. Journal of Clinical Microbiology 1988;26:2313-8.

[28] Teitelbaum R, Glatman-Freedman A, Chen B, et al. A mAb recognizing a surface antigen of Mycobacterium tuberculosis enhances host survival. Proceedings of the National Academy of Sciences of the United States of America 1998;95:15688-93.

[29] Hamasur B, Haile M, Pawlowski A, Schroder U, Kallenius G, Svenson SB. A mycobacterial lipoarabinomannan specific monoclonal antibody and its F(ab ')(2) fragment prolong survival of mice infected with Mycobacterium tuberculosis. Clinical and Experimental Immunology 2004;138:30-8.

[30] Pethe K, Alonso S, Biet F, et al. The heparin-binding haemagglutinin of M-tuberculosis is required for extrapulmonary dissemination. Nature 2001;412:190-4.

[31] Chambers MA, Gavier-Widen D, Hewinson RG. Antibody bound to the surface antigen MPB83 of Mycobacterium bovis enhances survival against high dose and low dose challenge. Fems Immunology and Medical Microbiology 2004;41:93-100.

[32] Mazanec MB, Kaetzel CS, Lamm ME, Fletcher D, Nedrud JG. Intracellular Neutralization of Virus by Immunoglobulin-A Antibodies. Proceedings of the National Academy of Sciences of the United States of America 1992;89:6901-5.

[33] Crottet P, Cottet S, Corthesy B. Expression, purification and biochemical characterization of recombinant murine secretary component: a novel tool in mucosal immunology. Biochemical Journal 1999;341:299-306.

[34] Stockert RJ, Kressner MS, Collins JC, Sternlieb I, Morell AG. Iga Interaction with the Asialoglycoprotein Receptor. Proceedings of the National Academy of Sciences of the United States of America-Biological Sciences 1982;79:6229-31.

[35] Moura IC, Centelles MN, Arcos-Fajardo M, et al. Identification of the transferrin receptor as a novel immunoglobulin (Ig)A1 receptor and its enhanced expression on mesangial cells in IgA nephropathy. Journal of Experimental Medicine 2001;194:417-25.

[36] Shibuya A, Sakamoto N, Shimizu Y, et al. Fc alpha/mu receptor mediates endocytosis of IgM-coated microbes. Nature Immunology 2000;1:441-6.

[37] Michetti P, Mahan MJ, Slauch JM, Mekalanos JJ, Neutra MR. Monoclonal Secretory Immunoglobulin-A Protects Mice Against Oral Challenge with the Invasive Pathogen Salmonella-Typhimurium. Infection and Immunity 1992;60:1786-92.

[38] Apter FM, Michetti P, Winner LS, Mack JA, Mekalanos JJ, Neutra MR. Analysis of the Roles of Antilipopolysaccharide and Anticholera Toxin Immunoglobulin A

(Iga) Antibodies in Protection Against Vibrio-Cholerae and Cholera-Toxin by Use of Monoclonal Iga Antibodies In-Vivo. Infection and Immunity 1993;61:5279-85.

[39] Pal S, Theodor I, Peterson EM, delaMaza LM. Monoclonal immunoglobulin A antibody to the major outer membrane protein of the Chlamydia trachomatis mouse pneumonitis biovar protects mice against a chlamydial genital challenge. Vaccine 1997;15:575-82.

[40] Blanchard TG, Czinn SJ, Maurer R, Thomas WD, Soman G, Nedrud JG. Urease-Specific Monoclonal-Antibodies Prevent Helicobacter-Felis Infection in Mice. Infection and Immunity 1995;63:1394-9.

[41] Phalipon A, Kaufmann M, Michetti P, et al. Monoclonal Immunoglobulin-A Antibody-Directed Against Serotype-Specific Epitope of Shigella-Flexneri Lipopolysaccharide Protects Against Murine Experimental Shigellosis. Journal of Experimental Medicine 1995;182:769-78.

[42] Falero-Diaz G, Challacombe S, Rahman D, et al. Transmission of IgA and IgG monoclonal antibodies to mucosal fluids following intranasal or parenteral delivery. International Archives of Allergy and Immunology 2000;122:143-50.

[43] Williams A, Reljic R, Naylor I, et al. Passive protection with immunoglobulin A antibodies against tuberculous early infection of the lungs. Immunology 2004;111:328-33.

[44] Sherman DR, Voskuil M, Schnappinger D, Liao RL, Harrell MI, Schoolnik GK. Regulation of the Mycobacterium tuberculosis hypoxic response gene encoding alpha-crystallin. Proceedings of the National Academy of Sciences of the United States of America 2001;98:7534-9.

[45] Yuan Y, Crane DD, Simpson RM, et al. The 16-kDa alpha-crystallin (Acr) protein of Mycobacterium tuberculosis is required for growth in macrophages. Proceedings of the National Academy of Sciences of the United States of America 1998;95:9578-83.

[46] Cunningham AF, Spreadbury CL. Mycobacterial stationary phase induced by low oxygen tension: Cell wall thickening and localization of the 16-kilodalton alpha-crystallin homology. Journal of Bacteriology 1998;180:801-8.

[47] Garton NJ, Waddell SJ, Sherratt AL, et al. Cytological and transcript analyses reveal fat and lazy persister-like bacilli in tuberculous sputum. Plos Medicine 2008;5:634-45.

[48] Lenaerts AJ, Hoff D, Aly S, et al. Location of persisting mycobacteria in a guinea pig model of tuberculosis revealed by R207910. Antimicrobial Agents and Chemotherapy 2007;51:3338-45.

[49] Lederer JA, Perez VL, DesRoches L, Kim SM, Abbas AK, Lichtman AH. Cytokine transcriptional events during helper T cell subset differentiation. Journal of Experimental Medicine 1996;184:397-406.

[50] Yoshida A, Koide Y, Uchijima M, Yoshida TO. Ifn-Gamma Induces Il-12 Messenger-Rna Expression by A Murine Macrophage Cell-Line, J774. Biochemical and Biophysical Research Communications 1994;198:857-61.

[51] Liew FY, Li Y, Severn A, et al. A Possible Novel Pathway of Regulation by Murine T-Helper Type-2 (Th2) Cells of A Th1 Cell-Activity Via the Modulation of the Induction of Nitric-Oxide Synthase on Macrophages. European Journal of Immunology 1991;21:2489-94.

[52] Reljic R, Stylianou E, Balu S, Ma JK. Cytokine interactions that determine the outcome of mycobacterial infection of macrophages. Cytokine 2010;51:42-6.

[53] Lehn M, Weiser WY, Engelhorn S, Gillis S, Remold HG. Il-4 Inhibits H2O2 Production and Antileishmanial Capacity of Human Cultured Monocytes Mediated by Ifn-Gamma. Journal of Immunology 1989;143:3020-4.

[54] Cooper AM, Dalton DK, Stewart TA, Griffin JP, Russell DG, Orme IM. Disseminated Tuberculosis in Interferon-Gamma Gene-Disrupted Mice. Journal of Experimental Medicine 1993;178:2243-7.

[55] Flynn JL, Chan J, Triebold KJ, Dalton DK, Stewart TA, Bloom BR. An Essential Role for Interferon-Gamma in Resistance to Mycobacterium-Tuberculosis Infection. Journal of Experimental Medicine 1993;178:2249-54.

[56] Pearl JE, Saunders B, Ehlers S, Orme IM, Cooper AM. Inflammation and lymphocyte activation during mycobacterial infection in the interferon-gamma-deficient mouse. Cellular Immunology 2001;211:43-50.

[57] Dorman SE, Holland SM. Mutation in the signal-transducing chain of the interferon-gamma receptor and susceptibility to mycobacterial infection. Journal of Clinical Investigation 1998;101:2364-9.

[58] Condos R, Rom WN, Schluger NW. Treatment of multidrug-resistant pulmonary tuberculosis with interferon-gamma via aerosol. Lancet 1997;349:1513-5.

[59] Reljic R. IFN-gamma therapy of tuberculosis and related infections. Journal of Interferon and Cytokine Research 2007;27:353-63.

[60] Rook GAW, Hernandez-Pando R, Dheda K, Seah GT. IL-4 in tuberculosis: implications for vaccine design. Trends in Immunology 2004;25:483-8.

[61] Bogdan C, Vodovotz Y, Paik J, Xie QW, Nathan C. Interleukin-4 and Transforming Growth Factor-Beta Suppress Inducible Nitric Oxide Synthase by Different Mechanisms. Biology of Nitric Oxide, Pt 4 1994;8:313-6.

[62] Nemoto Y, Otsuka T, Niiro H, et al. Differential effects of interleukin-4 and interleukin-10 on nitric oxide production by murine macrophages. Inflammation Research 1999;48:643-50.

[63] Hernandez-Pando R, Orozco-Esteves H, Maldonado HA, et al. A combination of a transforming growth factor-beta antagonist and an inhibitor of cyclooxygenase is an effective treatment for murine pulmonary tuberculosis. Clinical and Experimental Immunology 2006;144:264-72.

[64] Rook GAW, HernandezPando R. The pathogenesis of tuberculosis. Annual Review of Microbiology 1996;50:259-84.

[65] Reljic R, Clark SO, Williams A, et al. Intranasal IFN gamma extends passive IgA antibody protection of mice against Mycobacterium tuberculosis lung infection. Clinical and Experimental Immunology 2006;143:467-73.

[66] Reljic R, Williams A, Clark S, Marsh P, Ivanyi J. Intranasal IFN gamma and anti alpha-crystallin IgA inhibit Mycobacterium tuberculosis lung infection in mice. Immunology 2007;120:43.

[67] Buccheri S, Reljic R, Caccamo N, et al. IL-4 depletion enhances host resistance and passive IgA protection against tuberculosis infection in BALB/c mice. European Journal of Immunology 2007;37:729-37.

[68] Roy E, Lowrie DB, Jolles SR. Current strategies in TB immunotherapy. Current Molecular Medicine 2007;7:373-86.

[69] Buccheri S, Reljic R, Caccamo N, et al. Prevention of the post-chemotherapy relapse of tuberculous infection by combined immunotherapy. Tuberculosis 2009;89:91-4.

[70] Launay P, Grossetete B, Arcos-Fajardo M, et al. Fc alpha receptor (CD89) mediates the development of immunoglobulin A (IgA) nephropathy (Berger's disease): Evidence for pathogenic soluble receptor-IgA complexes in patients and CD89 transgenic mice. Journal of Experimental Medicine 2000;191:1999-2009.

[71] Otten MA, van Egmond M. The Fc receptor for IgA (Fc alpha RI, CD89). Immunology Letters 2004;92:23-31.

[72] Pleass RJ, Dunlop JI, Anderson CM, Woof JM. Identification of residues in the CH2/CH3 domain interface of IgA essential for interaction with the human Fc alpha receptor (Fc alpha R) CD89. Journal of Biological Chemistry 1999;274:23508-14.

[73] Balu S, Reljic R, Lewis MJ, et al. A Novel Human IgA Monoclonal Antibody Protects against Tuberculosis. Journal of Immunology 2011;186:3113-9.

[74] Reljic R, Crawford C, Challacombe S, Ivanyi J. Mouse monoclonal IgA binds to the galectin-3/Mac-2 lectin from mouse macrophage cell lines. Immunology Letters 2004;93:51-6.

[75] Beatty WL, Rhoades ER, Hsu DK, Liu FT, Russell DG. Association of a macrophage galactoside-binding protein with Mycobacterium-containing phagosomes. Cellular Microbiology 2002;4:167-76.

[76] Mallery DL, McEwan WA, Bidgood SR, Towers GJ, Johnson CM, James LC. Antibodies mediate intracellular immunity through tripartite motif-containing 21 (TRIM21). Proceedings of the National Academy of Sciences of the United States of America 2010;107:19985-90.

[77] Beyer T, Lohse S, Berger S, Peipp M, Valerius T, Dechant M. Serum-free production and purification of chimeric IgA antibodies. Journal of Immunological Methods 2009;346:26-37.

[78] Rogers KA, Scinicariello F, Attanasio R. Identification and characterization of macaque CD89 (immunoglobulin A Fc receptor). Immunology 2004;113:178-86.

[79] Rogers KA, Jayashankar L, Scinicariello F, Attanasio R. Nonhuman primate IgA: Genetic heterogeneity and interactions with CD89. Journal of Immunology 2008;180:4816-24.

[80] Misra A, Hickey AJ, Rossi C, et al. Inhaled drug therapy for treatment of tuberculosis. Tuberculosis 2011;91:71-81.

[81] Reljic R, Ivanyi J. A case for passive immunoprophylaxis against tuberculosis. Lancet Infectious Diseases 2006;6:813-8.

6

The Hidden History of Tuberculin

Cristina Vilaplana and Pere-Joan Cardona

Unitat de Tuberculosi Experimental, Fund. Institut Germans Trias i Pujol
Catalonia, Spain

1. Introduction

Robert Koch was an eminence on Tuberculosis and a german hero worldwide since he discovered and described the ethiologic cause of the white plague. Soon afterwards, he devoted his work to study the effect of inoculating *M.tuberculosis* bacilli (Mtb) to guinea pigs, either healthy or already infected. From his experiments, as reported by himself, he learnt the infection was able to develop protection against reinfection in some extent and that using small doses of dead bacilli could help to heal the tuberculous lesions in the infected animals, while large doses could kill them. The 4th of July, 1890, during the International Medical Congress in Berlin, he announced he might have found a cure, and pointed out it should not be used in severe cases as it could do more harm than good. However, tuberculosis was one of the main causes of death at that moment, and the word of Koch's finding its cure rapidly spread. Many physicians from all over the world traveled to Berlin to learn how to use the new remedy, called tuberculin for being obtained from Mtb bacilli, as Sir Conan Doyle did himself. Koch, probably scared of the great expectancy generated by his cure still not too well-known, decided to write a manuscript entitled "A further report on a remedy for tuberculosis" (Koch 1890), which was published on mid-November of the same year. With this paper, he intended to clarify and to give a review of the subject, in order to avoid the public to get distorted knowledge on the remedy proposed by him. In the manuscript, he tried to explain why tuberculin worked: he believed the treatment was able to destroy the necrotic tissue of the tuberculous lesions, and this was the cause for the bacilli to die subsequently. But still more important, he cautioned about the fact of existing reactions following the inoculation of tuberculin, which severity depended on the patients and their previous illness status, and suggested it should be applied as early as possible to obtain a positive outcome (Koch 1890).

2. Tuberculins

2.1 Koch's tuberculin

Tuberculin was fine powder of Mtb (obtained after mechanically comminuting the products from a tubercle culture) brought into suspension, used in dilutions and sterilised by heating it. T was injected subcutaneously in the back, between the shoulder-blades and the lumbar region, for being the location where less local reactions (including pain) were recorded(Koch 1890). High doses were given in a schedule based in the inoculation of increasing doses. The inoculation of tuberculin was followed by the so-called „Reactions", which in some cases were large and quite severe, sometimes leading to death.

There were three types of reactions depending on where did they happen: local, general (which we nowadays would call systemic) or focal reactions (in tuberculous lesions)(Riviere and Morland 1913).

At the injection site, if existing, the local reactions included redness, inflammatory swelling and pain, signs and symptoms which used to appear 2 or 3 days after the inoculation, were well-tolerated and tended to disappear. Fever was the more constant sign among the general reactions, followed by headache, malaise, lost of appetite and nausea. The amount of fever varied among the individuals, and didn't previewed any outcome, neither good or bad (Ross 19--?).

Focal reactions included haemoptysis, pleuritic pain, greater cough, râles and swelling of lymphatic glands. These were the most feared reactions but also the most wanted ones, as giving T was endeavoured to help to solve the tuberculous lesions. People well-reacting to the treatment reached, in a period in between 8 weeks and 4 months, a cessation of sweating, cough and expectoration, an improvement of the general condition and a clearing up of the moist rales, which meant the necrotic and ulcerating lesion to become cicatricial (Ross 19--?).

But due to the sudden and massive use of Koch's new remedy, lots of cases with negative outcome reached the mass media as well as the scientific community.

Only one year after presenting T, Koch himself commented the reactions observed by other physicians when using it (Pottenger 1913).

In spite of the recommendations of Koch's to carefully select the patients to be treated, tuberculin was given to any patient, including greatly advanced cases of tuberculosis, with large cavities. While some physicians praised for the benefits on some clinical forms of tuberculosis, specially when combined to surgery (tuberculosis of joints, bones and lupus) (Ross 19--?; Anonymous 1891; Morris 1893), many deaths were also reported. Due to them, and to the sensation of the adverse effects being much impressive than the positive effects obtained, soon all the hopes placed on Koch's remedy seemed to vanish (Ross 19--?). In 1891, a report was issued commenting the 55 trials undergone in Prussia between last 1890 and early 1891. This report, published in the Klinisches Jahrbuch, registered about 20% of patients getting better with the treatment and, in summary, more deaths than positive results.

T was discredited as fast as Koch's reputation, even if the political-social-personal context that surrounded him played an important role in that (Ross 19--?; Sahli 1912; Daniel 1997; Gradmann 2001). Koch intended to be eximed of his academic duties to develop and sell the tuberculin, but the Prussian Government seemed to have other plans for him: to rule an Institute able to compete the Pasteur's French one, as the two empires were rivals. Koch competed directly with von Behring, a disciple of him which had success selling antitoxins against diphtheria and tetanus and could replace him as director of the Hygiene Institute. Von Behring and Ehrlich (the last by collaborating with Hoetsch) worked with biotechnological companies, as was in vogue among the eminent scientists (also for representing a good income of money). Koch also needed the money of selling his remedy to pay his former wife to get a divorce from her, as he fell in love with a young girl (Hedwig

Freiberg) and wanted to marry her. After the report of the Prussian Government was fully published, in April 1891, tuberculin was discredited and Koch, pushed by the Government, renounced to receive any economical compensation and accepted to be proposed for directing the new institute (Gradmann 2001; Cardona 2007).

2.2 New Tuberculins and other similar products

The first attempt to avoid the reactions was to produce new tuberculins and similar products, a thing that Koch did himself, all of them being obtained from tubercle products and differing in the manufacture and/or the excipients. The Old Tuberculin, as was commonly called the original Koch's remedy, was based on human tubercle cultures grown on nutrient broth with a 5% of glycerin, sterilised by steam, evaporated, filtered and adding a 0,5% of phenol to be further refiltered. The New Tuberculin and the Koch's bacilli emulsion were the newest products developed by Koch, intending to ameliorate the first version of tuberculin. To generate the New Tuberculin, the steamed cultures were ground and mixed with glycerin to obtain only the insoluble parts of bacillary bodies, and it was developed in 1897. The Koch's bacilli emulsion was from 1901, and was based on powdered tubercle culture suspended in a mixture of half part of glycerin and half of distilled water, in order to obtain an emulsion.

Many other tuberculins were designed, generally classified in exotoxins or soluble products (mere filtered extracts of tubercle bacilli), endotoxins (containing the less soluble substance of microorganisms, also differing according to the process of extraction), and a third group, including both products, the soluble and insoluble (Wilkinson 1909; Riviere and Morland 1913). Some authors considered the albumose to be responsible for the reactions, thus albumose-free tuberculin from cultures grown in albumose-free medium were generated. Beraneck tuberculin was one of this, based on a mixture of filtered culture of tubercle bacilli grown in albumose-free medium plus an extract of bacillary bodies in 1% of phosporic acid (Riviere and Morland 1913). Wolff-Eisner refined the Koch' s New Tuberculin by filtering the powdered body-substance of tubercle bacilli through a Berkefeld candle to substract all fragments of bacilli (Sahli 1912). The products differed in the way they were obtained and treated, thus how the cultures were killed (by mechanical, physical or chemical means), how and how much they were filtrated, how they were dissolved and how and with what they were treated after.

New tuberculins appeared all over the world: Hunter's modification B, von Ruck's Watery Extract, Behring's TC, and many others (Trudeau 1907). With the promise of avoiding reactions also other products were commercialized, as the Partigens of Much of Hamburg. Even if they weren't considered as tuberculins, they could in fact be so-called, as were supposed to be partial antigens of M.tuberculosis bacilli extracted from the non-soluble part of the cultures, further treated by alcohol and ether to obtain them (Rothschild 1921).

Friedmann thought the reactions could be avoided if using cultures of other Mycobacteria, and developed a vaccine from M.chelonei cultures. He gave it therapeutically with success, but he failed in obtaining reactionless vaccination. However, he even went further, proving the vaccine to be quite useful if given post-exposure in selected cases and prophylactically (Belmes 1937; Vilaplana and Cardona 2010).

Even the Medical Research Council (MRC) had its own tuberculin, supposedly better than other candidates, they finally had to admit in 1924 it was not better than other products (Bryder 1988).

At the end, the best definition for tuberculin seems to be the one given by Pottenger: all products made from tubercle bacilli which contain their bacterial proteins (Pottenger 1913).

Some products produced more local reactions, mostly by a depôt effect, as did the Koch's Bacillary Emulsion and the New Tuberculin, as remained as insoluble deposit at the site of the injection for more time. The more soluble tuberculins, on the other hand, were supposed to generate more general reactions (Riviere and Morland 1913).

The main problem of the products was its preparation, as they all required dilutions and these were performed by the physicians themselves, a fact that the manufacturer of the Beraneck tuberculin improved (as its dilutions could be already provided) ensuring a better uniformity of concentration (Sahli 1912). The concentration was important to graduate the doses of the vaccines, and this was indispensable to be able to organize to time the injections (Wright 1902).

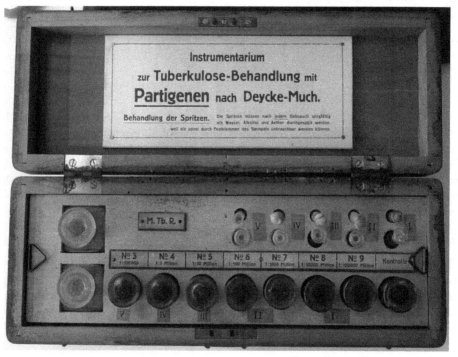

Fig. 1. Partigens of Deycke-Much.

The Old Tuberculin begun to be considered as the best for a diagnostic use. However, as pointed out Sahli, the therapeutic value of the treatment with different tuberculins were not comparable, as no standard existed (Sahli 1912).

Sahli also wrote that good responses could be obtained with all the products available if the right technique was used, but unfortunately, irrespective of which 'new' tuberculin was used, the reactions appeared to be similar, though varying somewhat in intensity (Sahli 1912).

The Partigens were tuberculin products, supposed to achieve good outcomes with less reactions, for being partial antigens instead of the former tuberculins. The Partigens were obtained from the insoluble parts of *M.tuberculosis* cultures after treating them with alcohol and ether, to obtain the 3 partial antigens: the fatty-acid-lipoids (soluble in alcohol); the neutral and highly molecular fats (soluble in ether) and the non-soluble residuum, supposed to belong to the group of proteins (Rothschild 1921). The picture shows how the Partigens were commercialized, providing diluted concentrations for better adjust the doses.

3. Dosage schedules

3.1 The clue of the dosage

It has already been said that no tuberculin was able to avoid reactions, and the difference between them was the intensity of the adverse effects. As soon as this became evident, the scientists and physicians devoted their efforts to find a safe schedule of inoculations. They were mainly two schools of therapists: those believing in true immunization, and thus only to be obtained by large tuberculin doses; and those believing in the recall of host immunity, and thus easily to be achieved by administering small doses of the remedy (as higher doses could do much harm and the effect of a stimulus is not always proportional to the intensity of the stimulus) (Sahli 1912; Pottenger 1913; Vilaplana and Cardona 2010).

Koch observed he needed high doses to obtain the effects he wanted in tuberculous focus, even if this implied reactions. For after each inoculation, a reaction happened, which was followed by tolerance. Consequently, next dose had to be higher to overcome this tolerance. This dosage method, consisting in small doses gradually incremented in short intervals, was developed by Ehrlich and coworkers on 1891, and was modified by the proposals of Goetsch in 1901 (introducing long treatment) and Petrushky later (proposing interrupted treatment in selected cases) (Vilaplana and Cardona 2010).

3.2 Sir Almroth Wright and the therapeutic vaccination

Back to 1896, Sir Almroth Wright, based on the observation of the agglutination of typhoid bacilli when being in contact with serum of someone's infected but not to someone's not infected, considered this a protective process and decided to use it to distinguish the typhoid fever from the Malta fever. It was known, from about 200 years before, human are able to generate resistance to infections, something already used by Jenner (vaccination with cowpox to prevent smallpox, 1796) and Pasteur (live attenuated bacilli to protect against anthrax, in 1870s) among others. But Wright feared using alive bacteria for this purpose could generate acute disease, and advocated for using dead bacilli instead, as he considered they should generate protective immunity as well (as did Dr. Ferran)(Vilaplana and Cardona 2010). Thus with these ideas he developed the typhoid vaccine to prevent typhoid fever, and demonstrated in vaccinated subjects a higher agglutinin levels similar to the levels found in those individuals who had survived an episode of the disease. Wright thought that if vaccination could generate protective substances in naïve subjects, it would probably boost the already existing protective substances if administered to infected individuals. From this assumption, he developed his idea of therapeutical vaccination: the vaccines wouldn't only be useful to prevent, but also to heal. With this purpose, he began to use heat-sterilized cultures of staphylococci to treat localized infections of staphylococcical nature. In 1902, he observed the agglutinin levels were decreased in the infected individuals but increased if these subjects were treated with dead bacterial cultures.

Therapeutical vaccinations also lead him to the observation of an immediate aggravation of the patient's condition, what he called the "Negative Phase"(Wright 1902).

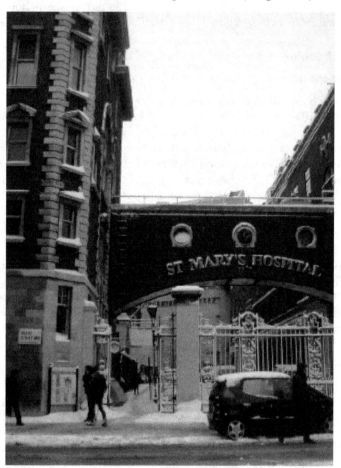

Fig. 2. Actual image of the St.Mary's Hospital in London, UK. Wright directed the former Inoculation Department of this hospital, devoted to administer the vaccines therapeutically.

Wright believed the reason for these Negative Phases was the vaccination exhausting the existing protective substances. Once the Negative Phase was overcome, a Positive Phase happened, with an increased well-being and healing tendency, in which the protective substances hypothetically increased and further decreased, but remaining in a certain amount of residual levels (Cope 1966). He also attributed the intensity of both phases to a problem of dosage, and established a general basis to treat localized infection with bacterial vaccines. If the dose was too low, the Negative Phase diminished, but the Positive Phase could not appear; if it was too high, the Negative Phase was too long, the Positive Phase appearing too late or not appear at all (Wright 1903). In two cases he treated of staphylococcia, he observed a considerable inflammatory swelling in the site of infection. He soon found a relationship between this reaction and the one described by the physicians when using Koch's tubercle vaccine. He also gave an explanation for this: he considered the infectious focus to be broken up, and he warned: if the patient is in a Negative Phase the tubercle bacilli are spread, being able to originate new infectious foci. He considered this to be because a bad-regulated dosage, and propose the rule for any therapeutical vaccination: to consider the resistance ability of both the invading microorganism and the host at the time of inoculation, to well-graduate the doses of the vaccine, timing the injections for any patient in a Negative Phase to be recovered (Wright 1902). Wright believed Koch's reactions were due to an accumulation of Negative Phases, while the true objective was to achieve successive Positive Phases to increase the immunity, thus introduced a new dosage method of tuberculin, based on the inoculation of small doses at spaced intervals (Gunter 1928), giving tuberculin in a 1000 times lower doses than in Koch's time (Riviere and Morland 1913).

3.3 Dosage schedules

In spite of the early discredit which tarnish the usefulness of tuberculin remedy, and even if the history has erased any trace of it, the fact is that its use was increased after Wright's contribution, all over Europe and even America. As previously pointed by Sahli, Pottenger also remarked the difference in the effect between the tuberculins was more quantitative than qualitative (Sahli 1912) (Pottenger 1913).

The administration regimens soon derived to only two (with variations). As after an inoculation tolerance came, only two things could be done: to give a higher next dose to overcome the tolerance or to wait the tolerance to pass. To give a higher next dose implied giving increasing doses at small intervals, and is linkable to Koch's idea of treatment administration. This method was widely used in Europe and America, and seems to be the best one to treat pthtisical forms of the disease.

Wright's method instead, intended to avoid tolerance, and implied the inoculation of constant small doses administered at long intervals. This method seems to have achieved more positive outcomes in disseminated tuberculosis, local tuberculosis, surface tuberculosis (typical of childhood), and especially if combined with surgery (Wright and Reid 1906; Vilaplana and Cardona 2010).

It is true that reactions continued to happen and scientists gave different explanations for this. Some believed a synergy existed between toxins contained in tuberculin and the toxins already existing in the infected body. There was a "difference theory", believing in the presence of antitoxins in the host, able to balance the disease, which effect could be overcome by the tuberculin administrated. Other theories more concrete believed in a direct effect of the remedy on the leucocytes or the fixation ability of the complement, the lysis of tuberculin into small toxins (Wolff-Eisner theory), antibody mediated allergy (Von Pirquet) and Hypersensitiveness (Sahli 1912; Vilaplana and Cardona 2009; Vilaplana and Cardona 2010).

But it is also described in literature the most important thing to avoid serious reactions was the ability of the physician to know when and which dose to apply to every single patient, depending on his condition.

Autopsies on fatal cases after administering tuberculin revealed the disease was that bad that no hope of cure or even improvement could be expected, no matter the remedy would have been given (Ross 19--?).

Physicians developed the sense to administer the remedy empirically without having many fatal results, and they had tools to do it.

No inoculation should be repeated before the fever to pass, according to the physicians' recommendation. The worst toxic effects were the cardiac toxic effect, with increase of the blood pressure and albuminuria, thus it is understandable that cardiac complications were among the contraindications of administering the remedy. Other contraindications were great loss of strenght, amyloid or other degeneration tissue, albuminuria and urea (Ross 19--?).

As appointed by Sahli, tuberculin seemed to not have any direct healing power, but enhancing in some way the host immune response. Healthy animals tolerated large doses which would be toxic and even fatal in tuberculous animals and humans. But either in healthy and tuberculous individuals, the tolerance could be increased up to a million times by gradual increase of dose (Sahli 1912).

As explained before, any inoculation of tuberculin was characterized by a local reaction in the site of injection (painfulness, inflammation and sometimes a little uneasiness at the site of injection), a focal reaction at the site of tubercular disease (haemoptysis, pleuritic pains, swelling of tuberculous glands, cough) and a general disturbance (basically fever and pain, loss of appetite and depression); but also to be followed by an immunizing response: with an improvement of tuberculosis symptomatology, a believed increase of the antibody content in the blood and a decrease on the response to the injected tuberculin (Riviere and Morland 1913). As it was no way to predict the effect (either good or bad) of the remedy on the infectious focus, physicians had to be guided by the effects on the symptomatology to infer the amount of the effect produced by a dose of tuberculin (Riviere and Morland 1913). The optimum therapeutic dose was the maximum amount of tuberculin which could be tolerated at any particular moment without producing any severe effects, and depended of each individual, as high interindividual variability existed (Sahli 1912).

Thus physicians used dosage tables to be helped to choose the right doses. They worked with 10% dilutions, beginning at 10000, the remedy given intradermically or subcutaneously. The most common schedule implied administering tuberculin once a week (twice a week at the most), during a minimum of a fortnight. The administration was adjusted according to the tolerance appeared, but being treated in public services or private practices also influenced this point. First, the physicians themselves prepared their tuberculins, but soon some pharmacists begun to produce and sell them at every point worldwide. Some of the products were sold as syringes with already prepared dilutions, which increased the uniformity of the preparation (Pottenger 1913) and avoided the variations in concentration of the active principle (Sahli 1912).

The physicians recommended the treatment and patients themselves bought the remedy to be administered, and even if it was cheap compared to other treatment, it still was expensive for the poor, which were the population collective more susceptible to need it (Salvat-Papasseit 2007).

"Tuberculin is quite harmless, if there is no tuberculosis". Wilkinson

"Tuberculin is not a poison". Pottenger

"The best rule to follow: better too little than too much tuberculin!". Sahli

"The physician of the future will, I foresee, take upon himself the rôle of an immunizator". Wright

Fig. 3. Quotes on tuberculin treatment, published in the manuscripts of that time.

4. Tuberculin and its historical context

4.1 Tuberculin's use

The scientists of that time tried to stick to every treatment which seemed to give any hope to the tuberculous patients, with the basic knowledge on medicine and immunology then available. Wright invented the use of the Opsonic Index as a biomarker for predicting good responses in tuberculin treatment (Wright and Douglas 1903-1904; Wright and Reid 1906; Ogilvy 1908), which years after revealed to be non-specific (Riviere 1914; Cope 1966) and brought the idea of "Autoinoculation". Wright called the Autoinoculation to some disturbance of the site of the disease, which supposedly generated a continuous periodic escape of bacilli or bacillary toxins to the blood stream, causing bursts of clinical symptoms as any chronic disease with acute episodes would do (Wright and Reid 1906). As the balance between the host response and the virulence of the infection would be the most important fact in the way the disease would develop, while certain amount of antigen was believed to be constantly needed to immunize, its excess could fatally overpower the host response. The source of antigens needed to maintain this residual host response needed could be provided by the infectious focus itself or externally, by inoculation of tuberculin (Riviere 1926), while rest would contribute to heal the infectious foci (Canetti 1955). English sanatoria, following this idea, combined resting hours with working hours at the fresh air, as part of the therapy (Bryder 1988).

Thus tuberculin treatment was administered combined to the hygienic measures commonly prescribed at that time: rest (which would favor the healing), fresh air and an improvement of nutrition (which would favor the immune system). At that time, sanatoria had flourished all over Europe and even America, and people with means attended them to be cured of tuberculosis or at least improve their hampered health status. On 1912, more than 200 institutions in UK and the 70% of the German ones used tuberculin as a standard regimen (Riviere and Morland 1913).

But sanatoria were expensive, and even if no one was safe of suffering tuberculosis, the truth is that the poor got the worst part. They lived in small overcrowded and poor-ventilated apartments in the cities, which favored the spread of the infection, and they were malnourished, which implied immunosupression. Charity sanatoria appeared in United Kingdom to cope with this big problem for public health, in order to both diminish the tremendous effect on the country's economy and to isolate the infectious sources (Bryder 1988). At 1921, the UK decided the remedy to be cofinanced depending on each family situation, but this measure had to be abandoned because it revealed to be non sustainable. Notes on 1937 already denounced the beneficence giving more money to cancer research to tuberculosis, as the last was considered a disease of the poor (Bryder 1988).

In 1912 it cost between 6,5 pences and 8 shillings depending on the tuberculin used (at that time, one pound was divided in 20 shillings, and each shilling into 12 pence), thus tuberculin was a cheap remedy (Riviere and Morland 1913). Receiving the treatment at non-charity sanatoria highly increased the cost of the remedy from a total of 2£ up to 32£ for the medical constant supervision, and other costs had to be added to this amount (the stay, food, etc) (Wilkinson 1909).

But the poor also had another problem: they couldn't lose their jobs, thus they didn't attend the charity sanatoria neither. With the aim of helping them considering this problem of them, Sir Robert Philip opened the Victoria Dispensary for Consumption and Diseases of the Chest in Edinburgh. Similar dispensaries appeared worldwide: in the period from 1912 and 1917 about 400 dispensaries existed in UK, 450 in America and 600 in Germany (Riviere 1926). Dispensaries were important not only because they permitted the patients to attend their jobs while being treated with tuberculin (Wilkinson 1909), but because the personnel teached the people to measure their temperature and basic guidelines on hygiene to improve their health status. Camac Wilkinson left a book devoted to these dispensaries, thoroughly describing his work at his Dispensary for the Poors in the Kennington Road of London. Besides administering tuberculin treatment and following-up the patients, the physicians in the dispensaries did screening and surveillance of contacts conducting epidemiological studies of undeniable value (Wilkinson 1909; Vilaplana and Cardona 2010). Tuberculin therapy continued to be used worldwide until the appearance of chemotherapy, when it was abandoned. Its efficacy being variable on the skills of each physician people feared the dangers of the reactions following its administration. However, a review of ancient documents provides an objective impression of the usefulness of the remedy: it was used for more than 50 years with more successes than failures, and thus even if it could be improved, it worked (Vilaplana and Cardona 2010).

The recent past years, research on tuberculosis has been focused on designing and developing new vaccines, mainly to be used prophylactically, but also therapeutic and to be given postexposure (Beresford and Sadoff 2010). The candidates are based on single antigens of Mycobacteria, obtained from cultures or by recombinant processes, or in whole organisms comminuted and/or sterilized, thus they call could be considered as tuberculins. Several candidates are in the pipeline for being used as immunotherapy, thus to be administered to a person once being exposed to the tubercle bacilli to prevent reactivation or progression to active tuberculosis, or to shorten or improve the response to chemotherapy (2009). Used as immunotherapy, all vaccines generate local reactions which intensity depends on the candidate (Johnson, Kamya et al. 2000; Sander, Pathan et al. 2009) (Vilaplana, Montané et al. 2010), and they could all be considered the local reactions described by Koch. No fatal reactions are encountered, but this could be due to the fact that nowadays infection can be easily discriminated from active disease by X ray assay, thus patients can be carefully selected, something non even envisageable at Koch's time. Moreover, nowadays we can follow-up the patients tightly, controlling general reactions and screening serious focal reactions with imaging. So should we fear that much Koch's reaction up to the point of avoiding using vaccines therapeutically? Probably not, especially if we do consider Wright's recommendation of sterilizing as much as possible the infectious foci before administering the vaccines (Wright 1904), something now possible with the help of chemotherapy, actually an advantage that some candidates have already used as a therapeutic strategy with success (Johnson, Kamya et al. 2000; Vilaplana, Montané et al. 2010).

5. References

(2009). TB Vaccines Pipeline, Stop TB Partnership Working Group on New TB Vaccines.

Anonymous (1891). "The value of Koch's tuberculin." JAMA XVI(19): 672-673.

Belmes, P. G. (1937). 1.500 casos de Tuberculosis tratados por la vacuna Friedmann. Buenos Aires, P.G. Belmes.

Beresford, B. and J. C. Sadoff (2010). "Update on research and development pipeline: tuberculosis vaccines." Clin Infect Dis 50 Suppl 3: S178-183.

Bryder, L. (1988). Below the magic mountain : a social history of tuberculosis in twentieth century Britain. Oxford, Clarendon.

Canetti, G. (1955). The tubercle bacillus in the pulmonary lesion of man. Histobacteriology and its bearing on the therapy of pulmonary tuberculosis. New York, Springer Publishing Company, Inc.

Cardona, P. (2007). "Robert Koch was right. Towards a new interpretation of tuberculin therapy." Enferm Infecc Microbiol Clin 24(6): 385-391.

Cope, Z. (1966). Almroth Wright: Founder of modern vaccine-therapy. London, Nelson.

Daniel, T. M. (1997). Captain of death : the story of tuberculosis. Rochester (New York), University of Rochester Press.

Gradmann, C. (2001). "Robert Koch and the pressures of scientific research: tuberculosis and tuberculin." Med Hist 45(1): 1-32.

Gunter, F. E. (1928). Tuberculin in practice. Its value in the treatment of early tuberculosis and asthma. London, The Gregg Publishing Company Ltd.

Johnson, J., R. Kamya, et al. (2000). "Randomized controlled trial of Mycobacterium vaccae immunotherapy in non-human immunodeficiency virus-infected ugandan adults with newly diagnosed pulmonary tuberculosis. The Uganda-Case Western Reserve University Research Collaboration." J Infect Dis 181(4): 1304-1312.

Koch, R. (1890). "A further communication on a remedy for tuberculosis." Br Med J 2: 1193-1199.

Morris, M. (1893). "The effects of Koch's tuberculin combined with surgical measures in the treatment of lupus." 1: 1154-1155.

Ogilvy, C. (1908). "A contribution to the study of tuberculin in orthopedic practice: the Calmette Ophtalmo-tuberculin test." J Bone Joint Surg Am(s2-6): 35-47.

Pottenger, F. M. (1913). Tuberculin in Diagnosis and Treatment. St. Louis, C. V. Mosby company.

Riviere, C. (1914). The early diagnosis of tubercle. London, Oxford Medical Publications.

Riviere, C. (1926). "A lecture on the principles of treatment of pulmonary tuberculosis." Br Med J 1(3409): 771-775.

Riviere, C. and E. Morland (1913). Tuberculin Treatment. London, Oxford Medical Publications.

Ross, G. (19--?). Study of Koch's treatment in Berlin. CIHM/ICMH Microfiche series. Montreal, Canadian Institute for Historical Microreproductions. 51097: 1 microfiche (9 frames).

Rothschild, M. (1921). "the treatment of tuberculosis with partigens (after much-deycke." Cal State J Med 19(6): 226-228.

Sahli, H. (1912). Sahli's Tuberculin Tratment. London, John Bale, Sons & Danielsson, Ltd.

Salvat-Papasseit, J. (2007). Poesia i Prosa. Obra completa.

Sander, C., A. Pathan, et al. (2009). "Safety and immunogenicity of a new tuberculosis vaccine, MVA85A, in Mycobacterium tuberculosis-infected individuals." Am J Respir Crit Care Med 179(8): 724-733.

Trudeau, E. L. (1907). Tuberculin Immunization in the treatment of pulmonary tuberculosis. New York, American Journal of the medical sciences.

Vilaplana, C. and P. J. Cardona (2010). "Tuberculin immunotherapy: its history and lessons to be learned." Microbes Infect 12(2): 99-105.

Vilaplana, C., E. Montané, et al. (2010). "Double-blind, randomized, placebo-controlled Phase I Clinical Trial of the therapeutical antituberculous vaccine RUTI." Vaccine 28(4): 1106-1116.

Wilkinson, W. C. (1909). The tuberculin dispensary for the poor. London, Nisbet & Co. Ltd.

Wright, A. E. (1902). "Notes on the treatment of furunculosis, sycosis and acne by the inoculation of a staphylococcus vaccine." Lancet 2: 874-884.

Wright, A. E. (1903). "A lecture on therapeutic inoculations of bacterial vaccines and their practical exploitation in the treatment of disease." Br Med J 1(2210): 1069-1074.

Wright, A. E. (1904). A lecture on the inoculation treatment of tuberculosis. London, The Medical Publishing Company, Limited.

Wright, A. E. and S. R. Douglas (1903-1904). An experimental investigation of the role of the blood fluids in connection with phagocytosis. Proceedings of the Royal Society of London, The Royal Society. 72: 357-370.

Wright, A. E. and S. Reid (1906). On spontaneous phagocytosis, and on the phagocytosis which is obtained with the heated serum of patients who have responded to tubercular infection, or, as the case may be, to the inoculation of a tubercle vaccine. Proceedings of the Royal Society of London. Series B, Containing Papers of a Biological Character, The Royal Society. 77: 211-225.

Wright, A. E. and S. Reid (1906). On the possibility of determining the presence or absence of tubercular infection by the examination of a patient's blood and tissue fluids. Proceedings of the Royal Society of London. Series B, Containing Papers of a Biological Character, Royal Society. 77: 194-211.

7

Therapy for Tuberculosis: *M. vaccae* Inclusion into Routine Treatment

Diana G. Dlugovitzky, Cynthia Stanford and John Stanford
Cátedra de Microbiologia, Virologia y Parasitologia, Facultad de Ciencias Medicas,
Universidad Nacional de Rosario, Santa Fe Rosario,
Centre for Infectious Diseases & International Health, Windeyer Institute of Medical
Sciences, University College London, London,
Argentina
UK

1. Introduction

Tuberculosis (TB) – an infectious airborne disease –is a re-emerging major global health problem. Each year, there are around nine million new cases of TB, and close to two million deaths among 14 million persons with active clinical disease. All countries are affected, but 85% of cases occur in Africa (30%) and Asia (55%), of which India and China alone represent 35% (World Health Organization, 2011).

Control and cure of tuberculosis has become a very serious problem in recent years because of its association with the Acquired Immune Deficiency Syndrome (AIDS) of the Human Immunodeficiency Virus (HIV) infection and its increasing resistance to generally used antituberculosis drugs (DOTS) (Ferreira Gonçalves, M. J.; Ponce de Leon, A. C. & Fernandez Penna, M. L., 2009).

The HIV epidemic has led to an increase in the incidence of tuberculosis globally, with an important increase in the mortality rate.

Despite this, TB is in most instances, a curable disease with 85% to 90% of people with newly diagnosed drug-susceptible TB cured in six months using combinations of first-line drugs (Nunn, P.; Williams, B.; Floyd, K.; Dye, C.; Elzinga, G. & Raviglione, M., 2005). Treatment of multidrug-resistant TB (MDR-TB), of which there are around 0.5 million cases each year, is more exigent and the use of newer therapies is required. Cure rates for MDR-TB are lower, typically ranging from around 50% to 70% (World Health Organization, 2011). Extensively drug-resistant TB has been reported in 45 countries, including countries with limited resources and a high TB burden (Mitnick, C. D.; Shin, S. S.; Seung, K. J.; et. al., 2008). When tuberculosis patients (TBP) are co-infected with HIV, have drug-resistant or relapsed TB, the commonly indicated drugs are less effectives. It takes between 12-24 months to cure such patients. In these cases second line drugs are required. This involves a significant increase in the cost of therapy, particularly important in poor countries (Arjanova, O. V.; Prihoda, N. D.; Yurchenko, L. V.; Sokolenko, N. I.; Frolov, V. M.; Tarakanovskaya, M. G.; Batdelger, D.; Jirathitikal, V. & Bourinbaiar, A. S., 2011).

Considerable labors are aimed at finding new drugs and vaccines against TB and several immune-based interventions have been proposed as adjunct immunotherapy to conventional treatment.

Thus, TB is considered a re-emerging global public disease, particularly in developing countries, where its incidence has reached alarming proportions. BCG, the only vaccine available for prevention in humans has been inefficient when tested in several field trials. It is therefore an urgent need for new vaccines against tuberculosis to be developed. A better understanding of the immune response induced during infection with *Mycobacyterium tuberculosis* (*M. tuberculosis, Mtb*) could help in a relatively short time to obtain the desired vaccine against this organism (García, M. A.; Sarmiento, M. E. & Acosta, A., 2009).

TB accounted for one in four deaths among HIV-positive people. Coinfection with HIV leads to difficulties in both the diagnosis and treatment of tuberculosis. Because of the poor performance of sputum smear microscopy in HIV-infected patients, more sensitive tests — such as liquid culture systems, nucleic acid amplification assays, and detection of mycobacterial products in various body fluids — are being investigated. The treatment of coinfected patients requires a combined therapy of antituberculosis and antiretroviral drugs administered concomitantly. Difficulties include pill burden and patient conformity, drug interactions, extending beyond the toxic effects, and immune reconstitution syndrome. Both multidrug-resistant and extensively drug-resistant tuberculosis can spread rapidly among an immunocompromised population, with resulting high mortality rates. Current guidelines recommend starting antiretroviral treatment within a few weeks of antituberculosis therapy for patients with CD4 cell counts <350 cells/μL. However, important problems concerning the drug regimens and timing of antiretroviral therapy still remain unresolved. Ongoing trials may answer many of these questions (Swaminathan. S.; Padmapriyadarsini, C. &, Narendran, G., 2010).

The risk of developing tuberculosis is estimated to be between 20-37 times greater in people living with HIV than among those without HIV infection. In 2009 there were 9.4 million new cases of TB, of which 1.2 (13%) million were among people living with HIV and of the 1.7 million people who died from TB 400,000 (24%) were living with HIV. With 13% of new TB cases and 24% of TB deaths being HIV associated, TB is a leading cause of morbidity and mortality among people living with HIV and as such TB remains a serious health risk for people living with HIV. The AIDS and Rights Alliance for Southern Africa (ARASA), in collaboration with WHO hosted a workshop to develop an advocacy toolkit on the *Three I's for HIV/TB* based on WHO policy for healthcare workers, HIV/TB advocates (World Health Orgamization, 2011). Several factors including previous therapeutic failure, duration of antiretroviral therapy, low CD4+ T-cell count at the initiation of HAART, severe manifestations of disease, low adherence to HAART, and previous treatment interruption are contributory of defective immune reconstitution. It was not definitively demonstrated that age, viral strain/clade, or host genetic factors play a role in these different responses to HAART (Aiuti, F. & Mezzaroma, I., 2006).

The roles of different T-cell subsets which participate in the protector mechanisms against *M. tuberculosis*, thymic function, and cytokines involved in immune response against the bacilli have been investigated. The increased T-cell activation or apoptosis has been associated with a deficiency of effective immunologic response. The continuous virologic replication in lymphoid tissues, regardless of the undetectable plasma viral load, has been proposed as the fundamental mechanism of cellular activation. This incoherent response probably can be associated with other procedures. Insufficient CD4+ T-cell repopulation of lymphoid tissues may be due to a thymus failure or a defect in bone marrow function. Permanent infection, the toxic effect of antiviral drugs on T- and B-cell precursors, the severity of disease, and the low number of CD4+ T-cells before HAART could also prime for thymus exhaustion and deficient T-cell renewal. Finally, an imbalance in the production of cytokines such as TNF-α, IL-2 and IL-7 may also be crucial for the induction of immune system failure. In patients in which CD4+ T-cells are not increased by HAART, therapeutic tactics aimed at increasing these cells and reducing the risk of infections are needed. IL-2 and/or other cytokines may be of benefit in this scene. Some antiviral drugs may be better than others in immunologic reconstitution. Protease inhibitors may have additional, independent positive effects on the immune system.

There may be little justification for using immunosuppressive agents such as cyclosporine or hydroxyurea in this subgroup of immunologic non responder patients, as these molecules may increase T-cell decline and/or favor susceptibility to infections

Different mechanisms are involved in the control of the tuberculosis dissemination such as granuloma.

Granulomas, the hallmark of the host response to mycobacterial infection, represent a strategy to physically contain infections that cannot otherwise be eradicated by host defenses. The successive recruitment of cells to the site of *M. tuberculosis* infection forms a physical barrier to mycobacterial propagation and creates a hostile microenvironment in which oxygen tension, pH, and micronutrient supply may all be reduced. In this environment, mycobacteria go through profound alterations in metabolism, biosynthesis, and replication.

This adaptation creates the basis of clinical latency in tuberculosis. Although these sequestered, semidormant bacilli have been much investigated, their paucity makes direct studies *in vivo* problematic, and multiple researches on this question have been performed such as *in vitro* oxygen deprivation or intracellular growth in macrophages (Wallis, R. S., 2005).

M. tuberculosis is an atypical member of its genus (Stanford, J. L.; Bahr, G. M.; Rook, G. A. W.; Shaaban, M. A.; Chugh, T.D.; Gabriel, M.; Al-Shimali, B.; Siddiqui, Z.; Ghardanis, F.; Shahin, A. & Behbehani, K., 1990). Apparently the capacity of *M. tuberculosis* to cause illness is due not only to the severity of the damage it causes to the host tissue but also to its aptitude to alter the immune response, to one that is inappropriate. It is evident that new alternative and improved treatment options are needed. In consequence, more efficient resources were considered crucial to improve the employed chemotherapy. Significant efforts have been directed at finding new drugs and vaccines against TB. (Small, P. M., 2009). Thus, the immunomodulatory effects of a heat killed *Mycobacterium vaccae* (*M. vaccae, Mv*) preparation have been investigated by Stanford, J. et. al. during the 1970´s.

It has been stated that the variation of disease expressions and severity was entirely inherent in the host and his surroundings, disease depending on human genetic control of the immunological response in interaction with environmental factors rather than to bacterial features. In the environment a free-living mycobacterium, the potentially beneficial *M. vaccae* was recognized as an important source for influencing the human immune response (Stanford, J.L. & Paul, R. C., 1973; Stanford, J. L. & Rook, G. A.W., 1983).

Several studies using an optional new therapy, which involved the addition of a preparation of inactivated *M. vaccae*, were carried out over the last twenty-five years with successful results. In those investigations it has been shown that the killed bacterium or its components are enhancers of the immune responses in opposition to different infectious agents. A number of pre-clinical studies of tuberculosis, bronchospasm, *Trypanosoma cruzi* infection, Leishmaniasis, autoimmune conditions and cancer have been also carried out in mice, demonstrating protection induced by this treatment. (Hernandez-Pando, R.; Pavon, L.; Arriaga, K.; Orozco, H.; Madrid-Marina, V. & Rook, G., 1997; Zuany-Amorim, C.; Sawicka, E.; Manlius, C.; Le Moine, A.; Brunet, L. R.; Kemeny, D. M.; Bowen, G.; Rook, G. & Walker, C., 2002; Valian, H. K.; Kenedy, L.K.A.; Rostami, M.N.; Mohammadi, A. M. & Khamesipour, A., 2008).

Some promising results have been reported of its immune stimulative action against *M. tuberculosis* infection, tumors such as melanoma and adenocarcinoma, and pollen-induced asthma (Hopkin, J.M.; Shaldon, S.; Ferry, B.; Coull, P. P. A.; Enomoto, T.; Yamashita, T.; Kurimoto, F.; Stanford, J.; Shirakawa, T. & Rook, G. A. W., 1998; Maraveyas, A.; Baban, B.; Kennard, D.; Rook, G. A.; Westby, M.; Grange, J. M.; Lydyard, P.; Stanford, J. L.; Jones, M.; Selby, P. & Dalgleish, A. G., 1999; Stanford, J. L.; Stanford, C. A.; O'Brien, M.; Grange, J. M., 2008; Hrouda, D.; Souberbielle, B. E.; Kayaga, J.; Corbishley, C. M.; Kirby, R. S. & Dalgleish, G., 1998).

2. Clinical trials of adjunctive immunotherapy

The concept of immunotherapy in tuberculosis is not new and many immune based interventions have been investigated as adjuncts to convenional chemotherapy. It is evident that the modulation of immune reactivity can be of great therapeutic value.

IFN-γ: As IFN-γ is central to antimycobacterial host defenses; it has been used in several clinical trials of adjunctive immunotherapy. In mice, IFN-γ enhances the mycobactericidal capacity of macrophages by increasing the production of reactive nitrogen intermediates, such as nitric oxide. Condos et al. reported in 1997 the first study of therapeutic IFN-γ in patients with tuberculosis without evident defects on IFN-γ production or responsiveness. In this investigation 500 μg of IFN-γ was administered 3 times per week by aerosol to 5 patients with MDR tuberculosis together with their previous therapy. The study found that sputum smear results became negative and the number of colony-forming units (CFU) tended to fall. Three similar successive studies performed by other investigators showed that differed in IFN-γ type, dose, and route of administration were not successful in inducing any hopeful results. The only randomized, placebo-controlled, multicenter trial of inhaled adjunctive IFN-γ for MDR tuberculosis was done by InterMune in 2000, and the trial was stopped because of a lack of efficacy and the data obtained have never been published. Subsequent investigations have indicated that IFN-γ–induced genes, such as *IP-10* and *iNOS*, are already upregulated in the lung in patients with tuberculosis and that therapeutic aerosol IFN-γ has a relatively minor additional effect. These findings indicate that the fairly small mycobactericidal capacity of lung macrophages cannot effectively be increased by therapeutic IFN-γ (Wallis, R. S., 2005).

IL-2 Considering that IL-2 is able to induce T cell replication and is essential for cellular immune function and granuloma formation, a small, unblinded study of 2 low-dose IL-2 regimens (daily or in 5-day "pulses") in patients with MDR tuberculosis demonstrated that the daily treatment produce a decrease of sputum counts of acid-fast bacilli (Johnson, B. J.; Bekker, L. G.; Rickman, R.; Brown, S.; Lesser, M.; Ress, S.; Willcox, P.; Steyn, L. & Kaplan, G., 1997; Wallis, R. S., 2005).

Taking into account this observation, a randomized, double-blind, placebo-controlled study of the effect of IL-2 on conversion of sputum culture was conducted by the Case Western Reserve University Tuberculosis Research Unit (Cleveland, OH) with 110 Ugandan, HIV-uninfected patients with drug-susceptible tuberculosis (Johnson, J. L.; Ssekasanvu, E.; Okwera, A.; Mayanja, H.; Hirsch, C. S.; Nakibali, J. G.; Drzayich Jankus, D.; Eisenach, K. D.; Boom, W. H.; Ellner, J. J. & Mugerwa, R. D., 2003; Wallis, R. S., 2005).

IL-2 or placebo was administered twice daily for the first month of standard therapy. Contrary to expectations, the study found significant delays in clearance of viable *M. tuberculosis* CFU and conversion of sputum culture results in the IL-2 treatment arm. This report suggested a possible antagonism during combined chemotherapy and immunotherapy for tuberculosis.

TNF-α: TNF-α, like IFN-γ, is crucial for host defenses against tuberculosis. TNF-α is a potent proinflammatory cytokine, expressed by macrophages and T cells, (Wallis, R.S.; Amir Tahmasseb, M. & Ellner, J. J., 1990; Black, R. A.; Rauch, C.T.; Kozlosky, C.J.; Peschon, J. J.; Slack, J. L.; Wolfson, M. F.; Castner, B.J.; Stocking, K. L.; Reddy, P.; Srinivasan, S.; Nelson, N.; Boiani, N.; Schooley, K. A.; Gerhart, M.; Davis, R.; Fitzner, J. N.; Johnson, R. S.; Paxton, R. J.; March, C. J. & Cerretti, D. P., 1997; Wallis, R. S., 2005). TNF-α stimulates the release of inflammatory cytokines, endothelial adhesion molecules, and chemokines, and is considered essential for the formation and conservation of granulomas.

Monocytes express TNF-α after phagocytosis of mycobacteria or after stimulation by mycobacterial proteins or glycolipids (Wallis, R.S.; Amir Tahmasseb, M. & Ellner, J. J., 1990; Wallis, R. S.; Paranjape, R. & Phillips, M., 1993; Valone, S.E.; Rich, E. A.; Wallis, R. S. & Ellner, J. J., 1988; Barnes, P. F.; Chatterjee, D.; Abrams, J. S.; Lu, S.; Wang, E.; Yamamura, M.; Brennan, P. J. & Modlin, R. L., 1992; Wallis, R. S., 2005). TNF-α is produced at the site of disease in patients with newly diagnosed tuberculosis (Ribeiro-Rodrigues, R.; Resende Co, T.; Johnson, J. L.; Ribeiro, F.; Palaci, M.; Sá, R. T.; Maciel, E. L.; Pereira Lima, F. E.; Dettoni, V.; Toossi, Z.; Boom, W. H.; Dietze, R.; Ellner, J. J. & Hirsch, C. S., 2002; Barnes, P. F.; Fong, S. J.; Brennan, P. J.; Twomey, P. E.; Mazumder, A. & Modlin, R. L., 1990; Bekker, L. G.; Maartens, G.; Steyn, L. & Kaplan, G., 1998; Wallis, R. S., 2005). It have been shown a small increase of TNF-α level occurs after initiation of antituberculosis therapy (Bekker, L. G.; Maartens, G.; Steyn, L. & Kaplan, G., 1998; Wallis, R. S., 2005), possibly attributed to microbial constituents that stimulate TNF-α production (Wallis, R. S.; Perkins, M.; Phillips, M.; Joloba, M.; Demchuk, B.; Namale, A.; Johnson, J. L.; Williams, D.; Wolski, K.; Teixeira, L.; Dietze, R.; Mugerwa, R. D.; Eisenach, K. & Ellner, J. J., 1998; Wallis, R. S.; Phillips, M.; Johnson, J. L.; Teixeira, L.; Rocha, L. M.; Maciel, E.; Rose, L.; Wells, C.; Palaci, M.; Dietze, R.; Eisenach, K. & Ellner, J. J., 2001; Aung, H.; Toossi, Z.; Wisnieski, J. J.; Wallis, R. S.; Culp, L.

A.; Phillips, N. B.; Phillips, M.; Averill, L. E.; Daniel, T. M. & Ellner, J. J., 1996; Wallis, R. S., 2005). Levels subsequently decrease as the bacillary burden is diminished by treatment (Ribeiro-Rodrigues, R.; Resende Co, T.; Johnson, J. L.; Ribeiro, F.; Palaci, M.; Sá, R. T.; Maciel, E. L.; Pereira Lima, F. E.; Dettoni, V.; Toossi, Z.; Boom, W. H.; Dietze, R.; Ellner, J. J. & Hirsch, C. S., 2002; Wallis, R. S., 2005). It was shown in experimental animals that neutralization of TNF-α interferes with the early recruitment of inflammatory cells to the site of *M. tuberculosis* infection and inhibits granulomas formation (Kindler, V.; Sappino, A. P.; Grau, G. E.; Piguet, P. F. & Vassalli, P., 1989; Algood, H. M.; Lin, P. L.; Yankura, D.; Jones, A.; Chan, J. & Flynn, J. L., 2004; Wallis, R. S., 2005), and TNF-α blockade also reduces the microbicidal activity of macrophages and natural killer (NK) cells (Roach, D. R.; Bean, A. G.; Demangel, C.; France, M. P.; Briscoe, H. & Britton, W. J., 2002; Hirsch, C. S.; Ellner, J. J., Russell, D. G. & Rich, E. A., 1994; Wallis, R. S., 2005).

The effects of potent immunosuppressive and/or anti-TNF-α therapies on microbiologic outcomes in tuberculosis have been investigated in two controlled clinical trials. Both were conducted with HIV-1–infected patients who had relatively well -preserved tuberculosis immune responses (based on the presence of high CD4 cell sum and cavitary lung disease). The studies shared a single placebo control arm (for tuberculosis therapy only). Their major aim was to examine the role of TNF-α in the HIV disease progression due to tuberculosis; as such, their main end points were CD4 cell count and plasma HIV RNA load. Nevertheless, both studies prospectively accrue clinical and microbiologic data as indicators of safety.

High-dose methylprednisolone: In a comparative study was reported (Mayanja-Kizza, H.; Jones-Lopez, E.; Okwera, A.; Wallis, R. S.; Ellner, J. J.; Mugerwa, R. D.; Whalen, C. C. & Uganda-Case Western Research Collaboration, 2005; Wallis, R. S., 2005) in which 189 subjects received either prednisolone (2.75 mg/kg/day) or placebo during the first month of conventional anti-TB therapy. The prednisolone dosage was selected on the basis of a phase I study indicating that it reduced the rate of tuberculosis-stimulated TNF-α production *ex vivo* by one-half. During the second month, the daily dose was reduced to 0 mg/kg; the average subject received a cumulative dose of 16500 mg. Though there is extensive experience with the use of corticosteroids to diminish tuberculosis symptoms, no previous studies have examined the microbiologic effects of doses of this magnitude. Unexpectedly, one-half of prednisolone-treated subjects had conversion of sputum culture results to negative after 1 month of treatment, compared with 10% of subjects in the placebo arm (*P*<0.001). This effect was bigger than that observed in the landmark study in which the addition of rifampin to a 6-month regimen of streptomycin and isoniazid reduced the relapse rate from 29% to 2% and increased the 2-month sputum culture conversion rate from 49% to 69% (East African-British Medical Research Councils, 1974; Wallis, R. S., 2005). The effect of prednisolone therapy was not due to reduced sputum production, which decreased similarly during treatment in both study arms. There were no serious opportunistic infections. However, prednisolone-treated subjects were more likely to experience other early serious adverse events, including edema, hyperglycemia, electrolyte disturbances, and severe hypertension.

Two other prospective, randomized trials of adjunctive corticosteroids administered at lower doses have observed similar, albeit smaller, effects on the kinetics of conversion of sputum culture results (Bilaceroglu, S.; Perim, K.; Buyuksirin, M. & Celikten, E., 1999; Wallis, Horne, N.W., 1960; R. S., 2005), but a third trial found no effect (Tripathy, S.P.;

Ramakrishnan, C.V.; Nazareth, O.; Parthasarathy, R.; Santha Devi, T.; Arumainayagam, D.C.; Balasubramaniam, R.; Rathasabapathy, S.V. & Manjula Datta, S., 1983; Wallis, R. S., 2005).

There have been no reports of deleterious effects of corticosteroids on microbiologic outcomes in patients withTB.

Early studies of immunotherapy for TB were those of Robert Koch who used injections of "old tuberculin" during the last 10 years of the 19th century (Koch, R., (a) 1890; Koch, R., (b) 1890).

In the early 20th century, Charles Stevens developed "Stevens cure" based on a root called Umckaloabo from South Africa (Sechehaye, A., 1920), recently shown to have potent anti-mycobacterial activity (Seidel, V. & Taylor, P. W., 2004; Kim, C. E.; Griffiths, W. J. & Taylor, P. W., 2009) and particularly to act as a TNF-α antagonist. In 1904 Friedrich Friedmann developed a turtle tubercle suspension of live *Mycobacterium chelonae*, which he later called "Anningzochin" which was available until recently from Laves-Arzneimittel GmbH, Barbarastr. 14, A-30952, Ronnenberg, Germany (Friedmann, F., 1904; Hart, C. A.; Beeching, N. J. & Duerden, B. I., 1996; Rosenau, M. J.& Anderson, J., 1915). Although Friedman investigated this mycobacterium species and showed that it was able of confer immunity against tuberculosis, he never considered that it might cause a limited tuberculous process. In the 1920s and 30s, Henry Spahlinger developed a serum from horses immunized with various extracts of tubercle bacilli (Spahlinger, H.; Macassey, L. & Saleeby, C. W., 1934). Even though many investigations supported the success of these different preparations in the treatment of tuberculosis, until very recently immunotherapy has not contributed significantly to its treatment (Sechehaye, A., 1920).

2.1 Immunomodulatory therapy in tuberculosis

Two problems confronted the early attempts of immunotherapy for tuberculosis. First, in the absence of drugs, the immunotherapy was directed towards the total destruction of the tubercle bacillus in the host. Secondly it was then thought that the triggering of immune reactivity in tuberculosis was synonymous with protection. The concept of immune reactivity in mycobacterial infections embraces both protective immunity and also tissue destruction. Distinguishing between them has been a controversial topic for many years (Stanford, J. L. & Rook, G. A.W., 1983). During the last decades it was resolved by the demonstration of two functional subpopulations of helper T cells - TH1 and TH2 (Flynn, J. L. & Ernst, J. D., 2000).

Immunotherapy, is directed to replace an inadequate immune reaction by an appropriate one. The keys to reaching success for immunotherapy arise from the evidence of the considerable variation in the efficacy of vaccination with BCG from one country to another. This is due to prior contact with environmental mycobacteria, which, depending on species, could provide some degree of protection or the antagonistic reaction of tissue necrosis.

Although the search for new vaccines and immunotherapies should continue, investigation of those already available to us is important and is the purpose of our investigations.

For many years it has been accepted that variation in clinical presentation and severity entirely rested in the host and his environment, disease depending on an interaction between human genetic control of the immunological response influenced by environmental factors. In the environment are the free-living mycobacteria and it was from amongst them that the potentially beneficial *M. vaccae* and the deleterious *M. scrofulaceum* were identified as important factors influencing the human immune response (Stanford, J. L. & Paul, R. C., 1973; Stanford, J. L. & Rook, G. A.W., 1983). It is now established that genetic diversity within *Mtb,* expressing significant phenotypic differences between clinical isolates, may also be important (Flynn, J. L. & Ernst, J. D., 2000).

BCG is commonly referred to as a vaccine but its effects are very different from those of other vaccines and it is better designated as an immune modulator influencing susceptibility to leprosy (Truoc, L. V.; Ly, H. M.; Thuy, N. K.; Trach, D. D.; Stanford, C. A. & Stanford, J. L., 2001) and malignant melanoma (Grange, J. M.; Stanford, J. L.; Stanford, C. A. & Kölmel, K. F., 2003) as well as tuberculosis. Indeed the concept of a vaccine in its commonly used sense against tuberculosis is a difficult one as illustrated by the difficulty in interpreting the Tuberculin test. A positive Tuberculin test can signify protection, susceptibility and the presence of disease (Stanford, J. L. & Lemma, E., 1983), thus attempting to vaccinate using the species-specific, group iv antigens of *Mtb* (Stanford, J.; Stanford, C.; Stansby, G.; Bottasso, O.; Bahr, G. & Grange, J., 2009) is unlikely to be successful.

3. Immunotherapy with *Mycobacterium vaccae* in the treatment of respiratory disease

3.1 *Mycobacterium vaccae* - a part of our environment

The idea of using a saprophytic mycobacterium that causes no harm, has few side effects and is unable to induce adverse reactions in patients, as a potential immunotherapeutic or vaccine has only been considered during the last few years. *Mycobacterium vaccae* (NCTC 11,659), is a rapidly growing scotocromogenic organism.

First isolated in Germany from the surroundings of cattle, the potential and the importance of the species was first appreciated from field studies in Uganda. A killed suspension of this strain was first added to BCG and investigated as a combined vaccine. Later it was recognized as an immunotherapeutic agent. Immunotherapy with *M. vaccae* improves immune recognition of common mycobacterial antigens and also regulates immune reactions away from necrotic processes. The re-introduction of cellular responsivness to common mycobacterial antigens indicates that *M. vaccae* should induce protective immunity and suppress antagonostic responses. Looked at in the opposite way, failure to make a response to common mycobacterial antigens is an attribute of diseases that should be responsive to treatment with heat-killed *M. vaccae.*

3.2 *M. vaccae,* its adjuvants

The cell walls of all mycobacteria possess potent adjuvant activity attributed to structural lipids and glyco-lipids.

The actions of these adjuvants vary between species. Thus BCG and most species of mycobacteria enhance the type of immune response for which the recipient is already primed, whereas *M. vaccae* and probably a small number of other Actinomycetales enhance the most beneficial cellular immune responses.

3.3 *M. vaccae*, its antigens

M. vaccae possesses the group i antigens shared by all mycobacteria and most other aerobic genera of the Actinomycetales.

Some of these antigens are partially cross-reactive with those expressed by mitochondria, when stressed, in animal tissues.

M. vaccae lacks the groups ii and iii antigens, and the group iv antigens of pathogenic mycobacterial species.

All the information obtained from several studies performed in countries around the world, from minor investigations to those made using a placebo control and a properly randomized trial, show that increased cure rates in newly diagnosed TB patients receiving *M. vaccae* is only associated with minimal side effects. Studies of immunotherapy with *M. vaccae* in drug-resitant, relapsed and chronic TB Patients have shown that it is also favorable under these conditions. The effects are more readily seen when specific chemotherapy is difficult to establish or ineffective because of low patient compliance, or resistance to multiple drugs.

Progress was suggested from the early work with irradiation-killed organisms in leprosy to the study in London of modulation of tuberculin skin-test responses, and the first comparative trials in The Gambia and Kuwait. In these successive investigations the dose of 10^9 heat-killed organisms, equivalent to 1 mg wet-weight of bacilli, has been used as a standard dose. A series of small trials in Argentina, India, Nigeria, Romania, South Africa, Uganda and Vietnam have shown that the method can be effective across wide-ranging geographic variability, with South Africa as the only country where almost no effects were recorded (Dlugovitzky, D.; Stanford, C. & Stanford, J., 2011).

Despite this wide geographical efficacy, it is likely that the schedule of treatment with *M. vaccae* should change with different environments. Thus single doses were effective in the Gambia, Nigeria, Kuwait, Romania and the UK, but further South in Africa the environment may necessitate multiple doses, just as some diseases such as cancer require repeated doses to overcome the drive towards Th2 exerted by the tumour.

Numerous studies have shown that certain patterns of cellular immunity are associated with active disease and others are associated with health and recovery from disease. Modulating the immune response from the one to the other is now possible with *M. vaccae* and this chapter records its successful achievement (Ottenhoff, T.H.; Verreck, F. A. & Lichtenauer-Kaligis, E. G., 2002; Dlugovitzky, D.; Torres-Morales, A.; Rateni, L.; Farroni, M.A.; Largacha, C.; Molteni, O. & Bottasso, O.A., 1997).

3.4 Our initial studies on immune response against *M. tuberculosis*

The purpose of the early series of studies that we have carried out to investigate the immune response of patients with pulmonary tuberculosis has been to make steps towards immunotherapy as an effective addition to standard short-course chemotherapy and to identify proper *in vitro* alternative markers of successful treatment for its evaluation. A good deal of the immunological work on TB has been done on murine models – animals that have short lives and do not normally suffer from this disease. And in consequence we wanted to make use of appropriate methods for and related to human patients.

Initial studies in our laboratory in Rosario, Argentina, have shown that the changes in cellular immune response in pulmonary tuberculosis patients are related to the severity of disease and to the administration of tuberculosis chemotherapy. We showed that increased levels of IL-8 in the pleural exudates of patients with pulmonary tuberculosis, in comparison with those patients with pneumonia-associated pleural effusions, was associated with different levels of expression of CD3, CD4, CD19, CD25 and CD68 markers on their cells (Dlugovitzky, D.; Rateni, L.; Torres-Morales, A.; Ruiz-Silva, J.; Piñesky, R.; Canosa, B.; Molteni, O. & Bottasso, O., 1997; Caruso, A. M.; Serbina, N.; Klein, E.; Triebold, K.; Bloom, B. R. & Flynn, J. L., 1999). This data suggested that increased IL-8 levels in pleural effusions plays a key role in initiation and maintenance of inflammatory reactions.

Patients with moderate to severe pulmonary tuberculosis showed a marked and significant decrease in their circulating levels of cells bearing these phenotypes when compared with those of healthy persons, with patients with pneumonia-associated pleural effusions or with patients with mild pulmonary tuberculosis. Differences between the levels of these cell markers on pleural and peripheral T-cells from pulmonary tuberculosis patients may be the consequence of an incursion of T-lymphocytes from the circulatory system to the pleural cavity, probably linked to the presence of chemokines within the pleural fluid including IL-8 (Fulton, S.A.; Reba, S. M.; Martin, T.D. & Boom, W. H., 2002).

In other assays in pulmonary tuberculosis, circulating immune complexes and the main peripheral blood T-cell subsets were evaluated (Dlugovitzky, D.; Luchesi, S.; Torres-Morales, A.; Ruiz-Silva, J.; Canosa, B.; Valentini, E. & Bottasso, O., 1995). This showed that immune complex levels in cases with severe disease are significantly higher, and expression of CD4 on T lymphocytes significantly lower than in cases of mild disease (Fiorenza, G.; Farroni, M. A.; Bogué, C.; Selenscig, D.; Martinel Lamas, D. & Dlugovitzky, D., 2007). Diverse studies of our group helped to explain the effective cellular immune response detected in less severe tuberculosis cases and simultaneously, the impaired cell-mediated immune response in severe cases. Several immune mechanisms within cell-mediated immunity generate a multifaceted response involving activated macrophages, T cells, and cytokines directed to manage mycobacterial infection. Other cell populations also take part in the immune response against mycobacteria and may be important in the development of the disease (Dlugovitzky, D.; Torres-Morales, A.; Rateni, L.; Farroni, M.A.; Largacha, C.; Molteni, O. & Bottasso, O.A., 1997; Dlugovitzky, D.; Bay, M. L.; Rateni, L.; Urízar, L.; Rondelli, C. F.; Largacha, C.; Farroni, M. A.; Molteni, O. & Bottasso, O. A., 1999; Dlugovitzky, D.; Bay, M. L.; Rateni, L.; Fiorenza, G.; Vietti, L.; Farroni, M. A. ; Bottasso, O. A., 2000).

Polymorphonuclear neutrophils (PMN) are the professional phagocytes first at the site of bacterial invasion and are able to play a protective role in opposition to M. tuberculosis in the early phase of infection controlled by T lymphocytes. Although recruitment of neutrophils to bronchoalveolar spaces has been described during active human tuberculosis and associated with local chemokine expression, it has not been clarified whether neutrophils have direct bactericidal or immunologic functions. In vitro studies suggest that human neutrophils are mycobacteriocidal and are activated by soluble mycobacterial antigens (Fiorenza, G.; Bottasso, O. A.; Rateni, L.; Farroni, M. A. & Dlugovitzky, D., 2003).

Several mechanisms including phagocytosis of bacteria and the subsequent generation of reactive oxygen intermediates during oxidative bursts are considered important instruments for destruction of mycobacteria (Jones, G. S.; Amirault, H. J. & Andersen, B. R., 1990). Several findings demonstrated a significant alteration in PMN functions in pulmonary tuberculosis. Production of reactive oxygen intermediates was reduced in severe disease and was significantly increased by antituberculosis chemotherapy (Denis, M. J., 1991). Recognition of Mtb by phagocytic cells leads to cell activation and production of cytokines, which in itself leads to further activation and cytokine production in a complex process of regulation and cross-regulation (Denis, M. J., 1991). Thus phagocytic cells are thought to contribute to the control of infection through the production of chemokines (Appelberg, R.; Castro, A. G.; Gomes, S.; Pedrosa, J. & Silva, M. T., 1995), the induction of granuloma formation (Riedel, D. D. & Kaufmann, S. H., 1997) and the transference of their own microbicidal molecules to infected macrophages (Ehlers, S., 2003). Levels of circulating cytokines correlate significantly with the severity of the disease, antibody concentration and the reduction of Th1 activities. We evaluated plasma cytokines of type-1 and type-2 in relation to humoral and cell-mediated responses in patients with different amounts of lung damage and with different clinical symptoms of tuberculosis. We found that patients with pulmonary tuberculosis of different levels of severity have higher serum levels of IFN-γ, IL-2, IL-4 and IL-10 when compared with those of healthy controls. Mean titers of IFN-γ, and IL-2, in mild and moderate patients were found to be greater than in those with severe disease, whereas moderate and advanced patients showed higher levels of IL-4 in comparison with mild cases. Raised levels of interleukin-10 were more prevalent in advanced disease, and statistically different from those in patients with mild disease. This cytokine pattern would explain the effective cellular immune responses found in patients with less severe tuberculosis in comparison with those of patients with advanced disease in whom cellular immunity is seriously damaged (Dlugovitzky, D.; Luchesi, S.; Torres-Morales, A.; Ruiz-Silva, J.; Canosa, B.; Valentini, E. & Bottasso, O., 1995).

We investigated the relationship between the competence of lymphocytes to proliferate and induce cytokine synthesis in vitro, in response to stimulation with antigens, and the amount of pulmonary involvement in tuberculosis patients. Higher levels of IFN-γ compared with IL-4 in culture supernatants of Peripheral Blood Monuclear Cells (PBMC) stimulated with Mtb antigens were observed in patients with mild tuberculosis (Bay, M. L.; Dlugovitzky, D.; Urízar, L., 1997). To amplify these results we assessed in vitro the synthesis of the cytokines - transforming growth factor beta (TGF-β) and IL-1β. Reduced concentrations of IFN-γ and IL-4 and an increased synthesis of TGF-β were observed in patients with moderate tuberculosis in comparison with those with mild disease.

In patients with severe disease, PBMC synthesize the highest levels of IL-4 and TGF-β, with low levels of IFN-γ synthesis, suggesting that in these cases an expressed Th2-type response suppresses the Th1 reaction in vitro (Dlugovitzky, D.; Bay, M. L.; Rateni, L.; Urízar, L.; Rondelli, C. F.; Largacha, C.; Farroni, M. A.; Molteni, O. & Bottasso, O. A., 1999).

Rook et al confirmed this type of response and demonstrated strong links between IL-4 and TGF-β. In their studies PBMC from patients with the most advanced TB showed the highest release of both IL-4 and TGF-β (Rook, G. A. W.; Lowrie, D. B. & Hernandez-Pando, R., 2007; Hernández-Pando, R.; Aguilar, D.; Orozco, H.; Cortez, Y.; Brunet, L. R. & Rook, G. A., 2008).

The immune system generally responds in a regulated way to microbes and eliminates them, but it does not respond to self-antigens unless regulatory mechanisms are impaired and unresponsiveness or tolerance to self-antigens is not maintained (Van Parijs, L. & Abbas, A. K., 1998). Such a disharmonic immune response may result in several autoimmune diseases. The altered Th1 and Th2 expression found in severe tuberculosis patients may lay them open to such diseases. To investigate this we inquired into the incidence of arthritic manifestations (Poncet's disease) in such patients. The kinds and distribution of T cell subsets in these cases and the presence of several auto-antibodies were also investigated. In the detected arthritic cases an augmented number of CD4+ Tcells was observed in comparison with CD8+ T cells and autoantibodies were detected. However, we could not rule out the presence of unknown factors that might be partly responsible for the reactive arthritis. (Dlugovitzky, D.; Torres, A.; Hourquescos, M. C.; Svetaz, M. J.; Quagliato, N.; Valentini, E.; Amigot, B.; Molteni, O. & Bottasso, O., 1995; Kroot, E. J.; Hazes, J. M.; Colin, E. M. & Dolhain, R. J., 2006)

In addition to these results it has been demonstrated that CD8+ cells also synthesize IL-4, and this cytokine profile correlates with cavitation (van Crevel, R.; Karyadi, E.; Preyers, F.; Leenders, M.; Kullberg, B. J.; Nelwan, R. H. & van der Meer, J. W., 2000).

Several studies have established that continuous IL-12 production is necessary for maintenance of the pulmonary Th1 cells required for host control of persistent *Mtb* infection and suggest that breakdown of this mechanism could be a contributing factor in the reactivation of disease (Feng, C. G.; Jankovic, D.; Kullberg, M.; Cheever, A.; Scanga, C. A.; Hieny, S.; Caspar, P.; Yap, G. S. & Sher, A., 2005).

The capacity of IL-12 to induce the differentiation of naive CD4+ T cells into Th1 cells and stimulate production of IFN-γ was investigated by studying the capacity of PBMNC from patients with different severities of tuberculosis to produce IFN-γ, IL-4 and IL-12. The production of IFN-γ is increased in patients with less severe tuberculosis rather than in those with severe disease (Dlugovitzky, D.; Bay, M. L.; Rateni, L.; Fiorenza, G.; Vietti, L.; Farroni, M. A. & Bottasso, O. A., 2000). In this study we also demonstrated that Tumour Necrosis Factor-alpha (TNF-α) production is increased in moderate and advanced tuberculosis patients and nitrite levels are augmented in severe tuberculosis cases, significantly different from those of healthy controls (Feng, C. G.; Jankovic, D.; Kullberg, M.; Cheever, A.; Scanga, C. A.; Hieny, S.; Caspar, P.; Yap, G. S. & Sher, A., 2005; Trinchieri, G., 2003; Casanova, J. L. & Abel, L., 2002; Fieschi, C. & Casanova, J. L., 2003). Several mycobactericidal and immunoregulatory mechanisms are developed by host cells including the production of NO and inflammatory cytokines, through extra- and intra-cellular mediated cytotoxicity, or cytostatic activity, which restrain a variety of pathogens including *Mtb* (Vouldoukis, I.; Riveros-Moreno, V.; Dugas, B.; Ouaaz, F.; Bécherel, P.; Debré, P.; Moncada, S. & Mossalayi, M. D., 1995; Kitabatake, A; Sakuma, I., 1999).

Our results suggest that the synthesis of nitric oxide by the host is not always associated with a favourable evolution since higher levels are synthesized in cases with severe tuberculosis. Other authors propose that this event may be related to the interaction of several cytokines and/or eicosanoids through disease related induction of immune reactions (Tunçtan, B.; Okur, H.; Calişir, C. H.; Abacioğlu, H.; Cakici, I.; Kanzik, I. & Abacioğlu, N., 1998). It has also been shown that an inverse correlation exists between TNF-α, TGF-β and NO concentrations in serum, behavior that could be a predominantly TGF-β effect (Fiorenza, G.; Rateni, L.; Farroni, M A.; Bogué, C. & Dlugovitzky, D. G., 2005).

The production of NO, TNF-α and IL-12 by the peripheral blood monocytes of patients suffering from MDR-TB has been investigated by others and NO production was found to be significantly depressed. A sub-cellular fraction of *Mtb* whole cell lysate, culture filtrate protein or lipoarabinomannan induced higher concentrations of NO to be released by peripheral blood monocytes from newly diagnosed tuberculosis patients in comparison with those from MDR-TB patients (Sharma, S.; Sharma, M.; Roy, S.; Kumar, P. & Bose, M., 2004).

Respiratory diseases treated with M. vaccae to date have been: Pulmonary tuberculosis, Bronchial aspects of hay-fever, Bronchial asthma, Lung cancer

Related conditions under investigation Chronic obstructive pulmonary disease (COPD) in man and recurrent airway obstruction (RAO) in horses.

Arterial disease.
Myocarditis.
(These are being investigated with related bacterial immuno-modulators)

4. Salient results of immunotherapy studies in treatment of tuberculosis

In a preliminary study conducted some years ago in Carrasco Hospital, 14 pulmonary tuberculosis patients receiving heat-killed, borate-buffered *M. vaccae* (SRL172) had a better outcome than did 7 patients who received placebo (Vacirca, A.; Dominino, J. C.; Valentín, E; Bottasso, O. & Stanford, J., 1993. Subsequently we have carried out three small studies of this immunotherapy. All were performed in newly diagnosed, moderate to severe, pulmonary tuberculosis patients. In the first of these, the effects of a single dose given by intradermal injection was monitored to evaluate the potential of the approach and assess the value of the selected investigations. Levels of IFN-γ rose and TNF-α fell, with decreases also in levels of IL-4, IL-10 and anti-hsp 70 kDa (Dlugovitzky, D.; Bottasso, O.; Dominino, J. C.; Valentini, E.; Hartopp, R.; Singh, M.; Stanford, C. & Stanford, J., 1999) (Table 1). From subsequent researches performed by our group, we concluded that immunotherapy with *M. vaccae* promotes changes in the immune response and improves patient recovery.

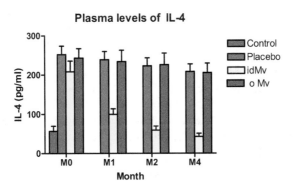

Fig. 1. Plasma levels of interleukin-4 for patients treated with placebo, intradermal or oral *Mycobacterium vaccae*. id: Intradermal, o: oral.

	Immunotherapy		Placebo	Controls
Hsp 65 kD	n=13		n=11	n=12
On admission	0.30±0.03		0.23±0.04	0.20±0.04[a]
	P<0.001		P<0.05	
After 1 month	0.19±0.02		0.2±0.02	
% decrease	32±5.5	P<0.05	15.6±5.4	
Hsp 70 kD				
On admission	0.59±0.05		0.62±0.06	0.25±0.06[b]
	P<0.001		n.s.	
After 1 month	0.31±0.03	P<0.001	0.53±0.06	
% decrease	48±3.6	P<0.0001	17±2.6	
IL-4				
On admission	685±77		586±63	69±9[b]
After 1 month	342±36	P<0.02	495±58	
% decrease	47±4.7	P<0.001	15±4.9	
IL-10				
On admission	3800±302		3863±270	35±6[b]
After 1 month	2292±187	P<0.002	3663±286	
% decrease	38±5.3	P<0.007	16.5±5.8	
IFN-γ				
On admission	524±76		553±57	157±7[b]
After 1 month	1172±173	P<0.05	700±99	
% increase	124±21	P<0.005	41±20	
TNF-α				
On admission	86±6		85.5±3.3	None detectable[b]
After 1 month	52±5	P<0.001	74±3.7	
% decrease	38±3.6	P<0.01	14±4.1	

[a] Different form immunotherapy group. P<0.02
[b] Different from immunotherapy and placebo groups. P<0.001 n.s., not significant

Table 1. Result of ELISA absorption measurements. ± SE of IgG antibodies to heat shock proteins 65 kD and 70 kD and of the serum cytokines interlukin-4 (IL-4), interleukin-10 (IL-10), interferon gamma (IFN-γ) and tumor necrosis factor alpha (TNF-α) in pg/ml

Salient results of serology and cell culture supernatant immunology of data drawn from all three studies of *M. vaccae*, injected or oral are shown. With the rise in serum IFN-γ and fall in serum IL-4 (Fig. 1), is seen a reduction in production of IgG antibodies to stress proteins and a reduction in circulating TNF-α (Fig. 2). Culture supernatants of both PBMC and PMN cells showed steady increases with time of IFN-γ and IL-2, and as the disease regressed production of TNF-α fell steeply.

In addition to these results it has been demonstrated that CD8+ cells also synthesize IL-4, and this cytokine profile correlates with cavitation (van Crevel, R.; Karyadi, E.; Preyers, F.; Leenders, M.; Kullberg, B. J.; Nelwan, R. H. & van der Meer, J. W., 2000).

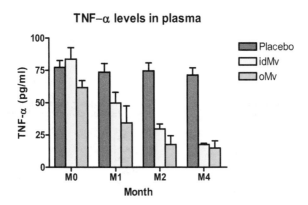

Fig. 2. Plasma TNF-α values for patients treated with placebo, intradermal or oral *Mycobacterium vaccae*. id: Intradermal, o: oral.

Respiratory Burst expression (Fig. 3) increased in the successives samples of intradermal and oral *M. vaccae* treated TBP, and it was higher in those patients receiving oral *M. vaccae* then in those receiving intradermal *Mv* in relation to placebo recipients.

IFN-γ (Fig. 4), TNF-α (Fig. 5), IL-6 and IL-10 (Fig. 6) levels in PBMC and PMN culture supernatants. and IL-6, IL-10 (Fig. 7) and TNF-α values in plasma (Fig. 2) also increased more in those receiving oral *M. vaccae* than in intradermal *M. vaccae* recipients.The immunomodulatory effect of both oral *M. vaccae* and intradermal. *M. vaccae* treatments was shown both by Respiratory Burst expression and cytokine increase in culture supernatants and plasma, with oral therapy the more effective.

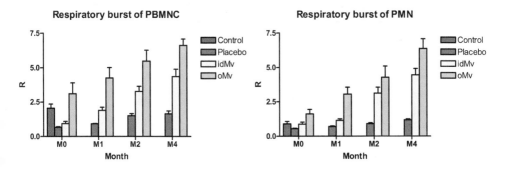

Fig. 3. Respiratory index for polymorphonuclear cells and for mononuclear cells, calculated by dividing the mean fluorescence value for H37Rv-stimulated cells by the mean fluorescence value for unstimulated cells.

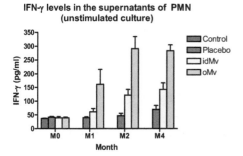

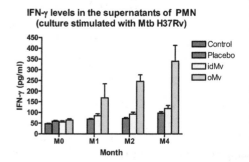

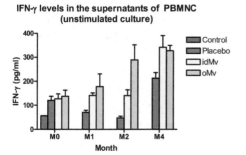

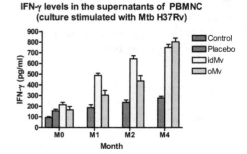

Fig. 4. IFN-γ levels in the supernatants of cultured cells

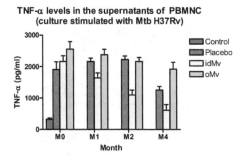

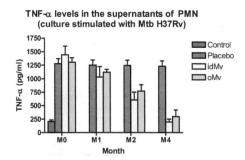

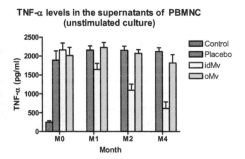

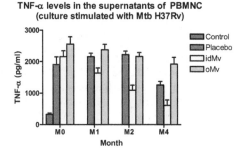

Fig. 5. TNF-α levels in the supernatants of cultured cells

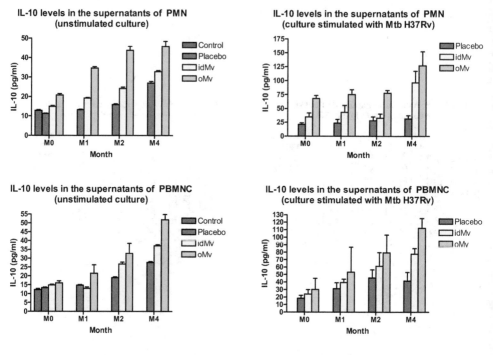

Fig. 6. IL-10 levels in the supernatants of cultured cells.

The data obtained with all 3 immunotherapy regimens produced significantly better results than those achieved with chemotherapy alone.

The data show that the addition of oral capsules of *M. vaccae* to a DOTS program in the treatment of drug-sensitive tuberculosis would have the clinical advantages of hastening sputum negativity and recovery from the disease. Such a strategy would reduce new infections, both among contacts and in the community at large and might allow shortening of the treatment period.

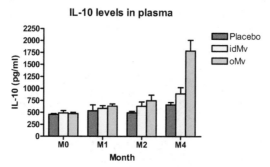

Fig. 7. Plasma IL-10 values for patients treated with placebo, intradermal or oral *Mycobacterium vaccae*. id: Intradermal, o: oral.

The mechanism of action of injected *M. vaccae* is thought to be via immunomodulating adjuvant activities of the mycobacterial cell envelope. The short amino acid-chain lengths of common mycobacterial antigens and sugars preserved by the borate buffer on dermal dendritic cells (Stanford, J. L. & Grange, J. M., 1974; Stanford, J.; Stanford, C.; Stansby, G.; Bottasso, O.; Bahr, G. & Grange, J., 2009; Hernández-Pando, R.; Aguilar, D.; Orozco, H.; Cortez, Y.; Brunet, L. R. & Rook, G. A., 2008) act to direct the modulated response to the sites of expression of host-cell stress proteins (Matzinger, P., 1994). This may be especially to those stress proteins of mitochondrial origin showing homologies with the common antigens of mycobacteria (Cohen, I. R. & Young, D. B., 1991) and the bacteriomimetic sugars expressed by rapidly replicating cells. The results reported in animals (Stainsby, K. J., 1989; Zuany-Amorim, C.; Sawicka, E.; Manlius, C.; Le Moine, A.; Brunet, L. R.; Kemeny, D. M.; Bowen, G.; Rook, G. & Walker, C., 2002; Hernandez-Pando, R.; Pavon, L.; Arriaga, K.; Orozco, H.; Madrid-Marina, V. & Rook, G., 1997) and our observations in man suggest that the same, or similar, beneficial immunomodulation can be stimulated via the mucosal immune system, where the multifold (M) cells (Gebert, A.; Rothkotter, H. J. & Pabst, R., 1996) of the intestine play a part analogous to that of the dermal dendritic cells in the skin.

In addition to the reported immunological results, the bacteriological findings indicated that the conversion to negative of both sputum smear and culture was significantly enhanced by injected or oral immunotherapy with *M. vaccae* above that achieved by chemotherapyalone.

Although this study deals with drug-sensitive tuberculosis, the reported immunological changes, which are paralleled in both injected and oral studies, allow confidence that the oral formulation will prove of similar efficacy in patients infected with drug-resistant bacilli (Stanford, J. L.; Stanford, C. A.; Grange, J. M.; Lan, N. N. & Etemadi, A., 2001). This would accord with our earlier experience of intradermal injection of *M. vaccae* in patients with a variety of drug resistance (Farid, R.; Etemadi, A.; Mehvar, M.; Stanford, J. L.; Dowlati, Y. & Velayati, A. A., 1994; Corlan, E.; Marica, C.; Macavei, C.; Stanford, J. L. & Stanford, C. A., 1997) in many countries (Stanford, J. L.; Stanford, C. A.; Grange, J. M.; Lan, N. N. & Etemadi, A., 2001), where excellent clinical results have already been obtained in the treatment of MDR-TB. As the immunological data obtained in the oral study, albeit with a more intensive schedule, paralleled that of the intradermal study it is logical to suppose that MDR-TB could also be treated successfully with oral *M. vaccae*. The properly functioning immune system recognizes and regulates the appropriate response to disease and would be capable of destroying both drug-sensitive and drug-resistant organisms quite impartially.

This approach to treatment at the outset would allow initial resistance to be treated early and at the same time discourage secondary resistance due to treatment inadequacy. As an example, at the chest hospital in Ho Chi Minh City, Vietnam, 12 patients accepted for immigration into the USA were subsequently found to be infected with highly drug-resistant organisms. They failed to be cured with the latest drugs provided from the USA, but following up to twelve injections of *M. vaccae* (administered on the initiative of the staff of the Chest Hospital) all were cured and allowed into the USA. Similar results have been obtained in several countries (Stanford, J. L.; Stanford, C. A.; Grange, J. M.; Lan, N. N. & Etemadi, A., 2001).

5. Conclusions of the 3 studies

The inclusion of immunotherapy with SRL-172 improved the results of DOTS chemotherapy and it led us to the conclusion that this therapy might allow a reduced period of chemotherapy without loss of efficacy and help to prevent the development of multi-drug-resistance. The three small studies of immunotherapy with heat-killed, borate-buffered, *M. vaccae* for drug-susceptible pulmonary TB developed in the department in Medicine Faculty of Rosario have produced successful results. It was demonstrated that the transformation of a Th2 response, towards Th1, is accompanied by clinical, bacteriological and radiological improvement in the immunotherapy recipients.

The results showed that three injected doses of *M. vaccae* were more effective than a single dose, and that ten oral doses scattered throughout the period of chemotherapy, were as effective, or more so, than was the injected preparation. The reagent deserves formal field trials, particularly in patients infected with highly drug-resistant strains of tubercle bacilli.

In conclusion, we have found that immunotherapy with *M. vaccae* in TB, whether by injection or by the oral route, hastens recovery, bacteriologically, clinically and radiologically, as well as returning immune responses towards those of healthy persons.

6. References

Aiuti, F. & Mezzaroma, I. (2006). Failure to reconstitute CD4+ T-cells despite suppression of HIV replication under HAART. *AIDS reviews*, 8, 2, (Jun 2006), 88-97, ISSN: 1139-6121.

Algood, H. M.; Lin, P. L.; Yankura, D.; Jones, A.; Chan, J. & Flynn, J. L. (2004). TNF-influences chemokine expression of macrophages in vitro and that of CD11b+ cells in vivo during Mycobacterium tuberculosis infection. *Journal of Immunology*, 172, 11, (Jun, 2004), 6846-6857. ISSN: 0022-1767.

Appelberg, R.; Castro, A. G.; Gomes, S.; Pedrosa, J. & Silva, M. T. (1995). Susceptibility of beige mice to Mycobacterium avium: role of neutrophils. *Infection and Immunity*, 63, 9, (Sep, 1995), 3381-3387, ISSN: 0019-9567.

Appelberg, R.; Castro, A. G.; Gomes, S.; Pedrosa, J. & Silva, M. T. (1995). Susceptibility of beige mice to Mycobacterium avium: role of neutrophils. *Infection and immunity*, 63, 9, (Sep, 1995), 3381-3387, ISSN: 0019-9567.

Arjanova, O. V.; Prihoda, N. D.; Yurchenko, L. V.; Sokolenko, N. I.; Frolov, V. M.; Tarakanovskaya, M. G.; Batdelger, D.; Jirathitikal, V. & Bourinbaiar, A. S. (2011). Adjunct oral immunotherapy in patients with re-treated, multidrug-resistant or HIV-coinfected TB. *Immunotherapy*, 3, 2, 181–191, ISSN: 1750-743X.

Aung, H.; Toossi, Z.; Wisnieski, J. J.; Wallis, R. S.; Culp, L. A.; Phillips, N. B.; Phillips, M.; Averill, L. E.; Daniel, T. M. & Ellner, J. J. (1996). Induction of monocyte expression of TNF-a by the 30-kD a antigen of *M. tuberculosis*, and synergism with fibronectin. *The Journal of clinical investigation*, 98, 5, (Sep, 1996), 1261–1268, ISSN: 0021-9738.

Barnes, P. F.; Chatterjee, D.; Abrams, J. S.; Lu, S.; Wang, E.; Yamamura, M.; Brennan, P. J. & Modlin, R. L. (1992). Cytokine production induced by Mycobacterium tuberculosis lipoarabinomannan: relationship to chemical structure. *Journal of immunology*, 149, 2, (Jul, 1992), 541–547, ISSN: 0022-1767.

Barnes, P. F.; Fong, S. J.; Brennan, P. J.; Twomey, P. E.; Mazumder, A. & Modlin, R. L. (1990). Local production of tumor necrosis factor and IFN-gamma in tuberculous pleuritis. *Journal of immunology*, 145, 1, (Jul, 1990), 149–154, ISSN: 0022-1767.

Bay, M. L.; Dlugovitzky, D.; Urízar, L. (1997). Lymphoproliferative response of tuberculosis patients to antigen specific or mitogen stimulation and their relation whit IL-1 b production. *Biocell*, 21–42, ISSN: 0327-9545.

Bekker, L. G.; Maartens, G.; Steyn, L. & Kaplan, G. (1998). Selective increase in plasma tumor necrosis factor–a and concomitant clinical deterioration after initiating therapy in patients with severe tuberculosis. *The Journal of infectious diseases*, 178, 2, (Aug, 1998), 580–584, ISSN: 0022-1899.

Bilaceroglu, S.; Perim, K.; Buyuksirin, M. & Celikten, E. (1999). Prednisolone: a beneficial and safe adjunct to antituberculosis treatment? A randomized controlled trial. *The international journal of tuberculosis and lung disease*, 3 1, (Jan, 1999), 47–54, ISSN: 1027-3719.

Black, R. A.; Rauch, C.T.; Kozlosky, C.J.; Peschon, J. J.; Slack, J. L.; Wolfson, M. F.; Castner, B.J.; Stocking, K. L.; Reddy, P.; Srinivasan, S.; Nelson, N.; Boiani, N.; Schooley, K. A.; Gerhart, M.; Davis, R.; Fitzner, J. N.; Johnson, R. S.; Paxton, R. J.; March, C. J. & Cerretti, D. P. (1997). A metalloproteinase disintegrin that releases tumour-necrosis factor–alpha from cells. *Nature*, 385, 6618, (Feb, 1997), 729–733, ISSN: 0028-0836.

Bogdan, C.; Röllinghoff, M. & Diefengach, A. (2000). Reactive oxygen and reactive nitrogen intermediates in innate and specific immunity. *Current Opinion in Immunology*, 12, 1, (Feb, 2000), 64-76, ISSN: 0952-7915.

Caruso, A. M.; Serbina, N.; Klein, E.; Triebold, K.; Bloom, B. R. & Flynn, J. L. (1999). Mice deficient in CD4 T cells have only transiently diminished levels of IFN-γ, yet succumb to tuberculosis. *Journal of Immunology*, 162, 9, (May, 1999), 5407–5416, ISSN: 0022-1767.

Casanova, J. L. & Abel, L. (2002). Genetic dissection of immunity to mycobacteria: the human model. *Annual review of immunology*, 20, 581-620, ISSN: 0732-0582.

Cohen, I. R. & Young, D. B. (1991). Autoimmunity, microbial immunity and the immunological homunculus (Immunculus). *Immunology today*, 12, 4, (Apr, 1991), 105-110, ISSN: 1471-4906.

Corlan, E.; Marica, C.; Macavei, C.; Stanford, J. L. & Stanford, C. A. (1997). Immunotherapy with Mycobacterium vaccae. 2. In the treatment of chronic or relapsed tuberculosis in Romania. *Respiratory medicine*, 91, 1, (Jan, 1997), 21–29, ISSN: 0954-6111.

Denis, M. J. (1991). Human neutrophils, activated with cytokines or not, do not kill virulent Mycobacterium tuberculosis. *The Journal of infectious diseases*, 163, 4, (Apr, 1991), 919-920, ISSN: 0022-1899.

Dlugovitzky, D.; Bay, M. L.; Rateni, L.; Fiorenza, G.; Vietti, L.; Farroni, M. A. & Bottasso, O. A. (2000). Influence of disease severity on nitrite and cytokine production by peripheral blood mononuclear cells from patients with pulmonary tuberculosis. *Clinical and experimental immunology*, 122, 3, (Dec, 2000), 343–349, ISSN: 0009-9104.

Dlugovitzky, D.; Bay, M. L.; Rateni, L.; Urízar, L.; Rondelli, C. F.; Largacha, C.; Farroni, M. A.; Molteni, O. & Bottasso, O. A. (1999). In vitro synthesis of interferon-γ, interleukin-4, transforming growth factor-β, and interleukin 1-β by peripheral blood mononuclear cells from tuberculosis patients. Relationship with the severity of pulmonary involvement. *Scandinavian journal of immunology*, 49, 2, (Feb, 1999), 210–217, ISSN: 0300-9475.

Dlugovitzky, D.; Bottasso, O. A.; Dominino, J. C.; Valentini, E.; Hartrop, R.; Mahavir, Dingh.; Stanford, C. & Stanford, J. L. (1999). Clinical and Serogical Studies of Tuberculosis Patients in Argentina receiving Immunotherapy with Mycobacterium vaccae. *Respiratory medicine*, 93,8, (Aug, 1999), 557-562, ISSN: 0954-6111.

Dlugovitzky, D.; Fiorenza, G.; Farroni, M.; Bogue, C.; Stanford, C.; & Stanford, J. (2006). Immunological consequences of three doses of heat-killed Mycobacterium vaccae in the immunotherapy of tuberculosis. *Respiratory medicine*, 100, 6, (Jun, 2006), 1079–1087, ISSN: 0954-6111.

Dlugovitzky, D.; Luchesi, S.; Torres-Morales, A.; Ruiz-Silva, J.; Canosa, B.; Valentini, E. & Bottasso, O. (1995). Circulating immune complexes in patients with advanced tuberculosis and their association with autoantibodies and reduced CD4+ lymphocytes. *Brazilian journal of medical and biological research*, 28, 3, (Mar, 1995), 331–335, ISSN: 0100-879X.

Dlugovitzky, D.; Notario, R.; Martinel-Lamas, D.; Fiorenza, G.; Farroni, M.; Bogue, C.; Stanford, C. & Stanford, J. (2010). Immunotherapy with oral heat-killed Mycobacterium vaccae in patients with moderate to advanced pulmonary tuberculosis. *Immunotherapy* 2, 2, (Mar, 2010), 159–169, ISSN: 1750-743X..

Dlugovitzky, D.; Rateni, L.; Torres-Morales, A.; Ruiz-Silva, J.; Piñesky, R.; Canosa, B.; Molteni, O. & Bottasso, O. (1997). Levels of interleukin-8 in tuberculous pleurisy and the profile of immunocompetent cells in pleural and peripheral compartments. *Immunology Letters*, 55, 1, (Jan, 1997), 35-39, ISSN: 0165-2478.

Dlugovitzky, D.; Stanford, C. & Stanford, J. (2011). Immunological basis for the introduction of immunotherapy with Mycobacterium vaccae into the routine treatment of TB. *Immunotherapy*, 3, 4, (Apr, 2011), 557-568, ISSN: 1750-743X.

Dlugovitzky, D.; Torres, A.; Hourquescos, M. C.; Svetaz, M. J.; Quagliato, N.; Valentini, E.; Amigot, B.; Molteni, O. & Bottasso, O. (1995). Low Occurrence of arthritic manifestations in patients with pulmonary tuberculosis. T-cell subsets and humoral Studies. *Memorias do Instituto Oswaldo Cruz*, 90, 5, (Sep, 1995), 623-628, ISSN: 0074-0276.

Dlugovitzky, D.; Torres-Morales, A.; Rateni, L.; Farroni, M.A.; Largacha, C.; Molteni, O. & Bottasso, O.A. (1997). Circulating profile of Th1 and Th2 cytokines in tuberculosis patients with different degree of pulmonary involvement. *FEMS immunology and medical microbiology*, 18, 3, (Jul, 1997), 203–207, ISSN: 0928-8244.

East African-British Medical Research Councils. (1974). Controlled clinical trial of four shortcourse (6-month) regimens of chemotherapy for treatment of pulmonary tuberculosis: third report. *Lancet*, 61, 2, (Jun, 1980), 237–240, ISSN: 0140-6736.

Ehlers, S. (2003). Pathomorphogenesis of tubercular histologic changes: mechanisms of granuloma formation, maintenance and necrosis. *Der Internist (Berl)*, 44, 11, (Nov, 2003), 1363-1673, ISSN: 0020-9554.

Etemadi, A.; Farid, R. & Stanford, J. L. (1992). Immunotherapy for drug resistant tuberculosis. *Lancet*, 340, 8831, (Nov, 1992), 1360-1361, ISSN: 0140-6736.

Farid, R.; Etemadi, A.; Mehvar, M.; Stanford, J. L.; Dowlati, Y. & Velayati, A. A. (1994). Mycobacterium vaccae immunotherapy in the treatment of multi-drug-resistant tuberculosis: a preliminary report. *Iranian Journal of Medical Science*, 19, 37–39. ISSN: 0253-0716.

Feng, C. G.; Jankovic, D.; Kullberg, M.; Cheever, A.; Scanga, C. A.; Hieny, S.; Caspar, P.; Yap, G. S. & Sher, A. (2005). Maintenance of pulmonary Th1 effector function in chronic tuberculosis requires persistent IL-12 production. *Journal of Immunology*, 174, 7, (Apr, 2005), 4185-4192, ISSN: 0022-1767.

Ferreira Gonçalves, M. J.; Ponce de Leon, A. C. & Fernandes Penna, M. L. (2009). Análisis multinivel de los factores asociados con Tuberculosis. *Revista de Salud pública*, 11, 6, (Dec. 2009), 918-930. ISSN: 0124-0064.

Fieschi, C. & Casanova, J. L. (2003). The role of interleukin-12 in human infectious diseases: only a faint signature. *European journal of immunology*, 33, 6, (Jun, 2003), 1461-1464, ISSN: 0014-2980.

Fiorenza, G.; Bottasso, O. A.; Rateni, L.; Farroni, M. A. & Dlugovitzky, D. (2003). Impaired neutrophil function in patients with pulmonary tuberculosis and its normalization in those undergoing specific treatment, except the HIV-coinfected cases. *FEMS immunology and medical microbiology*, 35, 2, (Mar, 2003), 159-164, ISSN: 0928-8244

Fiorenza, G.; Farroni, M. A.; Bogué, C.; Selenscig, D.; Martinel Lamas, D. & Dlugovitzky, D. (2007). Functional characteristics of neutrophils and mononuclear cells from tuberculosis patients stimulated in vitro with heat killed *M. tuberculosis*. *Archives of Medical Research*, 38, 5, (Jul, 2007), 526-533, ISSN: 0188-4409.

Fiorenza, G.; Rateni, L.; Farroni, M A.; Bogué, C. & Dlugovitzky, D. G. (2005). TNF-α, TGF-β and NO relationship in sera from tuberculosis (TB) patients of different severity. *Immunology Letters*, 98, 1, (Apr, 2005), 45-48, ISSN: 0165-2478.

Flynn, J. L. & Ernst, J. D. (2000). Immune responses in tuberculosis. *Current opinion in immunology*, 12, 4, (Aug, 2000), 432-436, ISSN: 0952-7915.

Friedmann, F. (1904). Zur frage der skitien immunisiering gegen Tuberculose. *Deutsche medizinische Wochenschrift*, 5, 166, ISSN: 0012-0472.

Fulton, S.A.; Reba, S. M.; Martin, T.D. & Boom, W. H. (2002). Neutrophil-mediated mycobactericidal immunity in the lung during Mycobacterium bovis BCG infection in C57BL/6 mice. *Infection and Immunity*, 70, 9, (Sep, 2002), 5322-5327, ISSN: 0019-9567.

García, M. A., Sarmiento M. E. & Acosta A. (2009). The anti-tuberculosis immunity and their implications in the vaccine candidates development. *Vaccimonitor*, 18, 1, (Jan-Apr, 2009), 25-34. ISSN 1025-028X.

Gebert, A.; Rothkotter, H. J. & Pabst, R. (1996). M cells in Peyer's patches in the intestine. *International review of cytology*, 167, 91–159, ISSN: 0074-7696.

Grange, J. M.; Stanford, J. L.; Stanford, C. A. & Kölmel, K. F. (2003). Vaccination strategies to reduce the risk of leukaemia and melanoma. *Journal of the Royal Society of Medicine*, 96, 8, (Aug, 2003), 389–392, ISSN: 0141-0768.

Hart, C. A.; Beeching, N. J. & Duerden, B. I. (1996). Tuberculosis into the next century. Proceedings of a symposium held on 4 February 1995 at the Liverpool School of Medicine. *Journal of medical microbiology*, 44,1, (Jan, 1996), 1–34, ISSN: 0022-2615.

Hernández-Pando, R.; Aguilar, D.; Orozco, H.; Cortez, Y.; Brunet, L. R. & Rook, G. A. (2008). Orally administered Mycobacterium vaccae modulates expression of immunoregulatory molecules in Balb-C mice with pulmonary tuberculosis. *Clinical and Vaccine Immunology*, 15, 11, (Nov, 2008), 1730–1736, ISSN: 1556-6811.

Hernandez-Pando, R.; Pavon, L.; Arriaga, K.; Orozco, H.; Madrid-Marina, V. & Rook, G. (1997). Pathogenesis of tuberculosis exposed to low and high doses of an environmental mycobacterial saprophyte before infection. *Infection and Immunity*, 65, 8, (Aug, 1997), 3317-3327, ISSN: 0019-9567.

Hirsch, C. S.; Ellner, J. J., Russell, D. G. & Rich, E. A. (1994). Complement receptor-mediated uptake and tumor necrosis factor–alpha-mediated growth inhibition of Mycobacterium tuberculosis by human alveolar macrophages. *Journal of Immunology*, 152, 2, (Jan, 1994), 743–753. ISSN: 0022-1767.

Hopkin, J.M.; Shaldon, S.; Ferry, B.; Coull, P. P. A.; Enomoto, T.; Yamashita, T.; Kurimoto, F.; Stanford, J.; Shirakawa, T. & Rook, G. A. W. (1998). Mycobacterial immunisation in grass pollen asthma and rhinitis. *Thorax*, 53,S63, ISSN: 0040-6376.

Horne, N.W. (1960). Prednisolone in treatment of pulmonary tuberculosis: a controlled trial. Final report to the Research Committee of the Tuberculosis Society of Scotland. *British Medical Journal*, 2, 5215, (Dec, 1960), 1751–1756, ISSN: 0959-8138.

Hrouda, D.; Souberbielle, B. E.; Kayaga, J.; Corbishley, C. M.; Kirby, R. S. & Dalgleish, G. (1998).Mycobacterium vaccae (SRL-172): a potential immunological adjuvant evaluated in rat prostate cancer. *British Journal of Urology*, 82, 6, (Dec, 1998), 870-876, ISSN: 1464-4096.

Johnson, B. J.; Bekker, L. G.; Rickman, R.; Brown, S.; Lesser, M.; Ress, S.; Willcox, P.; Steyn, L. & Kaplan, G. (1997). rhuIL-2 adjunctive therapy in multidrug resistant tuberculosis: a comparison of two treatment regimens and placebo. *Tubercle and Lung Disease*, 78, 3-4, 195–203, ISSN: 0962-8479.

Johnson, J. L.; Ssekasanvu, E.; Okwera, A.; Mayanja, H.; Hirsch, C. S.; Nakibali, J. G.; Drzayich Jankus, D.; Eisenach, K. D.; Boom, W. H.; Ellner, J. J. & Mugerwa, R. D. (2003). Randomized trial of adjunctive interleukin-2 in adults with pulmonary tuberculosis. *American journal of respiratory and critical care medicine*, 168, 2, (Jul, 2003), 185–191, ISSN: 1073-449X.

Jones, G. S.; Amirault, H. J. & Andersen, B. R. (1990). Killing of Mycobacterium tuberculosis by neutrophils: a nonoxidative process. *The Journal of infectious diseases*, 162, 3, (Sep, 1990), 700-704, ISSN: 0022-1899.

Kim, C. E.; Griffiths, W. J. & Taylor, P. W. (2009). Components derived from Pelagonium stimulate macrophage killing of Mycobacterium species. *Journal of applied microbiology*, 106, 4, (Apr, 2009), 1184–1193, ISSN: 1364-5072

Kindler, V.; Sappino, A. P.; Grau, G. E.; Piguet, P. F. & Vassalli, P. (1989). The inducing role of tumor necrosis factor in the development of bactericidal granulomas during BCG infection. *Cell*, 56, 5, (Mar, 1989), 731–740, ISSN: 0092-8674.

Kitabatake, A; Sakuma, I. (1999). *Recent advances on Nitric Oxide research*, Publisher: Springer Verlag, ISBN: 443170230X, Japan.

Koch, R. (a) (1890). An address on bacteriological research. Delivered before the International Medical Congress, held in Berlin. *British Medical Journal*, 2, 1546, (Aug, 1890), 380-383, ISSN: 0959-8138.

Koch, R. (b) (1890). A further communication on a remedy for tuberculosis. *British Medical Journal*, 2, 1560, (Nov, 1890), 1193-1199, ISSN: 0959-8138.

Kroot, E. J.; Hazes, J. M.; Colin, E. M. & Dolhain, R. J. (2006). Poncet's disease: reactive arthritis accompanying tuberculosis. Two case reports and a review of the literature. *Rheumatology (Oxford)*, 46, 3, (Mar, 2007), 484–489, ISSN: 1462-0324.

Maraveyas, A.; Baban, B.; Kennard, D.; Rook, G. A.; Westby, M.; Grange, J. M.; Lydyard, P.; Stanford, J. L.; Jones, M.; Selby, P. & Dalgleish, A. G. (1999). Possible improved survival of patients with stage IV AJCC melanoma receiving SRL-172 immunotherapy: correlation with induction of increased levels of intracellular interleukin-2 in peripheral blood lymphocytes. *Annals of Oncology*, 10, 7, (Jul, 1999), 817-824, ISSN: 0923-7534.

Matzinger, P. (1994). Tolerance, danger, and the extended family. *Annual review of immunology*, 12, 991–1045, ISSN: 0732-0582.

Mayanja-Kizza, H.; Jones-Lopez, E.; Okwera, A.; Wallis, R. S.; Ellner, J. J.; Mugerwa, R. D.; Whalen, C. C. & Uganda-Case Western Research Collaboration. (2005). Immunoadjuvant therapy for HIV-associated tuberculosis with prednisolone: a phase II clinical trial in Uganda. *The Journal of infectious diseases*, 191, 6, (Mar, 2005), 856–865, ISSN: 0022-1899.

Mitnick C. D.; Shin, S. S.; Seung, K. J.; Rich, M. L.; Atwood, S. S.; Furin J. J.; Fitzmaurice G. M.; Alcantara Viru, F. A.; Appleton, S. C.; Bayona, J. N.; Bonilla, C. A.; Chalco, K.; Choi, S.; Franke, M. F.; Fraser, H. S.F.; Guerra, D.; Hurtado, R. M.; Jazayeri, D.; Joseph, K.; Llaro, K.; Mestanza, L.; Mukherjee, J. S.; Muñoz M.; Palacios E.; Sanchez E.; Sloutsky, A. & Becerra M. C. (2008). Comprehensive Treatment of Extensively Drug-Resistant Tuberculosis. *The New Engand. Journal of Medicine*, 359, 6, (Aug, 2008), 563-574, ISSN: 0028-4793.

Nunn, P.; Williams, B.; Floyd, K.; Dye, C.; Elzinga, G. & Raviglione, M. (2005). Tuberculosis control in the era of HIV. *Nature Reviews. Immunology*, 5, 10 (Oct, 2005), 819-826, ISSN: 1474-1733.

Ottenhoff, T.H.; Verreck, F. A. & Lichtenauer-Kaligis, E. G. (2002). Genetics, cytokines and human infectious disease: lessons from weakly pathogenic mycobacteria and salmonellae. *Nature genetics*, 32, 1, (Sep, 2002), 97-105 ISSN: 1061-4036.

Pedrosa, J.; Saunders, B. M.; Appelberg, R.; Orme, I. M.; Silva, M. T. & Cooper, A. M. (2000). Neutrophils play a protective nonphagocytic role in systemic Mycobacterium tuberculosis infection of mice. *Infection and immunity*, 68, 2, (Feb, 2000), 577-583, ISSN: 0019-9567.

Pozniak, A.; Stanford, J. L. & Grange, J. M. (1991). Mycobacterium vaccae immunotherapy. *Lancet*, 338, 8781 (Dec, 1991), 1533-1534, ISSN: 0140-6736.

Ribeiro-Rodrigues, R.; Resende Co, T.; Johnson, J. L.; Ribeiro, F.; Palaci, M.; Sá, R. T.; Maciel, E. L.; Pereira Lima, F. E.; Dettoni, V.; Toossi, Z.; Boom, W. H.; Dietze, R.; Ellner, J. J. & Hirsch, C. S. (2002). Sputum cytokine levels in patients with pulmonary tuberculosis as early markers of mycobacterial clearance. *Clinical and diagnostic laboratory immunology*, 9, 4, (Jul, 2002), 818–823, ISSN: 1071-412X.

Riedel, D. D. & Kaufmann, S. H. (1997). Chemokine secretion by human polymorphonuclear granulocytes after stimulation with Mycobacterium tuberculosis and lipoarabinomannan. *Infection and Immunity*, 65, 11, (Nov, 1997), 4620-4623, ISSN: 0019-9567.

Roach, D. R.; Bean, A. G.; Demangel, C.; France, M. P.; Briscoe, H. & Britton, W. J. (2002). TNF- regulates chemokine induction essential for cell recruitment, granuloma formation, and clearance of mycobacterial infection. *Journal of Immunology*, 168, 9, (May, 2002), 4620–467. ISSN: 0022-1767.

Rook, G. A. W.; Lowrie, D. B. & Hernandez-Pando, R. (2007). Immunotherapeutics for Tuberculosis in Experimental Animals: Is There a Common Pathway Activated by Effective Protocols? *Journal of Infectious Diseases*, 196, 2, (Jul, 2007), 191–198, ISSN: 0022-1899.

Rosenau, M. J.& Anderson, J. (1915). The Friedmann treatment for tuberculosis. *The American journal of the medical sciences*, 149,3, (Mar, 1915), 324-465, ISSN: 0002-9629.

Sechehaye, A. (1920). *The treatment of tuberculosis with Umckeloabo (Steven's cure)*. B Frazer & Co., London, UK.

Seidel, V. & Taylor, P. W. (2004). In vitro activity of extracts and constituents of Pelagonium against rapidly growing mycobacteria. *International journal of antimicrobial agents*, 23, 6, (Jun, 2004), 613–619, ISSN: 0924-8579.

Shalekoff, S.; Tiemessen, C. T.; Gray, C. M. & Martin, D. J. (1998). Depressed Phagocytosis and Oxidative Burst in Polymorphonuclear Leukocytes from Individuals with Pulmonary Tuberculosis with or without Human Immunodeficiency virus Type 1 Infection. *Clinical and Diagnostic Laboratory Immunology*, 5, 1, (Jan, 1998), 41-44, ISSN: 1071-412X.

Sharma, S.; Sharma, M.; Roy, S.; Kumar, P. & Bose, M. (2004). Mycobacterium tuberculosis induces high production of nitric oxide in coordination with production of tumour necrosis factor-α in patients with fresh active tuberculosis but not in MDR tuberculosis. *Immunology and Cell Biology*. 82, 4, (Aug, 2004), 377–382, ISSN: 0818-9641.

Small, P. M. (2009). Tuberculosis: the new vision for the 21st century. *Kekkaku*, 84, 11, (Nov, 2009), 721-726, ISSN: 0022-9776.

Spahlinger, H.; Macassey, L. & Saleeby, C. W. (1934). *Spahlinger contra Tuberculosis 1908–1934. An International Tribute*, Publisher: John Bale, Sons & Danielsson Ltd, ISBN: B0017ZJGZM London, UK.

Sredni-Kenigsbuch, D.; Kambayashi, T. & Strassmann, G. (2000). Neutrophils augment the release of TNF-a from LPS-stimulated macrophages via hydrogen peroxide. *Immunology Letters*, 71,2, (Feb, 2000), 97-102, ISSN: 0165-2478.

Stainsby, K. J. (1989). Development of a tuberculosis vaccine for the badger. PhD Thesis. University of London.

Stanford, J. L. & Grange, J. M. (1974). The meaning and structure of species as applied to mycobacteria. *Tubercle*, 55, 2, (Jun, 1974), 143–152, ISSN: 1472-9792.

Stanford, J. L. & Lemma, E. (1983). The use of a sonicate preparation of Mycobacterium tuberculosis (new tuberculin) in the assessment of BCG vaccination. *Tubercle*, 64, 4, (Dec, 1983), 275–282, ISSN: 1472-9792.

Stanford, J. L. & Paul, R. C. (1973). A preliminary report on some studies of environmental mycobacteria. *Annales de la Societe Belge de Medecine Tropicale*, 53, 4, 389-393, ISSN: 0365-6527.

Stanford, J. L. & Rook, G. A.W. (1983). Environmental mycobacteria and immunisation with BCG. In: *Medical microbiology*, Editors: Easmon, C.S.F. & Jeljaszewicz, J., 2:43-69. Publisher: Academic Press, ISBN: 0122280024, London.

Stanford, J. L.; Bahr, G. M.; Rook, G. A. W.; Shaaban, M. A.; Chugh, T.D.; Gabriel, M.; Al-Shimali, B.; Siddiqui, Z.; Ghardanis, F.; Shahin, A. & Behbehani, K. (1990).Immunotherapy with Mycobacterium vaccae as an adjunct to chemotherapy in the treatment of pulmonary tuberculosis. *Tubercle* 71, 2, (Jun, 1990), 87-93, ISSN: 1472-9792.

Stanford, J. L.; Stanford, C. A.; Grange, J. M.; Lan, N. N. & Etemadi, A. (2001). Does immunotherapy with heat-killed Mycobacterium vaccae offer hope for the treatment of multi-drug-resistant pulmonary tuberculosis? *Respiratory medicine*, 95, 6, (Jun, 2001), 444-447, ISSN: 0954-6111.

Stanford, J. L.; Stanford, C. A.; O'Brien, M. & Grange, J. M. (2008). Successful immunotherapy with Mycobacterium vaccae in the treatment of adenocarcinoma of the lung. *European journal of cancer*, 44, 2, (Jan, 2008), 224-227, ISSN: 0959-8049.

Stanford, J.; Stanford, C.; Dlugovitzky, D.; Fiorenza, G.; Martinel-Lamas, D.; Selenscig, D. & Bogue, C. (2009). Potential for immunotherapy with heat-killed Mycobacterium vaccae in respiratory medicine. *Immunotherapy*, 1, 6, (Nov, 2009), 933-947, ISSN: 1750-743X.

Stanford, J.; Stanford, C.; Stansby, G.; Bottasso, O.; Bahr, G. & Grange, J. (2009). The common mycobacterial antigens and their importance in the treatment of disease. *Current Pharmaceutical Design*, 15, 11, 1248-1260, ISSN: 1381-6128.

Stanford, J.L. & Paul, R. C. (1973).A preliminary report on some studies of environmental mycobacteria. *Annals de la Societe Belge de Medecine Tropicale*, 53, 4, 389-393. ISSN: 1360-2276.

Swaminathan. S.; Padmapriyadarsini, C. &, Narendran, G. (2010). HIV-associated tuberculosis: clinical update. *Clinical infectious diseases*, 50, 10, (May, 2010), 1377-1386, ISSN: 1058-4838.

Trinchieri, G. (2003). Interleukin-12 and the regulation of innate resistance and adaptive immunity. *Nature reviews. Immunology*, 3, 2, (Feb, 2003), 133-146, ISSN: 1474-1733.

Tripathy, S.P.; Ramakrishnan, C.V.; Nazareth, O.; Parthasarathy, R.; Santha Devi, T.; Arumainayagam, D.C.; Balasubramaniam, R.; Rathasabapathy, S.V. & Manjula Datta, S. (1983). Study of chemotherapy regimens of 5 and 7 months' duration and the role of corticosteroids in the treatment of sputum-positive patients with pulmonary tuberculosis in South India. *Tubercle*, 64, 2, (Jun, 1983), 73–91, ISSN: 1472-9792.

Truoc, L. V.; Ly, H. M.; Thuy, N. K.; Trach, D. D.; Stanford, C. A. & Stanford, J. L. (2001). Vaccination against leprosy at Ben San Leprosy Centre, Ho Chi Minh City, Vietnam. *Vaccine*, 19, 25-26, (May, 2001), 3451-3458, ISSN: 0264-410X.

Tunçtan, B.; Okur, H.; Calişir, C. H.; Abacioğlu, H.; Cakici, I.; Kanzik, I. & Abacioğlu, N. (1998). Comparison of nitric oxide production by monocyte/macrophages in healthy subjects and patients with active pulmonary tuberculosis. *Pharmacological Research*, 37, 3, (Mar, 1998), 219-226, ISSN: 1043-6618.

Vacirca, A.; Dominino, J. C.; Valentín, E; Bottasso, O. & Stanford, J. (Rosario, 26-29 de Septiembre de 1993). La inmunización con Mycobacterium vaccae (Mv) en pacientes con tuberculosis pulmonar (TB) virgen de tratamiento. Un ensayo abierto. Congreso Argentino de Tisiología y Neumonología.

Valian, H. K.; Kenedy, L.K.A.; Rostami, M.N.; Mohammadi, A. M. & Khamesipour, A. (2008).Role of Mycobacterium vaccae in the protection induced by first generation Leishmania vaccine against murine model of leishmaniasis. *Parasitology Research*, 103,1, (Jun, 2008), 21-28, ISSN: 0932-0113.

Valone, S.E.; Rich, E. A.; Wallis, R. S. & Ellner, J. J. (1988). Expression of tumor necrosis factor in vitro by human mononuclear phagocytes stimulated with whole Mycobacterium bovis BCGand mycobacterial antigens. *Infection and immunity*, 56, 12, (Dec, 1988), 3313–3315, ISSN: 0019-9567.

van Crevel, R.; Karyadi, E.; Preyers, F.; Leenders, M.; Kullberg, B. J.; Nelwan, R. H. & van der Meer, J. W. (2000). Increased production of interleukin 4 by CD4+ and CD8+ T cells from patients with tuberculosis is related to the presence of pulmonary cavities. *Journal of Infectious Diseases*, 181, 3, (Mar, 2000), 1194-1197, ISSN: 0022-1899.

Van Parijs, L. & Abbas, A. K. (1998). Homeostasis and self-tolerance in the immune system: turning lymphocytes off. *Science*, 280, 5361, (Apr, 1998), 243–248, ISSN: 0036-8075.

Vouldoukis, I.; Riveros-Moreno, V.; Dugas, B.; Ouaaz, F.; Bécherel, P.; Debré, P.; Moncada, S. & Mossalayi, M. D. (1995). The killing of Leishmania major by human macrophages is mediated by nitric oxide induced after ligation of the Fc epsilon RII/CD23 surface antigen. *Proceedings of the National Academy of Sciences of the United States of America*, 92, 17, (Aug, 1995), 7804-7808, ISSN: 0027-8424.

Wallis, R. S. (2005). Reconsidering Adjuvant Immunotherapy for Tuberculosis. *Clinical Infectious Diseases*, 41, (Jul, 2005), 201-208, ISSN: 1058-4838.

Wallis, R. S.; Paranjape, R. & Phillips, M. (1993). Identification by two-dimensional gel electrophoresis of a 58-kilodalton tumor necrosis factor-inducing protein of Mycobacterium tuberculosis. *Infection and immunity*, 61, 2, (Feb, 1993), 627–632, ISSN: 0019-9567.

Wallis, R. S.; Perkins, M.; Phillips, M.; Joloba, M.; Demchuk, B.; Namale, A.; Johnson, J. L.; Williams, D.; Wolski, K.; Teixeira, L.; Dietze, R.; Mugerwa, R. D.; Eisenach, K. & Ellner, J. J. (1998). Induction of the antigen 85 complex of M. *tuberculosis* in sputum: a determinant of outcome in pulmonary tuberculosis. *The Journal of infectious diseases*, 178, 4, (Oct, 1998), 1115–1121, ISSN: 0022-1899.

Wallis, R. S.; Phillips, M.; Johnson, J. L.; Teixeira, L.; Rocha, L. M.; Maciel, E.; Rose, L.; Wells, C.; Palaci, M.; Dietze, R.; Eisenach, K. & Ellner, J. J. (2001). Inhibition of INH-induced expression of M. *tuberculosis* antigen 85 in sputum: a potential surrogate marker in TB chemotherapy trials. *Antimicrobial agents and chemotherapy*, 45, 4, (Apr, 2001), 1302–1304, ISSN: 0066-4804.

Wallis, R.S.; Amir Tahmasseb, M. & Ellner, J. J. (1990). Induction of interleukin 1 and tumor necrosis factor by mycobacterial proteins: the monocyte Western blot. *Proceedings of the National Academy of Sciences of the United States of America*, 87, 9, (May, 1990), 3348–3352, ISSN: 0027-8424.

World Health Orgamization (2011). *Guidelines for intensified tuberculosis case-finding and isoniazid preventive therapy for people living with HIV in resourceconstrained settings* World Health Organization, ISBN: 978 92 4 150070 8, Switzerland.

World Health Orgamization (2011). *The global plan to stop TB 2011–2015. Transforming the fight. Towards elimination of tuberculosis.* Avalaible from: http://www.stoptb.org/global/plan, Accessed: 2011-06-01.

Zuany-Amorim, C.; Sawicka, E.; Manlius, C.; Le Moine, A.; Brunet, L. R.; Kemeny, D. M.; Bowen, G.; Rook, G. & Walker, C. (2002). Suppression of airway eosinophilia by killed Mycobacterium vaccae-induced allergen-specific regulatory T-cells. *Nature Medicine*, 8, 6, (Jun, 2002), 625-629, ISSN: 1078-8956.

8

Biochemical and Immunological Characterization of the *Mycobacterium tuberculosis* 28 kD Protein

Elinos-Báez Carmen Martha[1] and Ramírez González[2]
*[1]Departamento de Medicina Genómica y Toxicología Ambiental, Edificio C, 2° piso
Instituto de Investigaciones Biomédicas, Circuito Exterior, UNAM,
Universidad Nacional Autónoma de México,
Ciudad Universitaria, México, D.F.
[2]Departamento de Farmacología, Facultad de Medicina, UNAM
Ciudad Universitaria, México, D.F.
México*

1. Introduction

Tuberculosis is currently a worldwide public health problem [Tiruviluamala, LB., 2002. World Health Organization, 2005]. Up to 33% of the world population may be infected due to the accelerated resurgence of the disease showing high resistance to drugs, which has been favored by the HIV epidemic [De Cock, KM., 2002], and to individual levels of susceptibility [Cooke, GS., 2001] and predisposition [Ogus, AC., 2004]. The unequal protection conferred by the BCG vaccine, which may range from 0% to 80% [Kipnis, A., 2005] depending on the individual, has led to the search for new vaccination strategies. Recent studies have focused on the identification of immunoprotective bacterial antigens [Zhang, Y., 2004].

Evidence has been forwarded which suggests that protective immunity against TB is closely related to the presence of CD4+ cells [Zhang, M. 1995]. Certain antigenic fractions of MW less than 10 kD with immunoprotective activity have been described [Boesen, H., 1995]. Other fractions of MW 45-64 and 61-80 kD [Harris, D.P., 1993] as well as a heat shock protein of 65 kD transfected to macrophages have been found to induce protective immunity [Cooper, A., 1995]. Moreover, CD8+ cells are known to lyse macrophages which express TB bacillus peptides on their surface [Flynn, JL., 1992]. Some bacillus proteins which induce protection are those of 30-31 and 19 kD [Méndez-Samperio, P., 1995], as well as the 38 kD fraction [Elinos, C.M., 2009]. Such observations suggest that the living microorganism releases certain protective and other potent immunosuppressive molecules. The specific activity of these molecules must therefore be determined before they can be suggested as vaccines.

The present study focused on a 28kD protein (Gp28). This fraction had not been characterized yet but is known to be immunogenic since it stimulates the production of

CD4+, CD8+ and TCRαβ, which in turn produce IL-2 and INFγ in healthy individuals [Elinos, C.M., 2009]. The present work determined certain biochemical and immunological characteristics of Gp28 obtained from the cultured strain H37Rv of *Mycobacterium tuberculosis*. A total protein extract (TPE) was obtained from which Gp28 was subsequently isolated. Anti-TPE hyper-immune serum (HIS) and monospecific polyclonal anti-p28 serum were prepared and used to determine p28 purity; as well as the number of peptides that form the protein; to identify the dominant immunoglobulin (IgG2a); to search for mannose-free radicals and classify it as a glycoprotein (Gp28); to determine the percentage of sugars that recognize the anti-Gp28 antibody, and the N-terminal amino acids, thus establishing the predictive nucleotides which form part of the gene. An *M. tuberculosis* strain H37Rv library was used to isolate the gene and confirm DNA purity. Studies were performed by analyzing phenotypic changes in peripheral mononuclear blood cells (PMBC) induced by Gp28 protein obtained from healthy subject involving the production of CD4+ helper T cells [van Crevel, R., et al. 2000] and CD8+ cytotoxic/suppressor cells [Lazarevic, J., 2002] in high risk healthy staff from the National Institute of Respiratory Diseases (INER) in Mexico, and from four TB patients.

2. Materials and methods

2.1 *M. tuberculosis* culture

Bacteria were sown in the Proskawer and Beck synthetic culture medium modified by Youmans (PBY) [Youmans, G.P., 1949], which was incubated for 6 weeks at 37°C to obtain a colony monolayer that completely covered the surface of the liquid culture medium.

2.2 *M. tuberculosis* Total Protein Extract (TPE)

The culture medium was sterilized by filtering through: 1) Whatman sterile #40 filter paper; 2) 1.2 μm micropore filter; 3) 0.45 μm micropore filter; 4) 0.22 μm micropore filter. A sterile filtrate was obtained and added with solid $(NH_4)_2SO_4$

to precipitate proteins and thus obtain the total protein extract (TPE) of *M. tuberculosis*. The TPE was then dialized with water.

2.3 *M. tuberculosis* 28 kD protein purification

The TPE was treated with the method described by Seibert [Seibert, F. B., 1949]. The acid-alcoholic fraction 2 was obtained enriched with 28 kD glicoprotein (Gp28) from which it was purified by SDS-PAGE. The gel was immersed for 15 min in 6M urea and was subsequently placed in a dark chamber. P28 was found to consist of 2 bands (peptids), which were then separated from the gel and dialized against water, thus obtaining the pure Gp28.

2.4 Anti-*M. tuberculosis* hyperimmune serum

One New Zealand rabbit was immunized with the TPE. Pre-immune serum was obtained, then 100 μl of EPT with 100 μl of complete Freund's adjuvant were administered i.d. on days 1, 10 and 20 thus obtaining the anti-*M. tuberculosis* hyperimmune serum (HIS).

2.5 Polyclonal monospecific anti-p28 serum

One New Zealand rabbit was immunized with p28 following the same protocol as described above. Polyclonal monospecific anti-Gp28 serum was thus obtained.

2.6 TPE and Gp28 purity determination by Western blot

Three SDS-PAGE gels were prepared. Gel 1 was stained with Coomassie blue and contained the following samples in the corresponding wells: a) MW control; b) TPE; c) Seibert fraction 2 enriched with p28; d) pure p28. Gel 2 was used for Western blot incubated with HIS, and contained the following samples in the corresponding wells: e) TPE; f) pure p28. Gel 3 was used for Western blot incubated with anti-p28 monospecific polyclonal serum, and contained the following samples in the corresponding wells: g) TPE and h) pure p28. The Western blots were incubated with alkaline phosphatase labeled anti-rabbit antibody for 1 h at room temperature and were developed with NBT/BCIP.

2.7 Electrofocusing assay for p28

Two dimensional gel electrophoresis would indicate if Gp28 consist of 2 peptides or is formed by more peptides. [Rosenkrands, I., 2000]. It is realized in two parts:

Part 1. The electrofocusing gel contained: 1.1 g urea; 30 µl 10% 30%-acrylamide-(0.8% bis-acrylamide); 400 µl 10% NP-40; 80 µl pH 5-7 ampholyte; 20 µl pH 3.5-10 ampholyte; 5 µl 10% ammonium persulfate; 2 µl Temed; water q.s.p. 400 µl. The sample buffer contained: 2.85 g urea; 1ml 10% NP-40; 80 µl pH 5-7 ampholyte; 20 µl pH 3.5-10 ampholyte; 250 µl β-mercaptoethanol; water q.s.p. 5ml.

Gel pre run: a capillary test tube was filled with recently prepared gel, placed vertically, and when the gel had polymerized the sample was added at the top together with 5 mg of urea per each 10 µl of sample. The gel was run at 400 V, for 12 h, with the cathode buffer (20 mM NaOH) at the top and the anode buffer (10 mM H_3PO_4) at the bottom.

Part 2. A 10% acrylamide larger gel (30%-acrylamide-(0.8% bis-acrylamide)) was prepared. The gel was extracted from the capillary test tube and placed on the surface of larger previously polymerized gel. The gel was run at 100 V for 1 h. The gel was transferred to nitrocellulose paper and incubated with anti-Gp28 serum for 3 h. It was subsequently incubated with alkaline peroxidase-labeled anti-rabbit antibody raised in mouse for 1 h at room temperature, and subsequently developed with ortho-chloronaphthol.

2.8 IgG1 and IgG2 in immun anti-p28 sera by ELISA

Pre immune serum was obtained from 6 month-old Balb/c mice immunized i.p. with Gp28 diluted 1:1 with Freund's complete adjuvant. Immune sera were obtained at 1, 4, 8, 12 and 16 weeks after immunization. Immunoglobulin expression times were determined for Gp28 using ELISA.

Microtitration plates were sensitized by overnight incubation with Gp28 protein antigen in carbonate buffer. Thereafter, the plate was blocked with PBS.BSA for 1 h. The first antibody (mouse anti-Gp28 of 1, 4, 8, 12 or 16 weeks) was added to the wells, and incubated for 3 h.

This was followed by the second antibody (rabbit anti-IgG1 or anti-IgG2) to which alkaline phosphatase-labeled anti-rabbit serum was added. This was later developed with a solution of p-nitrophenyl phosphate disodium in diethanolamine buffer and the reaction blocked with 2N NaOH. The plate was read with an ELISA reader using a 405 nm filter.

2.9 Free mannose radicals in p28

A 10% acrylamide gel (30%-acrylamide-(0.8% bis-acrylamide)) with Gp28 protein in a well was run and transferred to nitrocellulose paper. The nitrocellulose paper was first incubated for 1 h with Concanavaline A-biotin diluted 5:1000 in PBS.BSA at room temperature and then for 1 h with streptavidin peroxidase at room temperarure It was developed with ortho-chloronaphthol.

2.10 p28 amino acid sequence

The Gp28 amino acid sequence was determined by Joe Gray of the Molecular Biology Unit, and Catherine Cookson of the Medical School at the University of Newcastle Upon Tyne. Results showed that Gp28 is a doublet consisting of two Gp28 kD bands containing amino acids A(M) – P(C) – K(Y) – V(E) –A (Y or L).

The predictive nucleotides for the 2 peptides were determined as:

A   P   K   V   A   M   C   Y   E   Y   L

GCC CCC AAG GUC GCC   AUG UGC UAC GAG UAC CUG

These nucleotide sequences were not found in registered nucleotide banks and had not been previously identified.

2.11 Sodium periodate determination of sugar percentage in the anti-p28 antibody-recognizing epitope

ELISA method [Woodward, M. P., 1985]. The microtitration plate was sensitized with 5 µg Gp28 antigen per ml of PBS-BSA, placing 100 µl per well and incubating the plate overnight at 37°C. The plate was subsequently washed with 50 mM acetate buffer, pH 4.5. Recently prepared sodium periodate of 0.1, 1, 5 and 10 mM concentration in 50 mM acetate buffer, pH 4.5 was then added, each to a different well, and incubated in the darkness for 1 h at 37 °C. To block the aldehyde groups, the plate was incubated for 30 min at 37 °C with a recently prepared 1% glycine solution in PBS. The plate was washed with PBS-Tween 20 and immediately added 100 µl/well, with anti-Gp28 antibody and incubated for 1 h to 37°C, after which alkaline phosphate labeled anti-rabbit antibody was added and incubated for 1 h at 37°C. It was then developed with p-nitrophenyl phosphate disodium in diethanolamine buffer. The reaction was blocked with 2N NaOH and the plate was read in an ELISA reader at 405 nm.

2.12 Gene p28 from an *M. tuberculosis* library

The phage λgt11 was used to transfect lysogenic E. coli, strain Y1090hsdR, and construct a DNA expression library. Competent E. coli cell for λgt11 phage were incubated with 0.01 M

$MgSO_4$ for 1 h at 37°C. The phage carries the pMC9 plasmid that codes for the lac repressor, which, in turn, prevents the synthesis of fusion proteins potentially toxic for the β-galactosidase promoter. This plasmid carries the selective marker (amp^r). The HIS used was recognized by the strain H37Rv *Mycobacterium tuberculosis* library. The anti-p28 monospecific polyclonal serum was used to clone gene p28.

Titration of λgt11 phage. A 10 μl sample of the phage under study was added to a tube containing 1 ml dilution buffer, and a serial dilution was prepared in 10 tubes. The contens of each tube were next added to a tube containing Top agar a 50°C, and then transferred to a Petri dish containing Luria Bertani culture broth with ampicillin. Petri dishes were incubated at 37 °C for 24 h. Colonies were counted and those with 100 colonies were considered to contain $1x10^8$/ml λgt11 phage titre.

Titration of the M. tuberculosis library. A tube containing 1 ml of dilution buffer was added with 10 μl of λgt11 phage at $1x10^8$/ml titre and a serial dilution was prepared in 10 tubes. Each tube was added with 10 μl of the *M. tuberculosis* library. The contents of each tube were next added to a tube containing Top-agar at 50 °C and then transferred to a Petri dish containing Luria Bertani broth with ampicillin. They were then incubated at 37 °C for 24 h. Petri dishes with separate colonies were chosen and a nitrocellulose paper disc moistened with Isopropil-β-D-Thiogalactoside (IPTG) was placed in the dish marking its position and other nitrocellulose paper disc moistened with IPTG was placed in other dish marking its position These were then incubated for 1 h at 37 °C. The marked paper discs were then separated and one was incubated with HIS while the other was incubated with monoespecífic polyclonal anti-Gp28 for 3 h at 37°C, the two paper discs were incubated with alkaline peroxidase-labeled anti-rabbit anti-rabbit antibody for 1 h at room temperature.

Control. One tube containing 1 ml of dilution buffer was added with 10 μl of the studied phage. The contents of this tube were then added to a tube containing Top agar at 50°C and then transferred to a Petri dish containing Luria Bertini broth with amppicillin the dish was incubated for 24 h at 37°C. A nitrocellulose paper disk moistened with IPTG was placed in the dish marking its position, and it was then incubated for 1 h at 37°C. The disk was then separated from the Petri dish and incubated with HIS for 3 h at room temperature. Subsequently, it was incubated with alkaline peroxidase-labeled anti-rabbit serum for 1 h at room temperature and developed with NBT/BCIP. This served to prove that no protein from the *M. tuberculosis* library was recognized.

The Gp28 colonies were identified in the Petri dish and sown in Luria Bertani broth and ampicillin, incubated at 37 °C, 240 cycles/min for 20 h. Samples were then centrifuged, resuspended in lysis buffer centrifuged again and the supernatant was added with isopropanol to precipitate DNA, and incubated at 4 °C for 20 h. The samples were then centrifuged and the pellet was dissolved in 50 μl of Milli Q sterile water. A 2292 □g/μl concentration was determined by O.D. reading in a nanospectrophotometer; purity was established by the ratio of the values obtained at 260 nm = 52.697 and at 280 nm = 27.88 nm, which gave a value of 1.89 corresponding to DNA and of 0.11 corresponding to the protein. A 1% agarose gel with 1 μl/well of DNA diluted 1:10 was stained with ethidium bromide (10 μl/100 ml gel; obtained of 10mg/ml dilution) and run at 80 V for 50 min. Results were photographed.

2.13 Human Peripheral Blood Mononuclear Cells (PBMC)

PMBC were obtained from healthy subjects (PPD+, PPD-, with and without BCG vaccination), high risk subjects (staff from the Respiratory Disease Institute (Instituto de Enfermedades Respiratorias, INER)), and from tuberculosis patients (provided by INER) with the following characteristics:

Patient 1. Male, age 23, with untreated progressive tuberculosis; chest X-rays showing fibrosis in left lung and cavitary lesions in right lung.

Patient 2. Female, age 60, diabetic; chest X-rays showed unilateral and apical affliction .

Patient 3. Male, age 64, resistant to treatment with 6 years evolution.

Patient 4. Male, age 25, early infection; one brother died of tuberculosis at age 34, two sisters showed no infection.

Peripheral blood was obtained by venous puncture, subsequently it was treated with heparin (SIGMA, St. Louis Missouri, MO) at concentration of 10 U/ml of blood. An equal volume of RPMI medium was added. Samples of 8 ml of diluted blood were stratified with 4 ml of Ficoll-Hypaque. Tubes were centrifuged at 1500 rpm for 10 min to obtain PMBC and viability was determined with trypan blue.

2.14 T lymphocyte phenotype and antigen receptors

T lymphocytes were characterized by flow cytometry (FACScan, Becton Dickinson, San José, CA). PBMC were washed with RPMI medium and adjusted to 1×10^7 cells/ml per patient. Next, 100 µl/tube were used to determine the following surface molecules: CD3, CD4, CD8, TCR $\alpha\beta$. The corresponding tube was added with 200 µl of first antibody OKT3, OKT4, OKT8, anti TCR $\alpha\beta$. All antibodies were raised in mouse. Tubes were incubated for 40 min at 4 °C in the darkness. Then they were washed 3 times with PBS for FACS, centrifuged, and the pellet resuspended in 500 µl 1% paraformaldehyde. Finally they were read by flow cytometry

3. Results

Purification of Gp28 carried out from the Seibert fraction was sucessful as illustrated by the single band obtained in a PAGE gel eluted with urea 6M and stained with Coomasie Blue (Figure 1). Molecular weight standards (band a) confirm the presence of Gp28 in TPE (band b), and in the enriched Seibert fraction (c). Purified Gp28 is contained in only one band, as shown in (d). TPE immuneblot is shown in (e) and when purified Gp28 is incubated with HIS or with anti-Gp28 serum (in bands f and g and h, respectively) only one band of 28 kD can be observed.

Electrofocusing of Gp28 indicated that it contains two peptides (see Figure 2). This was also confirmed by the N-terminal aminoacid sequences observed by Joe Gray from the Unit of Molecular Biology at Newcastle University.

ELISA analysis indicated that after 1, 4, 8, 12 and 16 weeks after Gp28 treatment, IgG2a is the predominant immunoglobulin detected in mice sera (see Figure 3).

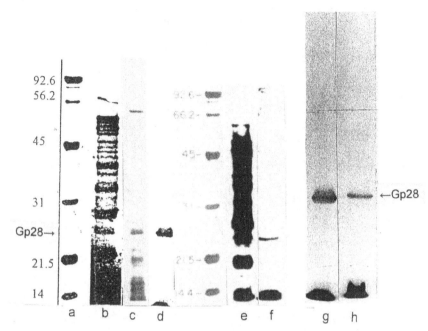

Fig. 1. Gels and immunoblots showing purification of the Gp28 protein isolated of *Mycobacterium tuberculosis* using TPE and Gp28 proteins. Gel stained with Coomassie blue contained the following sample, in **a**)MW; **b**) TPE; **C**) Seibert fraction 2; **d**) pure Gp28. Blot **e**) TPE; **f**) pure Gp28, In other blot **g**) TPE; **h**) pureGp28. Incubated with HIS or with monoespecific polyclonal anti-Gp28, showing pure Gp28

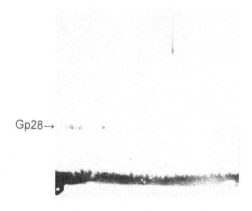

Fig. 2. Show than the protein is formed by only two peptides, which sequences was identified at the University of Newcastle Upon Tyne

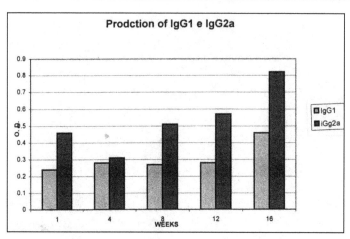

Fig. 3. Mice challenged with Gp28 showed that at 1, 4, 8, 12 and 16 weeks IgG2a predominate even after 16 weeks

The presence of free mannose residues is shown in the PAGE gel of Figure 4. Titration with NaIO3 indicates that Gp28 contains 43 % sugar residues, in the epitope that recognizes the antibody anti Gp28, and 57% peptide residues as shown in the ELISA assay in Figure 5.

Isolation of DNA coding for Gp28 was carried out using Luria Bertini plates blotted with nitrocellulose paper (Figure 6). Disc a presents staining attained when HIS prepared in our laboratory was incubated with a M. tuberculosis library. Disc b shows that HIS does not recognize any peptide when incubated only with λgt11 phage. When the policlonal monospecific anti-Gp28 is incubated with M. tuberculosis library only scattered staning is observed (Disc c). Figure 6d illustrates the electrophoresis of purified Gp28 DNA in an agarose gel that indicates the presence of 900 bp.

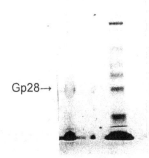

Gp28→

Fig. 4. 10 % acrilamida gel with Gp28 antigen in a well was run and transferred to nitrocellulose paper. This paper was incubated with Concanavaline A marked with Biotin and after it was incubated with streptavidin peroxidase and it is developed, showing that Gp28 is a glycoprotein, by the presence of free mannose radicals.

0.504
0.453
0.445
0.296
0.305

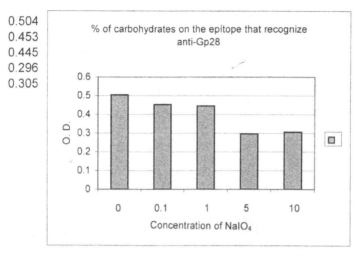

Fig. 5. The microtitration plate was sensitized with Gp28 antigens and incubating the plate overnight, The percentage of sugar in the epitope that recognize the anti-Gp28 was determined using sodium periodate of 0.1, 1, 5 and 10 Mm concentration in 50 mM acetate buffer pH 4.5. To block the aldehide groups with 1% glycine solution. Added with anti-Gp28. the Gp28 recognized the antigen a total of 43% of carbohydrates, leaving 57% of peptidic nature.

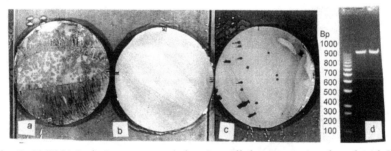

Fig. 6. The Gp28 DNA isolation process. **a)** the nitrocellulose paper incubated with HIS proved that *M. tuberculosis is recognized* in the library; **b)** no peptide of phago λgt11 was recognized in the nitrocellulose paper incubated with HIS; **c)** displays the nitrocellulose paper incubates with anti-Gp28 serum showing recognition of the Gp28; **d)** shows pure Gp28 DNA.

Incubation with pure Gp28 to induce specific cell lines in mononuclear cells obtained from venous human blood from non – vaccinated healthy subjects induced a significant increase of CD3+, CD4+ and TCRαβ+ (see Table 1). Vaccination of healthy subjects does not modify the CD3+, CD4+ nor CD8+ responses to Gp28, excepting for TCRαβ+ that is significantly higher when compared with the response observed in untreated patients with active TB: 92.5 – 94.7 versus 83.8 – 92.1 (IC 95%, P<0.05); this observation indicate which suggests that in active TB the response toGp28 appears to be significantly weakened. Otherwise the response to Gp28 of healthy subjects is not different from the one observed in untreated patients with active TB. The last line in Table 1 includes data from the literature for CD3+ (60 – 85), CD4+ (24 – 59) and CD8+ (18 – 48) that are consistent with the baseline values obtained in our laboratory in healthy subjects (Immunology Today, 1992). Considering the reduced number of patients analyzed, in Figure 7 are shown the individual responses to Gp28 observed in healthy subjects and untreated patients with active TB.

TABLE 1

Individual	CD3	CD4	CD8	CD4/CD8	TCRαβ
PPD+1	97.5	93.1	4.7	19.8	93.1
PPD-2	95.5	86.7	12.8	6.7	94.2
PPD+3	96.7	85.7	16 1	5.3	87.6
PPD-4	97.4	90.8	14.1	6.0	96.0

TABLE BASAL, NORMAL and CLASS

Individual	CD3	CD4	CD8	CD4/CD8	TCRαβ
PPD+3	51.1	34.6	23.0	1.5	52.3
PPD-4	59.5	50.4	18.3	2.7	62.7
Normal	73.0	44.0	33.0	1.2	95.0
Class	60-85	24-59	18-48		

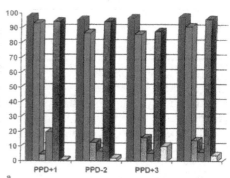

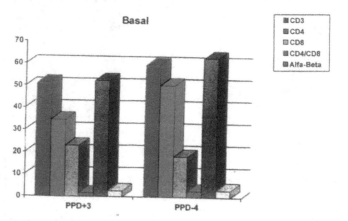

Fig. 7. and Table 1. *In vitro* production of CD3, CD4+, CD8+ and TCRαβ by the antigen specific cell lines induced with Gp28 protein obtained from healthy subjects high risk not vaccinated with BCG (PPD+1 and PPD-2) and vaccinated (PPD+3 and PPD-4), the phenotypic deviation were determined by FACS results confirmed that Gp28 induces proliferation of T helper (CD4+) by more than 90% in healthy.Table 1. bis. These results were compared with the same T cell type not treated with Gp28 of the same individuals, where they constituted approximately 50% of the total T lymphocytes.

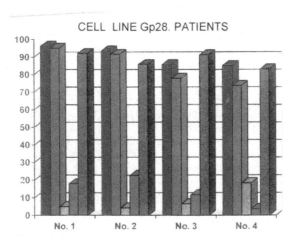

TABLE 2

Patient	CD3	CD4	CD8	CD4/CD8	TCRαβ
No. 1	96.3	94.9	5.1	18.0	92.0
No. 2	93.5	91.5	4.4	22.7	85.8
No. 3	85.7	77.8	6.7	11.6	91.1
No. 4	85.1	73.5	18.4	3.9	83.1

Fig. 8. and Table 2. In the studied tuberculosis patients CD4+ percentage increased by 90% in patients 1 and 2 and 73% in patients 3 and 4, these results are probably related with the severity of TB in these patients.

Value for cell cluster density	HS		TB
	Baseline values of non-vaccinated subjects (n=2)	Challenged with Gp28 (n=4)	Challenged with Gp28 (n=4)
CD3+	55.3 (47.1 – 63.5)*	96.8 (95.8 – 97.6)	90.1 (84.6 – 95.6)
CD4+	42.5 (27.1 – 57.9)*	89.1 (85.6 – 92.4)	84.4 (74.2 – 94.5)
CD8+	20.7 (16.0 – 25.2)	11.9 (7.0 – 16.8)	8.7 (2.2 – 15.0)
TCRαβ+	57.5 (47.3 – 67.6)*	92.7 (89.1 – 96.2)	88.0 (83.8 – 92.1)
CD4+/CD8+	2.1 (0.9 – 3.2)	9.4 (2.6 – 16.2)	14.1 (6.0 – 22.0)

Reference baseline values from (Immunology Today, 1992) for CD3+ (60 – 85), CD4+ (24 – 59), and CD8+ (18 – 48) are consistent with our findings. Data shown are mean value and confidence intervals estimated for a P value of 0.05 (IC 95%). *Indicates significant difference (P<0.05) when comparing baseline values of non-vaccinated HS with vaccinated or non-vaccinated HS challenged with Gp28. There is no significant difference between HS and TB when challenged with Gp28.

Statistic Values: confidence intervals P value of 0.05 (IC 95%).*significant diference P<0.05

Table 3. Effect of Gp28 on phenotype deviation of human peripheral monouclear cells obtained from venous blood of healthy subjects (HS) and from untreated patients with active tuberculosis (TB).

4. Conclusions

In view of the dissimilar protection conferred by the BCG vaccine, research has focused on the identification of immuneprotective antigens. This necessity has been recently magnified the increase in rates of TB, the appearance of bacilli resistant to multiple antituberculous drugs and the rise in the frequency of immunosupressor diseases [Olobo, JO., 2001]. The strategy followed in this study was first to purify the Gp28 antigen of a virulent strain of *Mycobacterium tuberculosis* from the culture medium and to examine its biochemical characteristics. The presence of the mannose radicals [Ehlers, MR., 1998. Heldwein, KA., 2002] was determined, which are identified by the complement receptors CR1, CR3 and CR5 of macrophages, inducing non-opsonic TB bacillus phagocytosis. Sugar and peptide porcentages in the epitope recognized by anti-Gp28 serum were investigated, and IgG2a was identified as the predominant immunoglobulin. The protein was found to consist of a peptide doublet. The N-terminal amino acids of the two peptides were determined as well as the predictive nucleotides, which had not been identified before. The interest in Gp28 was stimulated by its recognized capacity to induce IL2 and IFNγ and are know to be immunocompetent. Evidence has been obtained that protective immunity in tuberculosis is related to CD4+, CD8+ and TCRαβ [Zhan, M., 1995. Lazarevic, V., 2002] In the present experiment peripheral mononuclear blood cells (PMBC)from healthy individuals and TB patients were incubated with Gp28 to obtain cell lines and their phenotype and antigen receptors were determined by FACS. Results confirmed that Gp28 induces proliferation of T helper cells (CD4+) by more than 90% in healthy individuals, and TCRαβ also increased by more than 90%, with the single exception of one individual (PPD+3) who showed an 87% increase. These results were compared with the same T cell type not treated with Gp28 of the same individuals, where they constituted approximately 50% of the total T lymphocytes, In the studied tuberculosis patients CD4+ percentage increased by 90% in patients 1 and 2 and by 73% in patients 3 and 4. As to TCRαβ, these increased by 90% in patients 1 and 3 and by 83% in patients 2 and 4, these results are probably related with the severity of TB in these patients. Protein Gp28 exhibits an epitope capable of inducing the T response more intensely in healthy PPD+ than in PPD- individuals the application of BCG surely stimulated the adaptive immune response against the TB bacillus in PPD+ individuals than in PPD-individuals, the application of BCG surely stimulated the adaptative immune response against the TB bacillus in PPD+ individuals.

5. Acknowledgment

I want to thank Ing. M. en C. Mario Farías Elinos for excellent adviser in computation

6. References

Cooke. GS. & Hill. (2001). Genetics of susceptibility to human infection Disease. Nat Rev Genet, 2: 967-77.

Cosma, CL., Humbert, O., Ramakrishnan, L. (2004). Superinfective mycobacteria Home to established tuberculous granuloma. Nat Immunol. 5: 828-35.

De Cock K M., Mbori-Ngacha & Marum, E. (2002). Shadow on the continente Health and HIVIAIDDS in Africa in the 21st century. Lancet. 360: 67-72

Elinos-Báez. CM. & Ramírez González MD. 2009. Production of Limphocytes derived Cytokines in Response to Mycobacteriumtuberculosis Atigens in Humans. Research Journal of Bitechnology 4: 12-24..

Flynn, JL. & Goldstein, M. (1992). Major compatibility complex class I-restricted T cell are required for resistance to M. tuberculosis Infection. Proc Natl Acad Sci. 89: 12013-12017.

Heldwein, KA.,& Fenton, MJ. 2002. The role of toll-like receptors in immunity Against micobacterial infection. Nicrobes Infection. 4: 937-44.

Jacobsen, M., et. al. (2005). Ras associated small GTPasa 33A, a nobel T cell factor, is dawn-regulated in patients with tuberculosis. The Journal of Infectious Diseases. 19: 1211-8.

Kipnis, A., et al. (205). Memory T lymphocytes generated by Mycobacterium bovis BCG Vaccination reside within a CD4, CD44 CD62 ligandhi population. Infection and Immunity. 73: 7759-7764.

Kusner, DJ. & Adams J. (2000). ATP induced-killing of virulent Mycobacterium tuberculosis within human macrophages requires phospholipasa D. J Immunol. 164: 379-88.

Ougus, AC., et al. (2004). The Arg 753 Gln polymorphism of the human. Toll Like receptor 2 genes in tuberculosis disease. Eur Respir J. 23: 219-23.

Lazarevic, V., Flynn, J. (2002). CD8+ T cell in tuberculosis. Am J Respir Crit Care Med. 166: 1116-21

Melo MD., et al. (2000). Utilization CD4IIb knockout mice to characterize The role of complement receptor 3 (CR.CD11b/CD18) in the growth of *Mycobacterium tuberculosis* in macrophages. Cell Immunol. 205:13-23.

Seibert, FB. (1949). Isolation of three different proteins and two polysaccharides From tube)rculin by alcohol fractions their chemical and biological propiertes. Am Rev Tuberc. 59: 86-101.

Tiruviluamala, P.& Reichman. (2002). Tuberculosis. Annu Rev Public Health. 23: 403-26.)

Ulrichs, T., et al. (2005). Differential organization of the local immune respons in patients with active cavitary tuberculosis or with nonprogressive tuberculoma. The Journal of InfectionDisease. 192: 89-97.

Van Crvel, R., et al. (2000). Increased production of interleukin 4 by CD4+ and CD8+ T cell from patients with tuberculosis is related to the presence of pulmonary cavities. J Infect Dis. 181: 1194-7

World Health Organization. (2005). TB is a public health problem. Available at: http://www.whosea.org/tb/publishhealth.htm. Last accessed 15 August.

Youmans, GP. (1949). J. Bacterial. 51: 703.

9

Adjuvant Interferon Gamma in the Management of Multidrug - Resistant Tuberculosis

Idrian García-García et al.*

Center for Genetic Engineering and Biotechnology, Havana, Cuba

1. Introduction

Tuberculosis is an opportunistic infection, the minute it finds an immunocompromised host, it flourishes. The risk of tuberculosis is much higher in patients who are human immunodeficiency virus (HIV) positive. Drug resistance among microbes is testimony to their adaptive skills. In *Mycobacterium Tuberculosis* the resistance occurs due to random, single step, spontaneous mutation and is invariably induced by inadequate or incomplete therapy. This resistance was termed as Multidrug Resistant (MDR) tuberculosis when the organism was resistant to more than one anti-tuberculosis drug. The presence of MDR tuberculosis, in general population, exposes the immunodeficient patients to an MDR strain of tuberculosis, which has very serious consequences for them. The risk of tuberculosis is also higher in non-HIV immunocompromised patients such as those with genetic absence of Interferon (IFN) gamma receptors, or acquired immune defect in the elderly. In either these situations IFN gamma or its absence seems to play a major role. In addition to the pulmonary infection, immunocompromised patients (with or without HIV) fall victim to extrapulmonary tuberculosis.

IFN gamma belongs to a family of endogenously produced immunoregulators that induces an array of receptors for binding to pathogens and endothelia, degradative enzymes, transcription factors and cytokines involved in host defense. These agents have antibacterial activity against host of pathogens including *Mycobacteria* (*avium* complex, tuberculosis and *bovis*). Interferon gamma has also a potent antifibrotic effect and suggests that it can lead to pulmonary lesions improvement. Exogenously administered IFN gamma has demonstrated therapeutic effect against MDR Tuberculosis, atypical mycobacterial infections, and leprosy.

Attempts to control MDR tuberculosis, is a part of the overall strategy to finally eradicate the disease. Had it not been for the emergence of drug resistance, tuberculosis would in all

* María T Milanés-Virelles[2], Pedro A López-Saura[1], Roberto Suárez-Méndez[2],
Magalys Valdés-Quintana[2], Norma Fernández-Olivera[2], Carmen M Valenzuela-Silva[1],
Lidia González- Méndez[1], Yamilet Santos-Herrera[3], Gladys Abreu-Suárez[4] and Isis Cayón-Escobar[2]
[1] *Center for Genetic Engineering and Biotechnology, Havana, Cuba*
[2] *"Benéfico Jurídico" Hospital, Havana, Cuba*
[3] *"Amalia Simoni" Hospital, Camagüey, Cuba*
[4] *Pediatric Hospital of Centro Habana, Havana, Cuba*

probability been wiped off by this time. The advent of acquired immunodeficiency syndrome (AIDS) has provided new fodder for the *Mycobacterium*, which thrives in the immunocompromised and protects itself by acquired resistance. A consistent strategy to control MDR by using agents such as IFN gamma can control further spread of the disease and protect individuals at risk.

In this chapter we will focus on the role of IFN gamma as the principal macrophage-activating cytokine as well as their antifibrotic properties. Later on we will showed the results of several clinical trials which recombinant IFN gamma was used as immunoadjuvant to standard chemotherapy in patients with drug-resistant tuberculosis and other mycobacterial diseases.

2. Why can Interferon gamma be used for the treatment of Multidrug Resistant (MDR) tuberculosis?

Interferon (IFN) gamma, a dimeric protein composed of 146 amino acids and variable molecular weight depending of their glycosylation patterns, was discovered in 1965. The recombinant monomeric non glycosylated form has a molecular weight of 16-17 Kd, but it is twice when the active dimeric form is formed (Schreiber & Farrar, 1993). This cytokine is secreted by CD4+, CD8+ and Natural Killers (NK) cells. Nevertheless CD4+ Th1 lymphocytes, in response to an antigenic stimulus, are the main producers (Wang et al., 1999). IFN gamma is different to other interferons regarding its physiology, activation/modulation system and genetic regulation. The most striking differences between IFN gamma and other classes of interferons concern the immunomodulatory properties of this molecule. While gamma, alpha and beta interferons share certain biological properties (e.g. antiviral, antitumoral), IFN gamma, also known as immune IFN, has potent phagocyte-activating effects not seen with other IFN preparations. IFN gamma function has been strongly conserved throughout evolution and across multiple species. The biological response to IFN gamma is mediated by a cascade of complex cytoplasm and nuclear events that presuppose as first condition the binding of the ligand (IFN gamma) to their specific surface receptor (IFNGR). This receptor is a heterodimer, with IFNGR1 and IFNGR2 chains, and is present on the surface of many inflammatory cells. Binding of IFN gamma to IFNGR leads to modulation of nuclear gene expression via the Janus kinase (JAK)-STAT signaling pathway as follows. JAK associated with IFNGR phosphorylates STAT1. This enters the nucleus, where it binds to promoter regions of IFNG-inducible genes [Schroder et al., 2004]. The rationale of the use of exogenous IFN gamma for the treatment of MDR tuberculosis is based on:

2.1 Adjunctive immunotherapy may be particularly useful in the management of difficult-to treat tuberculosis or tuberculosis in the immunodeficient host

Tuberculosis (TB) is not yet a defeated affection. Although it is a controllable infection at community level and curable in an individual manner, its eradication seems distant. TB is an endemic disease in many parts of the world steadily decimating the population. At present, at least one third of the world population is infected with the *Mycobacterium tuberculosis*. The emergency of multidrug-resistant (MDR) strains has increased this world problem, leading to a high morbidity and mortality. Global estimates showed 9.27 million new cases of TB and 1.77 million deaths from TB in 2007 (WHO, 2009), which is the highest number of deaths attributable to a single infectious agent and corresponds to the 7th cause of death in the world. The World Health Organization (WHO) has estimated that in 2008 there were 440 000 people had MDR-TB worldwide and that a third of them died. Almost 50% of MDR-TB cases worldwide are estimated to occur in China and India (WHO, 2010). The mean survival of MDR-TB affected patients ranges from 2 to 14 months. The importance of treating MDR-TB can therefore not be overemphasized.

Directly Observed Treatment, Short-course chemotherapy (DOTS) strategy has helped prevent non-compliance and treatment failure. However drug resistance has been reduced though not eliminated, and what is been particularly worrisome is the MDR-TB. Multi drug resistance has different definitions in different countries. In the United States it is defined as resistance to rifampicin and isoniazid, while in South America it is resistance to one reserve drug in addition to rifampicin and isoniazid. It is therefore recommended that patients be classified as those resistant to the essential drugs, and those resistant to essential and reserve drugs (Mishin et al., 2002). A subset of MDR-TB strains has been identified as extensively (or extremely) drug-resistant (XDR-TB). These are now defined as being resistant not only to isoniazid and rifampin, but also to fluoroquinolones and to at least one of three injectable drugs usually employed in second-line therapy of MDR-TB: capreomycin, kanamycin and amikacin (Ginsberg, & Spigelman, 2007).

The increase in MDR-TB represents a serious set back to efforts in gaining control of tuberculosis. Resistance to drugs means a greater chance for an infected person remaining infectious and spreading the disease. It is thus imperative to control MDR-TB if we are to ever eradicate this disease. Patients of MDR-TB are difficult to treat, and mortality is significantly higher than in TB caused by susceptible organisms, as is the rate of re-infection. MDR tuberculosis poses a threat to both, the patient and the society. The patient is at risk of losing if not the life, a part of the lung permanently, while the society is at a risk of an MDR-TB epidemic (Yew, 2011). Such an epidemic is a serious threat to the life of individuals with a compromised immune system. The number of people with co-infection of HIV and TB is rising by leaps and bounds. This is a population at very high risk since, TB is the largest single cause of death in HIV infected persons (Daikos et al., 2003).

The infection is mainly transmitted by inhalation of the bacilli coming from infected secretions of the respiratory airways. Once inhaled, the bacilli are subjected to phagocytosis within the alveolar macrophages, where they can be destroyed. Nevertheless, *Mycobacterium tuberculosis* has developed mechanisms to adapt to the noxious intracellular environment of macrophages and escapes the host's innate immunity. It uses several strategies to avoid their destruction, including inhibition of the acidification/maturation of the phagosomes and phagosomal-lysosomal fusion (Pietersen et al., 2004) or by a directly inhibition of the human T cell IFN gamma production and proliferation in response to stimulation (Peng et al., 2011). Thus the *mycobacteria* can persist, replicate and disseminate, leading to new infectious foci. The emergence of resistance depends on several factors such as bacillar initial load, inadequate or incomplete chemotherapy administration, and the patient's immune condition.

Chemotherapy is successful in most cases given that they follow thoroughly the treatment schedule, which is prolonged, costly, and needs to be directly observed. Otherwise it is inadequate to kill all the bacilli and drug resistance emerges. Toxicities are frequent as well.

Treatment for MDR-TB typically requires 18–24 months of combination therapy with second-line drugs that are less efficacious, more toxic and much more expensive than the four first-line drugs. TB treatment in HIV-positive patients is further complicated by drug-drug interactions between some of the antiretroviral agents and key antituberculous drugs, especially rifampin. As *Mycobacterium tuberculosis* drug resistance is increasing worldwide, there is an urgent need for novel interventions in the fight against tuberculosis. The main goal consist in improving capacity to treat existing drug-resistant cases effectively, in order to provide patients with the greatest opportunity for a successful outcome (Ginsberg, & Spigelman, 2007). At the global level, the rational use of existing compounds must be urgently promoted to preserve their utility in treating the most difficult tuberculosis cases and intensify efforts to develop novel interventions (including new drugs and vaccines) to fight tuberculosis more effectively.

The immunologic approach to TB treatment can be promising since only 10 - 20% of infected people develop the disease and many of them have spontaneous remission. Therefore, an alternative therapeutic target can be directed to the manipulation of the host's defenses. In patients with active tuberculosis, *M. tuberculosis*-specific T-cell responses are low, and tissue-destructive and macrophage-deactiviting cytokines are upregulated. These patients have a relative weakness of production of the Th1-like cytokines Interleukin (IL-2) and IFN gamma. By contrast, the production of the immunosuppressive/macrophage-deactiviting cytokines Transforming Growth Factor (TGF) beta and IL-10 is upregulated (Tomioka, 2004). These immune dysfunctions correlate with the extent of pulmonary tuberculosis, more markedly in HIV-infected patients (Zhang et al., 1994). TGF beta is produced in excess by monocytes of patients with tuberculosis, and is present at sites of tuberculous granulomas (Aung et al., 2000).

Therapies that would upregulate the host immune response and/or attenuate the effects of tissue-damaging, macrophage-deactivating and/or T-cell-suppressive cytokines may prove to be helpful in the treatment of tuberculosis, particularly MDR-TB and tuberculosis among patients with HIV infection. Enhancing host immune responses by adjunctive immunotherapy may truncate the duration of chemotherapy, and thereby abolish the need for administration of and compliance with complex drug regimens. In that sense, T helper 1 cytokines, such as IFN gamma, IL-2, and IL-12 through increment of T-cell function and macrophage activation may prove to be potent immunotherapeutic agents.

Interferons are endogenous immunomodulators that play an active role in protecting the individuals from opportunistic infections. They were first used for the treatment of hard to treat virus and fungal infections, now with the availability of recombinant IFN it is possible to use this agent for the treatment of infections caused by drug resistant organisms. IFN gamma activates macrophages and also promotes a range of host immune responses. It helps in decreasing the bacterial load by a number of intermediate messengers such as the superoxide moiety, hydrogen peroxide, etc (Mata-Espinosa & Hernández-Pando, 2008).

2.2 IFN gamma plays a key role in the modulation of immune response and is responsible for the defense against intracellular *mycobateria*

Due to their pleiotrophic effects on the immune system, IFN gamma was thought to have great promise as an immunomodulatory drug. IFN gamma has been shown to be important for the function and maturation of multiple immune cells. It is essential for Th1 immune responses and regulates T cell differentiation, activation, expansion, homeostasis, and survival. Killing of intracellular pathogens requires IFN gamma production by T cells showing to be a critical cytokine in the resistance of infected macrophages. T regulatory cell (Treg) generation and activation requires IFN gamma. This cytokine stimulates dendritic cells and macrophages to upregulate the immune response. NK cells secrete IFN gamma early in host infection, facilitating immune cell recruitment and activation. IFN gamma also activates NK cells and enhances the antibody-dependent cellular cytotoxicity (ADCC). It recruits neutrophils, stimulates them to upregulate chemokines and adhesion molecules, and triggers rapid superoxide production and respiratory burst (Miller et al., 2009).

As most of the intracellular infections, immunity to tuberculosis depends on the development of CD4+ T cells- and macrophages-mediated Th1 response. The proper formation and function of granulomas at sites of *Mycobacterium tuberculosis* infection depends on the collective activity of several cytokines. Enough evidences exist related to the action of IFN gamma on the immunoregulatory activity of macrophages, including alveolar macrophages, which are important in host immunity against *M. tuberculosis* (Tomioka, 2004). There is present certain heterogeneity in human IFN gamma responses to *M. tuberculosis* according to specific strain sensibility (Cabral et al., 2010).

The role of IFN gamma as the main macrophage–activator Th1 cytokine has been clearly established in animal models infected with *M. tuberculosis* since it was able to produce bacilli destruction. Mice rendered incapable of IFN gamma production by gene targeting develop widespread mycobacterial infection with very poor granulomatous response and succumb rapidly. Exogenously supplied IFN gamma has not able to restore normal mycobacterial resistance in these mice, suggesting that IFN gamma plays a critical development role as well (Flynn et al., 1993).

IFN gamma action on the macrophages leads to kill intracellular *Mycobacteria*. Their broad range of biological activities include stimulation of macrophages to produce Tumor Necrosis Factor (TNF) alpha, oxygen free radicals (superoxide anion and H_2O_2) and nitric oxide, increases MHC surface antigens and Fc receptors display, increases expression of costimulatory molecules and decreases lysosomal pH. IFN gamma and TNF alpha cooperate in the induction of phagocytic activity in the mononuclear cells and are also involved in the regulation of the inflammatory response. IFN gamma downregulates the production of the macrophage-inhibitory cytokines IL-4 and IL-10. Additionally, IFN gamma increases the intracellular concentration of certain antibiotics among then macrolides and quinolones (Herbst, 2011; Holland, 2001; Tomioka, 2004). Therefore, its use as adjuvant is justified since existent multidrug therapy, despite its limited efficacy, must be offered to the patients.

The general involved pathway is the following: IL-12 and the pro-inflammatory cytokines (IL-1, TNF alpha and IL-6) are produced early after the interaction of *Mycobacterium tuberculosis*-infected macrophages and CD4+ T cells, and upregulate CD4+ T-cell production of IFN gamma and IL-2. IFN gamma upregulates macrophage ability to contain the growth of *M. tuberculosis*, and IL-2 is key in the clonal expansion of specific CD4+ T cells. IL-10 and TGF beta are later products of these macrophages, and both inhibit the CD4+ T cell cytokine (IL-2, IFN gamma) response and interfere with the effects of IFN gamma. TGF beta is also auto-induced (Figure 1).

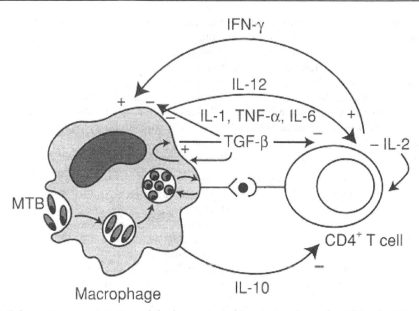

Fig. 1. Schematic representation of the known cytokine network produced by the interaction between CD4+ T cells and *Mycobacterium tuberculosis* (MTB)-infected macrophages.

IFN gamma and TNF alpha are present *in situ* in the paucibacillary pleural form of tuberculosis, in which the host successfully contains the replication of *M. tuberculosis*. In contrast, TGF beta increases the intracellular growth of *M. tuberculosis*. Also, neutralizing antibody to TGF beta reduce the intracellular growth of *M. tuberculosis* in monocites. TGF beta interferes with the production of TNF alpha and IFN gamma and it also downmodulates the bactericidal effect of both cytokines in *M. tuberculosis*-infected monocytes (Hirsch et al., 1994).

The Th1 cells-mediated generation of toxic oxygen metabolites within phagocytes *in vitro* is also capable of mediating the intracellular killing of other selected bacterial or parasites microorganisms such as *Staphylococcus aureus*, *Toxoplasma gondii*, *Leishmania donovani*, *Listeria monocytogenes*, *Mycobacterium avium intracellulare*, *Mycobacterium Leprae*, *Mycobacterium ulcerans* and *Trypanosoma cruzi* (Billiau et al., 1998; El Ridi et al., 2006; Silva et al., 2009).

Mice models confirm the requirement of T CD4+ cells for immunity to *M. avium* strains with low or intermediate virulence. Addition of IL-4 or IL-10 to macrophages culture tried with IFN gamma inhibited the generation of oxygen free radicals (Holland, 2001; Tomioka, 2004). On the other hand, IFN gamma plays an important role in the resistance to *M. leprae* infection (Lima et al., 2000). Those individuals who present absence of IFN gamma and live in endemic areas of visceral leishmaniasis have disease progression (Carvalho et al., 1992).

The concept that IFN gamma can be useful in mycobacterial infections is supported by individuals with impaired IFN gamma action. Lack of production of this cytokine or expression of its receptor increase susceptibility to develop the disease or is associated to the infection's most lethal forms or disease progression. Recurrences or development of the serious forms of infections with atypical *mycobacteria* have been detected in certain families that present mutations in the gene encoding for the IFN gamma receptor binding chain (IFNGR1) (Sexton & Harrison, 2008). Patients with defects in the production of IFN gamma or partial deficiencies of IFN gamma receptor can obtain benefits with IFN gamma treatment (Hallstrand et al., 2004). Similar outcome could be obtained in patients with dysfunctions related to other Th1 cytokines and their receptors (Alangari, et al., 2011). Additionally, patients without genetic disorders but with serum anti-IFN gamma autoantibodies have a higher susceptibility to develop Mycobacteriosis (Kampitak et al., 2011). IFN gamma production appears to decline with age, and this may contribute to the increased susceptibility of the elderly to mycobacterial infection (Rink et al., 1998).

Although for many years IFN gamma have been considered as a pro-inflammatory cytokine, sometimes associated with the pathogenesis of inflammatory and autoimmune diseases, more and more evidences of their anti-inflammatory actions appeared nowadays, supposing a dual effect. It unregulated several pro-inflammatory parameters such as IL-12, TNF alpha, IFN-inducible protein 10 (IP-10), among others, but it also induces anti-inflammatory molecules as IL-1 receptor antagonist (IL-1Ra) or IL-18 binding protein (IL-18BP), modulates the production of pro-inflammatory cytokines, and induces suppressive pathways of the inflammation (Mühl & Pfeilschifter, 2003).

2.3 Interferon gamma has also a potent antifibrotic effect

Extensive tissue destruction, formation of cavities, and fibrosis are characteristic of the pathology of human tuberculosis. Although some components of the *mycobacteria* may be directly associated in activating cellular proteases, most of the affection induced by the organism is probably cytokine-mediated.

The molecular biology of the fibrosis is characterized by a shift to increased production of Th2 cytokines and decreased production of Th1 cytokines. Th1 cytokines promote cell-mediated immunity and remove cellular antigens; decrease fibroblast procollagen mRNA, fibroblast proliferation, and fibroblast-mediated angiogenesis; and downregulate the growth mediator TGF beta. Contrarily, Th2 cytokines promote humoral immunity and produce antibody responses that can lead to fibroblast activation and fibrosis. The Th1 response is characterized by increased expression of IFN gamma, IL-2, IL-12, and IL-18. The net effect of a predominantly Th1 response is tissue restoration. The Th2 response is characterized by increased expression of IL-4, IL-5, IL-10, and IL-13. The net effect of a predominantly Th2 response is fibroblast activation and matrix deposition, leading to fibrosis (Figure 2). IFN gamma appears to restore the balance between Th1 and Th2 responses.

Enough evidences demonstrate the relevant role of IFN gamma to control the disease, since its antifibrotic properties. IFN gamma inhibits lung fibroblast proliferation and chemotaxis in a dose dependent manner. In the bleomycin-induced model of lung fibrosis, IFN gamma downregulates the transcription of the gene for TGF beta but production of IFN gamma may be decreased in patients with Idiopathic Pulmonary Fibrosis (IPF). IFN gamma reduces collagen synthesis and increases the activity of the collagenase (Tredget et al., 2000; Williams et al., 2008). Furthermore, IFN gamma contributes to the tissue repair and their remodeling (Pilette et al., 1997). This antifibrotic action agrees with that obtained with IFN gamma in IPF patients (see last paragraph on this section) and suggests that FN gamma may have a potential therapeutic role in the management of pulmonary fibrotic diseases, including tuberculosis (Williams & Wilson, 2008; Zhang & Phan, 1996).

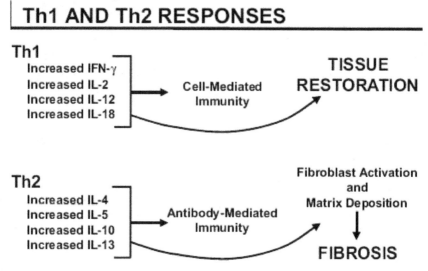

Th1 AND Th2 RESPONSES

Fig. 2. Th1 and Th2 Responses and pulmonary fibrosis.

TGF beta and IFN gamma have opposite effects on diverse cellular functions and the fibrotic events are not an exception. The excessive production of TGF beta is associated with extensive fibrosis and tissue damage. TGF beta is a strong inhibitor of epithelial and endothelial cell growth, and while it promotes the production and deposition of collagen matrix, it has also shown to increase the production of macrophage collagenases. Mice injected intraperitoneally with TGF beta develop generalized fibrosis (Xu et al. 2003). IFN gamma is a potent antagonist of TGF beta (Tredget et al., 2000), involved directly in the pathogenesis of many fibrotic lung diseases (e.g. IPF, bleomycin-induced fibrosis and sarcoidosis) (Zhang & Phan, 1996).

TGF beta signals through a receptor serine kinase that phosphorylates and activates the transcription factors Smad2 and Smad3, whereas the IFN gamma receptor and its associated protein tyrosine kinase Jak1 mediate phosphorylation and activation of the transcription factor Stat1. IFN gamma inhibits the TGF beta–induced phosphorylation of Smad3 and its attendant events: the association of Smad3 with Smad4, the accumulation of Smad3 in the cell nucleus, and the activation of TGF beta–responsive genes. IFN gamma, acting through Jak1 and Stat1, induces the expression of Smad7, an antagonistic SMAD, which prevents Smad3 from interacting with the TGF beta receptor. The results indicate a mechanism of transmodulation between the STAT and SMAD signal-transduction pathways and suggest a role for IFN gamma in the treatment of pulmonary fibrosis (Ulloa et al., 1999).

The first report about the use of IFN gamma in IPF demonstrated a considerable clinical improvement in these patients treated during one year compared to those that received placebo (Ziesche et al., 1999). Afterward, a phase III study was carried out, but no significant advantages in progression-free survival, pulmonary functionality or quality of life were observed. Nevertheless, patients with an initial less deteriorate pulmonary function impairment showed better survival (Raghu et al., 2004). Other authors indicate that IFN gamma can slow or arrested the loss of lung function, increase longevity and make possible lung transplantation (Nathan et al., 2004). Long-term treatment with this cytokine may improve survival and outcome in patients with mild-to-moderate IPF (Antoniou et al., 2006). However, the members of the recent INSPIRE trial declared that they cannot recommend one-year treatment with IFN gamma-1b since the drug did not improve survival in this disease (King et al., 2009). Our group found that in IPF a rapid clinical response could be obtained with a therapeutic schedule with IFN gamma combined with decreasing-dose prednisone (Cayón et al., 2010).

3. Clinical application of recombinant IFN gamma in multidrug – resistant tuberculosis and other mycobacterial diseases

There are reported several clinical trials where IFN gamma was used in combination with anti-TB drugs for the treatment of pulmonary TB. Some of these trials were conducted in drug-susceptible patients. Therefore, in our opinion these last studies have lower relevance or clinical impact than MDR-TB cases; despite in some of them combined treatment yielded better results than chemotherapy alone. In this review we include, in chronological order, several uncontrolled or controlled trials in patients with MDR-TB. Available communications of case report will be also included. Different routes of administration, subcutaneous, intramuscular, aerosol, have been evaluated for this immunoadjuvant cytokine. The aerosol route of administration has been proposed as organ specific delivery method, obtaining a high release to infected alveoli (Condos et al., 2004).

In spite of their high heterogeneity most of the studies refer as primary outcome the sputum negative conversion (sputum smear and/or *M. tuberculosis* culture) at a specific number of months after therapy. The secondary outcomes included chest radiographic improvement and severe adverse events. Chest radiographic improvement was defined as a decrease in the extent of lesions in the lungs, and some cases as a >50% decrease in the cavity size at a specific number of months after treatment. Other outcomes included biochemical variables reflecting immune function, and bacteriological relapse after completion of treatment. Nevertheless all trials did not have remarkably large sample sizes, which made it difficult to obtain definitive evidences.

Systemic or aerosolized IFN gammas have been reported as satisfactory in other similar intracellular infections, including other mycobacterial infections (e.g. intrinsically resistant *Mycobacterium avium*). At the end of this chapter we also show the most relevant reports regarding these species. The majority of the clinical trials here presented have been performed using Actimmune® (InterMune) or IFN gamma-1b, a genetically engineered form of human IFN gamma.

3.1 Clinical trials and case report of aerosolized or systemically administered IFN gamma in patients with drug-resistant tuberculosis

In a first report (Condos et al., 1997) safety and tolerability of aerosolized IFN gamma was investigated in patients with MDR-TB in an open-label trial. In addition, its efficacy in terms of sputum-smear grades was assessed. Aerosolized IFN gamma was given to five patients with smears and cultures positive for pulmonary MDR-TB, despite documented adherence to therapy. The patients received 500 micrograms three times a week for 1 month. IFN gamma was well tolerated by all patients. In all five, bodyweight stabilized or increased. Sputum acid-fast-bacillus smears became negative in all patients, and the time to positive culture increased (from 17 to 24 days, not significant), which suggested that the mycobacterial burden had decreased. The size of cavitary lesions was reduced in all patients, 2 months after treatment had ended. These preliminary, encourage data suggested that IFN gamma may be useful as adjunctive therapy in patients with MDR-TB who are otherwise not responding well to therapy.

Later on, a randomized, placebo-controlled, multicenter trial of inhaled adjunctive IFN gamma for MDR-TB was initiated by InterMune in 2000 (InterMune, 2000). The trial was halted prematurely because of a lack of efficacy, but its findings have never been published.

We carried out an open-label, non-randomized, non-controlled, pilot trial with the aim to evaluate IFN gamma effect on drug resistant pulmonary TB patients regarding their clinical, bacteriological and radiological evolutions (Suárez-Méndez et al., 2004). The study population was constituted by Cuban patients, both sexes, more than eighteen years old, with diagnosis of TB without a favorable response to the usual therapy, who gave their written, informed consent to participate. Patients received 1 x 10^6 IU of human recombinant IFN gamma (Heberon Gamma R®, Heber Biotec, Havana, produced in *Escherichia coli*, specific activity of 10^7 IU/mg protein), intramuscularly, daily during 4 weeks and then 3 times per week for the next 20 weeks. They received anti-TB drugs (WHO schemes) (Crofton et al., 1997), according to the resistance detected in each case by the antibiogram. After the end of the 6-months IFN gamma treatment period, chemotherapy continued up to 9 months if the scheme included rifampin and 18 months otherwise. Complete response was defined as total disappearance of all signs and symptoms, negative sputum acid-fast-bacilli smear and culture, and pulmonary lesions improvement at X-ray. Partial response included signs and symptoms decrease, negative sputum smear and culture and stable X-ray lesions. No response consisted in signs and symptoms persistence, positive bacteriological examinations, and lesions stabilization or progression.

Five of the eight included patients were men, six of them non-white. The age ranged between 23 and 54 years old, and Body Mass Index (BMI) between 13.2 and 22.0 Kg/m^2. Their main symptoms were cough, expectorations, dyspnea, stertors, distal cyanosis, and finger clubbing. Bacteriological tests codification was mostly high and all patients showed active lesions at thorax radiography. A rapid favorable evolution was obtained after treatment with IFN gamma (Table 1).

Clinical improvement was evident since the first month of treatment, when all signs and symptoms (except for finger clubbing) had disappeared in all patients and BMI increased in all but one of them. Sputum acid-fast-bacilli smears and cultures were negative since the 1 - 3 months of treatment. The eight patients had radiological improvement, with lesions size reduction (total disappearance in one case) (Figure 3). This radiological effect cannot be attributable to the antibiotics, since it is well known that DR-TB patients only develop radiological improvement long time after sputum smears and culture become negative. In many cases extensive fibrotic lesions never improve, and stay stable for life. Globular sedimentation rates decreased (2 of them normalized) in five out of 6 patients who had abnormal values at inclusion. At the end of the IFN gamma treatment all the patients were evaluated as complete responders (Suárez-Méndez et al., 2004).

Patient	1	2	3	4	5	6	7	8
Drug regimen	ETB ETN PRZ CPF KAN	RIF ETB PRZ KAN	ETB ETN PRZ CPF KAN	ETB ETN PRZ CPF AMK	RIF ETB PRZ KAN	ETB ETN PRZ CPF KAN	RIF ETB PRZ KAN	RIF ETB PRZ KAN
Gain BMI (Kg/m^2)	1.8	0.4	0.4	0.4	0.3	2.2	1.8	- 2.1
Sputum smear status	Negative	Negative	Negative	Negative	Negative	Negative	Negative	Negative
Sputum culture status	Negative	Negative	Negative	Negative	Negative	Negative	Negative	Negative
Conversion time	2 mo.	3 mo.	3 mo.	1 mo.	3 mo.	2 mo.	2 mo.	3 mo.
Thorax X-ray	Residual fibrosis	Reabsorption and residual fibrosis	Residual bilateral fibrosis.	Lesions resolution	Residual fibrosis	Lesions size reduction	Residual fibrosis	Lesions size reduction
GSR (mm/h)	5	48	26	40	42	20	23	77

BMI: Body Mass Index, GSR: Globular sedimentation rate. RIF: Rifampin; ETB: Ethambutol; ETN: Ethionamide; PRZ: Pyrazinamide; CPF: Ciprofloxacin; KAN: Kanamycin; AMK: Amikacin.

Table 1. Six months follow-up data of DR-TB patients treated with IFN gamma.

The treatment with Heberon Gamma R® was safe and well tolerated. The adverse events were arthralgias, fever, headache and asthenia. All adverse events were mild, except for one moderate fever, which was efficiently controlled with acetaminophen. Significant differences were not detected in other clinical laboratory tests. Seven of the eight patients remained bacteriologically, clinically and radiologically negative at least twelve months after the treatment with IFN gamma concluded. Clinical practice demonstrates that these results are very difficult to obtain in such a short period of time with the chemotherapy alone. None of previous historical controls at the same hospital reached culture conversion at three months of treatment with chemotherapy and less than half had converted at six months. Their clinical outcome was also worse (Suárez-Méndez et al., 2004).

The same IFN gamma was evaluated with a similar trial design in a MDR-TB Indian outpatient setting (unpublished data). Ten patients were included, 60% were men, with a mean age of 29 years. Previous treatment all the isolations were resistant to rifampicin and isoniazid. A reduction in the number of patients with positive sputum was recorded. A significant increment (1.6 g/dL) in hemoglobin values took place. The percent of damaged left lung decreased significantly (twice). Right lung and total fibrosis were also reduced but not significantly. At the end of treatment a complete clinical response and radiological improvement was obtained in most of the cases. All the patients presented adverse events, headache prevailed (50%). All the events were mild or moderate, and no case stop the treatment because intolerability.

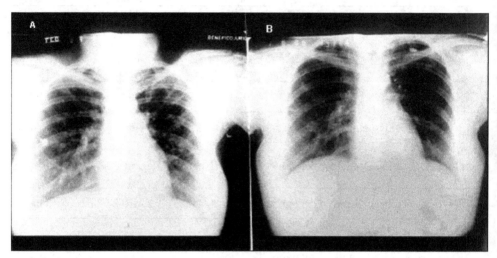

Fig. 3. Radiological improvement with IFN gamma treatment (ray-x of one patients are shown). Legend: (A), left-lung fibroexudative lesions, and (B) complete resolution after IFN gamma treatment. (Picture taken from Suárez-Méndez et al., 2004)

Aerosolized IFN gamma was given to six MDR-TB Korean patients with persistent positive smears and cultures despite long-term medical treatment (Koh et al., 2004). The patients received aerosolized 2×10^6 IU of IFN gamma three times a week for 6 months while they continued on identical antituberculous chemotherapy. Before IFN gamma inhalation therapy, the patients received a median of 6.5 (range, 4 to 7) antituberculous drugs for median duration of 29 months (range, 7 to 76). After IFN gamma inhalation therapy, sputum smears remained persistently positive in all patients throughout the study period. Sputum cultures were transiently negative at the 4th month in two patients, but became positive again at the end of 6 months of IFN gamma therapy. Five patients had radiological improvement including three patients who showed a decrease in the size of the cavitary lesions. Resectional surgery could be performed in one patient in whom substantial clinical and radiological improvement was noted after IFN gamma inhalation therapy (Figure 4).

In contrast, adjunctive subcutaneous therapy not improved the sputum culture conversion of refractory or advanced MDR-TB (Park et al., 2007). The authors evaluated the clinical and laboratory effects of subcutaneously administered IFN gamma in this class of patients. Eight patients with sputum smear and culture persistently positive MDR-TB were subcutaneously administered 2×10^6 IU of recombinant human IFN gamma three times a week for 24 weeks (72 doses total). Subjects also received a customized drug regimen containing second- and third-line antituberculosis agents based upon drug susceptibility testing and previous treatment history. Body weight remained stable or slightly decreased in all subjects during the study period, and none displayed radiographic improvement on serial chest computed tomography scanning. Sputum smears and cultures remained positive for all patients, and there was no increase in the mean time to yield a positive culture (from 16.5 to 11.8 days). There was no enhancement of cell-mediated immune responses in terms of production of IFN gamma or IL-10, or of composition of lymphocytes among peripheral blood mononuclear cells. In four patients, therapy was discontinued because of adverse reactions. In conclusion they did not obtain improvement in clinical, radiologic, microbiologic, or immunologic parameters.

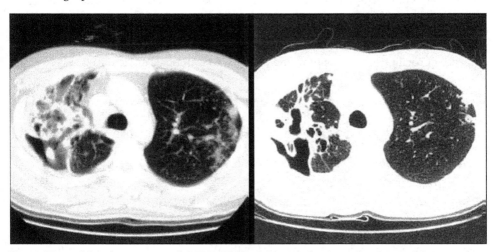

Fig. 4. 27-yr-old male patient with MDR-TB. (Left image) Computed tomographic scan of the chest showed multiple cavities in the right upper lobe and big nodular infiltrations in the left upper lobe. (Right image) After 6 months of IFN gamma inhalation therapy, computed tomographic scan showed reduction in the size of cavitary lesions and improvement of nodular infiltrates. (Picture taken from Koh et al., 2004).

In another protocol, four MDR-TB patients were treated with aerosolized recombinant IFN gamma twice weekly for 8 weeks and anti-tuberculosis drugs. Patients were monitored clinically and T-cell subpopulations were analyzed. The treatment was well tolerated. All sputum smears cleared within 6–8 weeks, and radiological signs of recovery lasted in all patients for 73–106 months (the entire follow-up period). Before treatment, a patient with a 20+ year history of TB showed no γδ T-cells; these cells appeared during treatment. The proportion of natural killer (NK) cells was enhanced during treatment and remained elevated. The proportion of CD4+/CD25+ T-cells in the blood rose after treatment and remained elevated at 2 and 10 months afterwards. No significant change in T-cell levels appeared in patients with a shorter history of TB, except for a tendency toward a slight increase in γδ T-cells during treatment (Grahmann & Braun, 2008).

At least two controlled clinical studies were carried out in Chinese MDR-TB patients (Yang et al., 2009; Yao, & Liu, 2003). These trials directly compared aerosolized IFN gamma plus anti-TB drugs with the same anti-TB drugs. The sample size was around 30 patients per group. Human recombinant IFN gamma was administered by aerosol at 1×10^6 IU per dose, three times weekly for 2 - 3 months. Anti-TB drug regimens varied in the trials. The follow-up time ranged from 9 to 12 months. Both trials were open-labeled. One trial (Yang et al., 2009) was randomized and the other (Yao, & Liu, 2003) was unclear. Both studies reported higher smear conversion rates in the IFN gamma-treated group compared with the control group after 3 months of treatment or at the completion of chemotherapy, although there were no statistically significant differences. Chest radiographs demonstrated cavitary lesion reduction after 2 months of treatment.

Gamma interferon therapy in patients co-infected with HIV and tuberculosis receiving TB medications is safe, improves clinical outcome and enhances host defense mechanism (Yola et al., 2006). Recombinant IFN gamma-1b adjuvant therapy plus DOTS in cavitary pulmonary tuberculosis can reduce inflammatory cytokines at the site of disease, improve clearance of bacilli from the sputum, and improve constitutional symptoms (Dawson et al., 2009).

The results of all these trials need to be viewed from both the individual patient's and the society's perspective. A patient of MDR-TB continues downhill, even in the presence of therapy, to finally lose a lung or even his life. From the point of view of the society, the conversion of patients from infective to non-infective is a major achievement (Noeske & Nguennko, 2002; Subhash et al., 2003).

In the literature can be also found the adjunctive treatment with IFN gamma of an immunocompromised patient who had refractory MDR-TB of the brain and spinal cord (Raad et al., 1996). Despite treatment with six antituberculous drugs for 11 months, there was no appreciable clinical or radiological improvement in the patient's condition. Within 5 months of initiating adjunctive therapy with IFN gamma and granulocyte colony stimulating factors, substantial neurological and radiological improvement was noted. Therapy with IFN gamma was continued for 12 months, resulting in complete resolution of the lesions in the brain and spinal cord.

3.2 Results from different trials and case report in other mycobacterial diseases or similar

IFN gamma has been effective as adjuvant in AIDS patients co-infected with *Mycobacterium avium* complex (MAC), where a clear decrement in the bacteremia was verified. These results were obtained in patients with low CD4+ lymphocytes counts, suggesting a non T cell-mediated effect (Squires et al., 1992). Holland and colleagues treated non-HIV patients with refractory disseminated nontuberculous mycobacterial infections. Three patients were from a family predisposed to the development of MAC infections; four patients had idiopathic CD4+ T-lymphocytopenia. Their infections were culture- or biopsy-proved, involved at least two organ systems, and had been treated with the maximal tolerated medical therapy. IFN gamma was administered subcutaneously two or three times weekly in a dose of 25 to 50 μg/m^2 in addition to antimycobacterial medications. In response to phytohemagglutinin, the production of IFN gamma by mononuclear cells from the patients was lower than in normal subjects (P<0.001). Within eight weeks of the start of IFN gamma therapy, all seven patients had marked clinical improvement, with abatement of fever, clearing of many lesions and quiescence of others, radiographic improvement, and a reduction in the need for paracentesis (Holland et al., 1994).

Around one year later was reported a 38-yr-old man negative for HIV, with silicosis and advanced cavitary lung disease due to *Mycobacterium avium intracellulare*, who failed to improve despite 3 yr of continuous medical therapy with three or more drugs. He received three courses of aerosolized IFN gamma (500 micrograms 3 d per week for 5 wk in two courses and 200 micrograms 3 d a week for 5 wk after a short single trial of subcutaneous IFN gamma). The numbers of bacilli decreased in the sputum during therapy, but cultures of the organism remained positive at the same level for the first two treatment periods. The patient's sputum became smear negative and the number of colonies decreased significantly after the third course of IFN gamma therapy. Cessation of IFN gamma was associated with a rapid increase in the numbers of bacilli (Chatte et al., 1995).

Fifteen patients with disseminated MAC and other nontuberculous mycobacteria infections were treated with subcutaneous IFN gamma during one year or more, 13 of them had clinical improved and 7 had even apparent disease eradication (Holland, 1996). Two human immunodeficiency virus–infected patients with refractory disseminated MAC infection were treated with recombinant IFN gamma given subcutaneously for 3 and 4 months, respectively. Although both patients demonstrated some clinical improvement initially, IFN gamma therapy did not produce sustained benefit (Lauw et al, 2001). It has been reported that a randomized trial testing this option was stopped early due to lack of efficacy (Lam et al, 2006).

A randomized, double-blind, placebo-controlled trial was done with the objective to assess the immunoadjuvant IFN gamma effect in patients with pulmonary atypical Mycobacteriosis regarding their clinical, bacteriological and radiological evolutions. Additionally, several immune response and oxidative stress markers were measured. The diagnosis comprised isolation and classification of any of the atypical Mycobacteria species three or more times in sputum-culture samples, symptoms such as cough and expectoration, and tuberculosis-like pulmonary lesions at thorax radiography. Patients were distributed to receive intramuscular IFN gamma as adjuvant to oral chemotherapy (IFN group) or chemotherapy plus placebo (placebo group) during 6 months (Milanés-Virelles et al., 2008). Patients received 1 x 10⁶ IU of Heberon Gamma R® or placebo intramuscularly. The schedule of administration and the response criteria were similar to the referred TB study (see Suárez-Méndez et al., 2004). All the patients received the same conventional daily antibiotic schedule, as follows: azithromycin 500 mg, ciprofloxacin 1000 mg, rifampin 600 mg, and ethambutol 2000 mg.

Thirty-two patients were enrolled. Eighteen patients were included in the IFN group and 14 received placebo. Groups were homogeneous at entry; average age was 60 years, 75% men, 84% white; MAC infection prevailed (94%). At the end of treatment, 72% of patients treated with IFN gamma were evaluated as complete responders, but only 36% in the placebo group (Table 2). The difference was maintained during follow-up. A more rapid complete response was obtained in the IFN group (5 months before), with a significantly earlier improvement in respiratory symptoms and pulmonary lesions reduction. Disease-related deaths were 35.7% of the patients in the placebo group and only 11.1% in the IFN group. Three patients in the IFN group normalized their globular sedimentation rate values. Although differences in bacteriology were not significant during the treatment period, some patients in the placebo group converted again to positive during a one-year follow-up. Significant increments in serum TGF beta and advanced oxidation protein products were

Evaluation	Month		IFN gamma	Placebo	P (test)
			Overall response		
Responders [a]	6		13/18 (72.2%)	5/14 (35.7%)	0.037 (χ^2)
(intention-to- treat)	18		12/18 (66.7%)	4/14 (28.6%)	0.030 (χ^2)
Responders (last evaluation)			15/18 (83.3%)	5/14 (35.7%)	0.005 (χ^2)
			Clinical		
	0		15/18 (83.3%)	13/14 (92.9%)	
Dyspnea	6		1/15 (6.7%)	3/9 (33.3%)	0.27 (FE)
	18		1/13 (7.7%)	3/8 (37.5%)	0.25 (FE)
Good general status	0		3/18 (16.7%)	4/14 (28.6%)	
(intention-to-treat)	6		13/18 (72.2%)	5/14 (35.7%)	0.037 (χ^2)
	18		12/18 (66.7%)	4/14 (28.6%)	0.03 (χ^2)
Improvement [b]	6		13/18 (72.2%)	5/14 (35.7%)	0.037 (χ^2)
(intention-to-treat)	18		12/18 (66.7%)	4/14 (28.6%)	0.03 (χ^2)
			Radiological		
		Adv	12 (66.7%)	11(78.6%)	
	0	Mod	5 (27.8%)	3 (21.4%)	
		Min	1 (5.6%)	0	
		Adv	2 (13.3%)	5 (55.6%)	
Lesion extension	6	Mod	12 (80.0%)	3 (33.3%)	1.00 [c] (FE)
		Min	1 (6.7%)	1 (11.1%)	
		Adv	1 (7.7%)	2 (25.0%)	
	18	Mod	5 (38.5%)	5 (62.5%)	0.085 [c] (FE)
		Min	7 (53.8%) [d]	1 (12.5%)	
Improvement	6		12/18 (66.7%)	6/14 (42.8%)	0.32 (χ^2)
(intention to treat)	18		13/18 (72.2%)	4/14 (28.6%)	0.036 (χ^2)
Cavitary lesions disappearance			5/12 (41.7%)	1/12 (8.3%)	0.15 (FE)
			Bacteriological		
	0		14/18 (77.8%)	10/14 (71.4%)	
	Cod.		7 ± 4	8 ± 8	
	6		1/15 (6.7%)	2/10 (20.0%)	0.54 (FE)
Sputum- Direct (+)	Cod.		0 ± 0	0 ± 2	0.28 (MW)
	18		1/13 (7.7%)	3/8 (37.5%)	0.253 (FE)
	Cod.		0 ± 0	0 ± 7	0.112 (MW)
	Relapse		1/13 (7.7%)	3/8 (37.5%)	0.25 (FE)
	0		18 (100%)	14 (100%)	
	Cod.		8 ± 2	9 ± 4	
	6		2/15 (13.3%)	2/10 (20.0%)	1.00 (FE)
Sputum- Culture (+)	Cod.		0 ± 0	0 ± 2	0.60 (MW)
	18		1/13 (7.7%)	4/8 (50.0%)	0.11 (FE)
	Cod.		0 ± 0	0 ± 8	0.042 (MW)
	Relapse		1/13 (7.7%)	3/8 (37.5%)	0.25 (FE)

(St): Student's t test; (MW): Mann-Whitney's U test; all binary variable comparisons were with the Fisher's exact test. [a] All overall responses were complete except for one IFN group case at month 6 with partial response. [b] General clinical status improvement if the patient passed from "bad" to "moderate" or from "moderate" to "good". Adv: Advanced; Mod: Moderate; Min: Minimum; [c] Combining advanced-moderate; [d] One of them had lesions disappearance at this time.

Table 2. Clinical, radiological, bacteriological and overall outcomes during the trial.

observed in the placebo group but not among IFN receiving patients. Treatments were well tolerated. Flu-like symptoms predominated in the IFN gamma group. No severe events were recorded. This report constituted the first and largest randomized, controlled clinical study, using an immunomodulating agent systemically in pulmonary or disseminated atypical Mycobacteriosis (Milanés-Virelles et al., 2008).

Use of a combination of IFN gamma and IL-2 resulted in a remarkable improvement in a 5-year-old girl presented with disseminated *Mycobacterium avium* complex infection during advanced HIV infection, together with an increase in circulating CD4+ T cells (Sekiguchi et al., 2005). A highly unusual case suggests that IFN gamma may be effective in patients with *M. chelonae* infection that fails to respond adequately to antimicrobials (Jousse-Joulin et al., 2007). Short-term IFN gamma-1b and IL-2 might be considered as therapeutic options in refractory mycobacterial infections in patients with idiopathic CD4 lymphopenia (Sternfeld et al., 2010).

The disseminated mycobacterial infection after *Bacillus Calmette-Guerin* (BCG) vaccination is a very rare disorder that appears mainly in immunocompromised patients. Two pediatric patients with adverse reactions induced by the BCG vaccine, both expressed by suppurative and abscessed regional lymphadenitis, one month after birth, were successfully treated with recombinant IFN gamma (6 months as minimum) after failed courses of chemotherapy (Abreu-Suárez et al., 2008). They showed a marked improvement of lesions after IFN gamma treatment. The evolution of the lesions in the case No.1 is showed in Figure 5. She had imperceptible lesions after 6 months of treatment.

During IFN gamma treatment, only few febrile episodes occurred, well-controlled with antipyretic medication. Both children conserved good general status, normal bodyweight, and no other adenopathies or visceromegaly appeared. During or after IFN gamma treatment no other infections were detected. The first case had a familiar history of tuberculosis (maternal great-grandfather, maternal grandmother and mother), which clearly increases susceptibility to mycobacterial infections by inherited recessive genetic defects. However, the second case did not present those antecedents and an IFNGR1 deficiency was not perceived (Abreu-Suárez et al., 2008).

IFN gamma has been shown efficacy (decrease in acid-fast bacilli) and safety in the treatment of patients with *Mycobaterium leprae*, where immunological pathways for killing intracellular pathogen are similar (Gallin et al., 1995; Nathan et al., 1986). In the 90s IFN gamma was administered to Cuban patients with lepromatous leprosy. Five patients received 1 x10^6 IU of IFN gamma three times per week during six months and other five received placebo solution with the same schedule. Those patients treated with IFN gamma showed better clinical and histological evolution. These patients remained with sensibility damage but all the infiltrated cutaneous lesions were clarified. They had less granuloma and reduced greatly the number of bacilli, which look mostly fragmented. Lepromin skin test and lymphoblastic proliferation test didn't have changes in these patients (unpublished data).

In visceral leishmaniasis, patients treated with short courses of recombinant IFN gamma and pentavalent antimony exhibit favorable results such as decrease of the splenic parasitic load, improvement of the symptoms, gain of body weight and reduction of the spleen size, without relapses after several months of follow-up. Doses up to 8 x 10^6 UI/m^2 of body surface has been used for 20 days without important toxic effects (Badaro et al., 1990; Squires et al., 1993; Sundar et al., 1994).

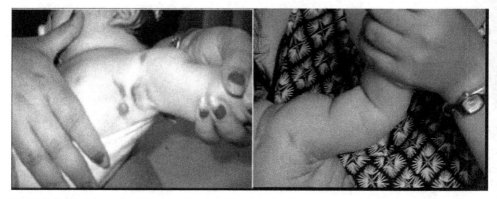

Fig. 5. BCGitis Case No.1: Suppurative axillary and supraclavicular adenopathies after BCG vaccination in a nursing girl. (Left photo): before IFN gamma treatment, (Right photo): complete healing after only 3 months of treatment. (Picture taken from Abreu-Suárez et al., 2008).

4. Conclusions

There is a scientific rationale for the use of recombinant IFN gamma in difficult-to treat cases of tuberculosis and other mycobacterial diseases. By activating macrophages and promoting a range of host immune and antifibrotic responses, IFN gamma may provide an effective adjunct to antimycobacterials in patients not responding to conventional courses of therapy.

Clinical and laboratory experience suggest that adding IFN gamma to established treatment regimens may upregulate macrophage function and decrease mycobacterial load in pulmonary, disseminated and cutaneous infections. Prospective, randomized, more extensive, controlled clinical trials are necessary to confirm previous clinical reports.

Combination with second-line drugs can reduce the time of treatment, diminishing toxicities and possible relapses; in many cases could reduce the application of recessional surgery. Adjunctive immunotherapies, including IFN gamma, will likely play a role in the treatment of mycobacterial disease in the years ahead.

5. References

Abreu-Suárez, G., García-García, I., Fuentes-Fernández, G., Ramos-Gómez, TI., Martínez-Grau, I., González-Méndez,L., & López-Saura, PA. (2008). Suppurative Lymphadenitis Caused by Bacillus Calmette-Guerin Treated with Recombinant Interferon Gamma. Two-Cases Report. *Revista Cubana de Pediatría*, Vol. 80, No. 3, (July-September, 2008), ISSN: 0034-7531

Alangari, AA., Al-Zamil, F., Al-Mazrou, A., Al-Muhsen, S., Boisson-Dupuis, S., Awadallah, S., Kambal, A., & Casanova, JL. (2011). Treatment of disseminated mycobacterial infection with high-dose IFN-γ in a patient with IL-12R□1 deficiency. *Clinical & developmental immunology*, Vol. 2011, (2011), pp. (691956), ISSN: 1740-2522

Antoniou, KM., Nicholson, AG., Dimadi, M., Malagari, K., Latsi, P., Rapti, A., Tzanakis, N., Trigidou, R., Polychronopoulos, V., & Bouros, D. (2006). Long-term clinical effects of interferon gamma-1b and colchicine in idiopathic pulmonary fibrosis. *European Respiratory Journal*, Vol. 28, No. 3, (September, 2006), pp. (496-504), ISSN: 0903-1936

Aung, H., Toossi, Z., McKenna, SM., Gogate, P., Sierra, J., Sada, E., & Rich, EA. (2000). Expression of transforming growth factor-beta but not tumor necrosis factor-alpha, interferon-gamma, and interleukin-4 in granulomatous lung lesions in tuberculosis. *Tubercle and Lung Disease*, Vol. 80, No. 2, (2000), pp. (61-67), ISSN: 0962-8479

Badaro, R., Falcoff, E., Badaro, FS., Carvalho, EM., Pedral-Sampaio, D., Barral, A., Carvalho, JS., Barral-Netto, M., Brandely, M., & Silva, L. Treatment of visceral leishmaniasis with pentavalent antimony and interferon gamma. (1990). *The New England Journal of Medicine*, Vol. 322, No. 1, (January, 1990), pp. (16-21), ISSN: 0028-4793

Billiau, A., Heremans, H., Vermeire, K., & Matthys, P. (1998). Immunomodulatory properties of interferon-gamma. An update. *Annals of the New York Academy of Sciences*, Vol. 856, (September, 1998), pp. (22-32), ISSN: 0077-8923

Cabral, VR., Souza, CF., Guimarães, FL., & Saad, MH. (2010). Heterogeneity in human IFN-γ responses to clinical Mycobacterium tuberculosis strains. *Jornal Brasileiro de Pneumologia*, Vol. 36, No. 4, (August, 2010), pp. (494-497), ISSN: 1806-3713

Carvalho, EM., Barral, A., Pedral-Sampaio, D., Barral-Netto, M., Badaró, R., Rocha, H., & Johnson, WD Jr. (1992). Immunologic markers of clinical evolution in children recently infected with Leishmania donovani chagasi. *The Journal of Infectious Diseases*, Vol. 165, No. 3, (March, 1992), pp. (535-540), ISSN: 0022-1899

Cayón, I., González, L., García, I., Rosas, C, Gassiot, C., García, E., Valenzuela, C., Oramas, M., Sánchez, R., & López, P. (2010). Gamma Interferon and prednisone decreasing-dose therapy in patients with Idiopathic Pulmonary Fibrosis. *Biotecnología Aplicada*, Vol. 27, No. 1 (January-March, 2010), pp. (29-35), ISSN: 1027-2852

Chatte, G., Panteix, G., Perrin-Fayolle, M., & Pacheco, Y. (1995). Aerosolized interferon gamma for Mycobacterium avium-complex lung disease. *American Journal of Respiratory and Critical Care Medicine*, Vol. 152, No. 3, (September, 1995), pp. (1094-1096), ISSN: 1073-449X

Condos, R., Rom, WN., & Schluger, NW. (1997). Treatment of multidrug-resistant pulmonary tuberculosis with interferon-gamma via aerosol. *Lancet*, Vol. 349, No. 9064, (May, 1997), pp. (1513-1515), ISSN: 0140-6736

Condos, R., Hull, FP., Schluger, NW., Rom, WN., & Smaldone, GC. (2004). Regional deposition of aerosolized interferon-gamma in pulmonary tuberculosis. *Chest*, Vol. 125, No. 6, (June, 2004), pp. (2146-2155), ISSN: 0012-3692

Crofton, J., Chaulet, P., & Maher, D. (1997-09). *Guidelines for the management of Drug-Resistant Tuberculosis* (1st Ed.), Word Health Organization, WHO:TB:96.210(Rev.1), ISBN: 0119517698, Geneva, Switzerland

Daikos, GL., Cleary, T., Rodriguez, A., & Fischl, MA. (2003). Multidrug-resistant tuberculous meningitis in patients with AIDS. *The International Journal of Tuberculosis and Lung Disease*, Vol. 7, No. 4, (April, 2003), pp. (394-398), ISSN: 1027-3719

Dawson, R., Condos, R., Tse, D., Huie, ML., Ress, S., Tseng, CH., Brauns, C., Weiden, M., Hoshino, Y., Bateman, E., & Rom, WN. (2009). Immunomodulation with Recombinant Interferon-gamma1b in Pulmonary Tuberculosis. *PloS One*, Vol. 4, No. 9, (September, 2009), pp. (e6984), ISSN: 1932-6203

El Ridi, R., Salem, R., Wagih, A., Mahana, N., El Demellawy, M., & Tallima, H. (2006). Influence of interleukin-2 and interferon-gamma in murine schistosomiasis. *Cytokine*, Vol. 33, No. 5, (March, 2006), pp. (281-288), ISSN: 1043-4666

Flynn, JL., Chan, J., Triebold, KJ., Dalton, DK., Stewart, TA, & Bloom, BR. (1993). An essential role for interferon gamma in resistance to Mycobacterium tuberculosis infection. *The Journal of Experimental Medicine*, Vol. 178, No. 6, (December, 1993), pp. (2249-2254), ISSN: 0022-1007

Gallin, JI., Farber, JM., Holland, SM., & Nutman, TB. (1995). Interferon-gamma in the management of infectious diseases. *Annals of Internal Medicine*, Vol. 123, No. 3, (August, 1995), pp. (216-224), ISSN: 0003-4819

Ginsberg, AM., & Spigelman, M. (2007). Challenges in tuberculosis drug research and development. *Nature Medicine*, Vol. 13, No. 3, (March, 2007), pp. (290-294), ISSN: 1078-8956

Grahmann, PR., & Braun, RK. (2008). A new protocol for multiple inhalation of IFN-γ successfully treats MDR-TB: a case study. *The International Journal of Tuberculosis and Lung Disease*, Vol. 12, No. 6, (June, 2008), pp. (636-644), ISSN: 1027-3719

Hallstrand, TS., Ochs, IID., Zhu, Q., & Liles, WC. (2004). Inhaled IFN-gamma for persistent nontuberculous mycobacterial pulmonary disease due to functional IFN-gamma deficiency. *European Respiratory Journal*, Vol. 24, No. 3, (September, 2004), pp. (367-370), ISSN: 0903-1936

Herbst, S., Schaible, UE., & Schneider, BE. (2011). Interferon gamma activated macrophages kill mycobacteria by nitric oxide induced apoptosis. *PloS One*, Vol. 6, No. 5, (May, 2011), pp. (e19105), ISSN: 1932-6203

Hirsch, CS., Yoneda, T., Averil,l L., Ellner, JJ., & Toossi, Z. (1994). Enhancement of intracellular growth of Mycobacterium tuberculosis in human monocytes by transforming growth factor-beta 1. *The Journal of Infectious Diseases*, Vol. 170, No. 5, (November, 1994), pp. (1229-1237), ISSN: 0022-1899

Holland, SM., Eisenstein, EM., Kuhns, DB., Turner, ML., Fleisher, TA., Strober, W., & Gallin, JI. (1994). Treatment of refractory disseminated nontuberculous mycobacterial infection with interferon gamma. *The New England Journal of Medicine*, Vol. 330, No. 19, (May, 1994), pp. (1348-1355), ISSN: 0028-4793

Holland, SM. (1996). Therapy of mycobacterial infections. *Research in Immunology*, Vol. 147, No. 8-9, (October-December, 1996), pp. (572-581), ISSN: 0923-2494

Holland, SM. (2001). Immunotherapy of mycobacterial infections. *Seminars in Respiratory Infections*, Vol. 16, No. 1, (March, 2001), pp. (47-59), ISSN: 0882-0546

InterMune investor relations press release. (2000). *InterMune enrolls first patient in phase III trial in multidrug-resistant tuberculosis.* 18.05.2010. Available from http://www.hopkins-tb.org/news/ 7-31-2000.shtml

Jousse-Joulin, S., Garre, M., Guennoc, X., Destombe, C., Samjee, I., Devauchelle-Pensec, V., & Saraux, A. (2007). Skin and joint infection by Mycobacterium chelonae: rescue treatment with interferon gamma. *Joint Bone Spine*, Vol. 74, No. 4, (July, 2007), pp. (385-388), ISSN: 1297-319X

Kampitak, T., Suwanpimolkul, G., Browne, S., & Suankratay, C. (2011). Anti-interferon-γ autoantibody and opportunistic infections: case series and review of the literature. *Infection*, Vol. 39, No. 1, (February, 2011), pp. (65-71), ISSN: 0300-8126

King, TE Jr., Albera, C., Bradford, WZ., Costabel, U., Hormel, P., Lancaster, L., Noble, PW., Sahn, SA., Szwarcberg, J., Thomeer, M., Valeyre, D, & du Bois, RM. (2009). Effect of interferon gamma-1b on survival in patients with idiopathic pulmonary fibrosis (INSPIRE): a multicentre, randomized, placebo-controlled trial. *Lancet*, Vol. 374, No. 9685, (July, 2009), pp. (222-228), ISSN: 0140-6736

Koh, WJ., Kwon, OJ., Suh, GY., Chung, MP., Kim, H., Lee, NY., Kim, TS., & Lee, KS. (2004). Six-month therapy with aerosolized interferon-gamma for refractory multidrug-resistant pulmonary tuberculosis. *Journal of Korean Medical Science*, Vol. 19, No. 2, (April, 2004), pp. (167-171), ISSN: 1011-8934

Lam, PK., Griffith, DE., Aksamit, TR., Ruoss, SJ., Garay, SM., Daley, CL., & Catanzaro, A. (2006). Factors Related to Response to Intermittent Treatment of Mycobacterium avium Complex Lung Disease. *American Journal of Respiratory and Critical Care Medicine*, Vol. 173, No. 11, (June, 2006), pp. (1283-1289), ISSN: 1073-449X

Lauw, FN., van Der Meer, JT., de Metz, J., Danner, SA., & van Der Poll, T. (2001). No beneficial effect of interferon-gamma treatment in 2 human immunodeficiency virus-infected patients with Mycobacterium avium complex infection. *Clinical Infectious Diseases*, Vol. 32, No. 4, (February, 2001), pp. (e81-e82), ISSN: 1058-4838

Lima, MC., Pereira, GM., Rumjanek, FD., Gomes, HM., Duppre, N., Sampaio, EP., Alvim, IM., Nery, JA., Sarno, EN., & Pessolani, MC. (2000). Immunological cytokine correlates of protective immunity and pathogenesis in leprosy. *Scandinavian Journal of Immunology*, Vol. 51, No. 4, (April, 2000), pp. (419-428), ISSN: 0300-9475

Mata-Espinosa, DA., & Hernández-Pando, R. (2008). Gamma interferon: basics aspects, clinic significance and therapeutic uses. *Revista de Investigación Clínica*, Vol. 60, No. 5, (September-October, 2008), pp. (421-431), ISSN: 0034-8376

Milanés-Virelles, MT., García-García, I., Santos-Herrera, Y., Valdés-Quintana, M., Valenzuela-Silva, CM., Jiménez-Madrigal, G., Ramos-Gómez, TI., Bello-Rivero, I., Fernández-Olivera, N., Sánchez-de la Osa, RB., Rodríguez-Acosta, C., González-Méndez, L., Martínez-Sánchez, G., & López-Saura, PA. (2008). Adjuvant interferon gamma in patients with pulmonary atypical Mycobacteriosis: a randomized, double-blind, placebo-controlled study. *BMC Infectious Diseases*, Vol. 8, (February, 2008), pp. (17), ISSN: 1471-2334

Miller, CH., Maher, SG., & Young, HA. (2009). Clinical Use of Interferon-gamma. *Annals of the New York Academy of Sciences* Vol. 1182, (December, 2009), pp. (69-79), ISSN: 0077-8923

Mishin, VIu., Chukanov, VI., & Vasil'eva, IA. (2002). Efficacy of treatment for pulmonary tuberculosis with multidrug mycobacterial resistance. *Problemy tuberkuleza*, Vol. 12, (2002), pp. (18-23), ISSN: 0032-9533

Mühl, H., & Pfeilschifter, J. (2003). Anti-inflammatory properties of pro-inflammatory interferon-gamma. *International Immunopharmacology*, Vol. 3, No. 9, (September, 2003), pp. (1247-1255), ISSN: 1567-5769

Nathan, CF., Kaplan, G., Levis, WR., Nusrat, A., Witmer, MD., Sherwin, SA., Job, CK., Horowitz, CR., Steinman, RM., & Cohn, ZA. (1986). Local and systemic effects of intradermal recombinant interferon-gamma in patients with lepromatous leprosy. *The New England Journal of Medicine*, Vol. 315, No. 1, (July, 1986), pp. (6-15), ISSN: 0028-4793

Nathan, SD., Barnett, SD., Moran, B., Helman, DL., Nicholson, K., Ahmad, S., Shorr, AF. (2004). Interferon gamma-1b as therapy for idiopathic pulmonary fibrosis. An intrapatient analysis. *Respiration*, Vol. 71, No. 1, (January-February, 2004), pp. (77-82), ISSN: 0993-9490

Noeske, J., & Nguennko, PN. (2002). Impact of resistance to anti tuberculosis drugs on treatment using World Health Organization standard regimens. *Transactions of the Royal Society of Tropical Medicine and Hygiene*, Vol. 96, No. 4, (July-August, 2002), pp. (429-433), ISSN: 0035-9203

Park, SK., Cho, S., Lee, IH., Jeon, DS., Hong, SH., Smego, RA Jr., & Cho, SN. (2007). Subcutaneously administered interferon-gamma for the treatment of multidrug-resistant pulmonary tuberculosis. *International Journal of Infectious Diseases*, Vol. 11, No. 5, (September, 2007), pp. (434-440), ISSN: 1201-9712

Peng, H., Wang, X., Barnes, PF., Tang, H., Townsend, JC., & Samten, B. (2011). The Mycobacterium tuberculosis early secreted antigenic target of 6 kDa inhibits T cell interferon-gamma production through the p38 mitogen-activated protein kinase pathway. *Journal of Biological Chemistry*, Vol. 286, No. 27, (July, 2011), pp. (24508-24518), ISSN: 0021-9258

Pietersen, R., Thilo, L., & de Chastellier, C. (2004). Mycobacterium tuberculosis and Mycobacterium avium modify the composition of the phagosomal membrane in infected macrophages by selective depletion of cell surface-derived glycoconjugates. *European Journal of Cell Biology*, Vol. 83, No. 4, (May, 2004), pp. (153-158), ISSN: 0171-9335

Pilette, C., Fort, J., Rifflet, H., & Calès, P. (1997). Anti-fibrotic effects of interferons. Mechanisms of action and therapeutic prospects. *Gastroentérologie Clinique et Biologique*, Vol. 21, No. 6-7, (1997), pp. (466-471), ISSN: 0399-8320

Raad, I., Hachem, R., Leeds, N., Sawaya, R., Salem, Z., & Atweh S. (1996). Use of adjunctive treatment with interferon-gamma in an immunocompromised patient who had refractory multidrug-resistant tuberculosis of the brain. *Clinical Infectious Diseases*, Vol. 22, No. 3, (March, 1996), pp. (572-574), ISSN: 1058-4838

Raghu, G., Brown, KK., Bradford, WZ., Starko, K., Noble, PW, Schwartz, DA, & King, TE Jr. (2004). A placebo-controlled trial of interferon gamma-1b in patients with idiopathic pulmonary fibrosis. *The New England Journal of Medicine*, Vol. 350, No. 2, (January, 2004), pp. (125-133), ISSN: 0028-4793

Rink, L., Cakman, I., & Kirchner, H. (1998). Altered cytokine production in the elderly. *Mechanisms of Ageing and Development*, Vol. 102, No. 2-3, (May, 1998), pp. (199-209), ISSN: 0047-6374

Schreiber, RD., & Farrar, MA. (1993). The biology and biochemistry of interferon-gamma and its receptor. *Gastroenterologia Japonica*, Vol. 28, Suppl. 4, (March, 1993), pp. (88-94), ISSN: 0435-1339

Schroder, K., Hertzog, PJ., Ravasi, T., & Hume, DA. (2004). Interferon-gamma: an overview of signals, mechanisms and functions. *Journal of Leukocyte Biology*, Vol. 75, Suppl. 2, (February, 2004), pp. (163-189), ISSN: 0741-5400

Sekiguchi, Y., Yasui, K., Yamazaki, T., Agematsu, K., Kobayashi, N., & Koike, K. (2005). Effective combination therapy using interferon-gamma and interleukin-2 for disseminated Mycobacterium avium complex infection in a pediatric patient with

AIDS. *Clinical Infectious Diseases*, Vol. 41, No. 11, (December, 2005), pp. (e104-e106), ISSN: 1058-4838

Sexton, P., & Harrison, AC. (2008). Susceptibility to nontuberculous mycobacterial lung disease. *European Respiratory Journal*, Vol. 31, No. 6, (June, 2008), pp. (1322-1333), ISSN: 0903-1936

Silva, MT., Portaels, F., & Pedrosa, J. (2009). Pathogenetic mechanisms of the intracellular parasite Mycobacterium ulcerans leading to Buruli ulcer. *The Lancet Infectious Diseases*, Vol. 9, No. 11, (November, 2009), pp. (699-710), ISSN: 1473-3099

Squires, KE., Brown, ST., Armstrong, D., Murphy, WF., & Murray, HW. (1992). Interferon-gamma treatment for Mycobacterium avium-intracellulare complex bacillemia in patients with AIDS. *The Journal of Infectious Diseases*, Vol. 166, No. 3, (September, 1992), pp. (686-687), ISSN: 0022-1899

Squires, KE., Rosenkaimer, F., Sherwood, JA., Forni, AL., Were, JB., & Murray, HW. (1993). Immunochemotherapy for visceral leishmaniasis: a controlled pilot trial of antimony versus antimony plus interferon-gamma. *The American Journal of Tropical Medicine and Hygiene*, Vol. 48, No. 5, (May, 1993), pp. (666-669), ISSN: 0002-9637

Sternfeld, T., Nigg, A., Belohradsky, BH., & Bogner, JR. (2010). Treatment of relapsing Mycobacterium avium infection with interferon-gamma and interleukin-2 in an HIV-negative patient with low CD4 syndrome. *International Journal of Infectious Diseases*, Vol. 14, Suppl. 3, (September, 2010), pp. (e198-e201), ISSN: 1201-9712

Suárez-Méndez, R., García-García, I., Fernández-Olivera, N., Valdés-Quintana, M., Milanés-Virelles, MT., Carbonell, D., Machado-Molina, D., Valenzuela-Silva, CM., & López-Saura, PA. (2004). Adjuvant interferon gamma in patients with drug - resistant pulmonary tuberculosis: a pilot study. *BMC Infectious Diseases*, Vol. 4, (October, 2004), pp. (44), ISSN: 1471-2334

Subhash, HS., Ashwin, I., Jesudason, MV., Abharam, OC., John, G., Cherian, AM., & Thomas, K. (2003). Clinical characteristics and treatment response among patients with multidrug-resistant tuberculosis: a retrospective study. *The Indian Journal of Chest Diseases & Allied Sciences*, Vol. 45, No. 2, (April-Jun, 2003), pp. (97-103), ISSN: 0377-9343

Sundar, S., Rosenkaimer, F., & Murray, HW. (1994). Successful treatment of refractory visceral leishmaniasis in India using antimony plus interferon-gamma. *The Journal of Infectious Diseases*, Vol. 170, No. 3, (September, 1994), pp. (659-662), ISSN: 0022-1899

Tredget, EE., Wang, R., Shen, Q., Scott, PG., & Ghahary, A. (2000). Transforming growth factor-beta mRNA and protein in hypertrophic scar tissues and fibroblasts: antagonism by IFN-alpha and IFN-gamma in vitro and in vivo. *Journal of Interferon and Cytokine Research*, Vol. 20, No. 2, (February, 2000), pp. (143-151), ISSN: 1079-9907

Tomioka, H. (2004). Adjunctive immunotherapy of mycobacterial infections. *Current Pharmaceutical Design*, Vol. 10, No. 26, (2004), pp. (3297-3312), ISSN: 1381-6128

Ulloa, L., Doody, J., & Massagué, J. (1999). Inhibition of transforming growth factor-beta/SMAD signaling by the interferon-gamma/STAT pathway. *Nature*, Vol. 397, No. 6721, (February, 1999), pp. (710-713), ISSN: 0028-0836

Wang, J., Wakeham, J., Harkness, R., & Xing, Z. (1999) Macrophages are a significant source of type 1 cytokines during mycobacterial infection. *The Journal of Clinical Investigation*, Vol. 103, No. 7, (April, 1999), pp. (1023-1029), ISSN: 0021-9738

Williams, TJ., & Wilson, JW. (2008). Challenges in pulmonary fibrosis: 7--Novel therapies and lung transplantation. *Thorax*, Vol. 63, No. 3, (March, 2008), pp. (277-284), ISSN: 0040-6376

World Health Organization. WHO report. (2009). *Global tuberculosis control: epidemiology, strategy, financing. WHO/HTM/TB/2009.411.* Accessed 2011, Available from: http://www.who.int/tb/publications/global_report/2009/en/index.html.

World Health Organization. WHO report. (March, 2010). *Multidrug and extensively drug-resistant TB (M/XDR-TB): 2010 global report on surveillance and response* (1st Ed.), WHO, ISBN: 978 92 4 159919 1, Geneva

Xu, YD., Hua, J., Mui, A., O'Connor, R., Grotendorst, G., & Khalil, N. (2003). Release of biologically active TGF-beta1 by alveolar epithelial cells results in pulmonary fibrosis. *American Journal of Physiology. Lung Cellular and Molecular Physiology*, Vol. 285, No. 3, (September, 2003), pp. (L527-L539), ISSN: 1040-0605

Yang, Z., Wang, L., Guo, L., Lin, M., & Chen, X. (2009). A short-term efficacy on aerosolizing inhalation recombinant human gamma interferon in multidrug-resistant pulmonary tuberculosis. *The Journal of the Chinese Antituberculosis Association*, Vol. 31, No. 11, (2009), pp. (660-663), ISSN: 1000-6621

Yao, YX., & Liu, CY. (2003). Effects of interferon for the treatment of multidrug-resistant tuberculosis. *The Journal of the Chinese Antituberculosis Association*, Vol. 25, No. 1, (2003), pp. (43-44), ISSN: 1000-6621

Yew, WW. (2011). Management of multidrug-resistant tuberculosis and extensively drug-resistant tuberculosis: current status and future prospects. *Kekkaku*, Vol. 86, No. 1, (January, 2011), pp. (9-16), ISSN: 0022-9776

Yola, A., Sologub, T., Nechaev, V., & Ivanov, A. (2006). Immune-based therapy using gamma interferon ingaron in the treatment of HIV/AIDS patients with active pulmonary tuberculosis (PTB) not previously highly active antiretroviral therapy (HAART). *Retrovirology*, Vol. 3, Suppl. 1, (December, 2006), pp. (S38), ISSN: 1742-4690

Zhang, K., & Phan, SH. (1996). Cytokines and pulmonary fibrosis. *Biological Signals*, Vol. 5, No. 4, (July-August, 1996), pp. (232-239), ISSN: 1016-0922

Zhang, M., Gong, J., Iyer, DV., Jones, BE., Modlin, RL., & Barnes, PF. (1994). T cell cytokine responses in persons with tuberculosis and human immunodeficiency virus infection. *The Journal of Clinical Investigation*, Vol. 94, No. 6, (December, 1994), pp. (2435-2442), ISSN: 0021-9738

Ziesche, R., Hofbauer, E., Wittmann, K., Petkov, V., & Block, LH. (1999). A preliminary study of long-term treatment with interferon gamma-1b and low-dose prednisolone in patients with idiopathic pulmonary fibrosis. *The New England Journal of Medicine*, Vol. 341, No. 17, (October, 1999), pp. (1264-1269), ISSN: 0028-4793

10

P27-PPE36 (Rv2108) *Mycobacterium tuberculosis* Antigen – Member of PPE Protein Family with Surface Localization and Immunological Activities

Vincent Le Moigne[1] and Wahib Mahana[1,2]
[1]Université de Bretagne Occidentale
[2]Endotoxines, IGM, Université Paris sud, Orsay
France

1. Introduction

The largest and most distinctive class of mycobacteria-specific genes encode a group of 167 proteins of repetitive sequence belonging to the *pe* and *ppe* families. The uniqueness of the *ppe* genes is illustrated by the fact that these genes are restricted to mycobacteria (Cole et al., 1998; Voskuil et al., 2004 (b)). The *Rv2108* gene belongs to this family and furthermore is highly specific for the *Mycobacterium tuberculosis* (*Mtb*) complex group of mycobacterium (containing notably *Mycobacterium africanum, Mycobacterium canettii, Mycobacterium microti, Mycobacterium pinnipedi, Mycobacterium bovis* and *M. bovis* BCG strain). This gene was described by Chevrier et al., (2000) and used as a molecular probe to develop a rapid test for the detection and identification of this group of mycobacteria. *Rv2108* is a gene coding for the protein P27-PPE36, member of the PPE protein family of *Mycobacterium tuberculosis*, a group of protein thought to be of immunological significance despite the fact that the exact role of the PPE proteins stills unknown.

The P27-PPE36 protein was produced as a recombinant protein in *Escherichia coli*. The expressed protein is immunologicaly active and recognized by sera from infected patients. It was used to generate specific polyclonal and monoclonal anti-P27-PPE 36 antibodies. These antibodies were used to study the immunochemical characterization of P27-PPE36, to verify its presence in *Mycobacterium bovis* BCG and clinical *Mtb* isolates, and to characterize and localize it in a parietal position in *M. tuberculosis* cells.

Using an ELISA test we found that the antibody immune response to P27-PPE36 in the sera of patients was dominated by an IgA antibody response accompanied by the absence of IgG response.

The immune response against the P27-PPE36 protein was investigated in mice. It was studied in the context of different pathogen associated molecular patterns (PAMPs). BALB/c mice were immunized either with the P27-PPE36 recombinant protein in Freund's adjuvant or in phosphate saline buffer (PBS), with a pcDNA3 plasmid containing the gene encoding the P27-PPE36 protein, or with the *Escherichia coli* bacteria expressing the P27-

PPE36 protein genetically fused into the flagellin. We found that P27-PPE36 expressed into the flagellin led to the strongest cellular responses, where we obtained the highest production of IFN-γ and cell proliferation, an indication of specific Th1-like orientation of the immune response.

2. Early works on Rv2108 and genetic analysis

2.1 *Mtb* PCR-based assay detection test

The *Rv2108* gene belongs to the *pe* and *ppe* families and furthermore is highly specific for the *Mycobacterium tuberculosis* (*Mtb*) complex group of mycobacterium. This gene was described by Chevrier et al., (2000) and was used as a molecular probe to develop a rapid test for the detection and identification of this group of mycobacteria. PCR targeting the insertion sequence IS 6110 has been considered specific for identification of *M. tuberculosis* and mycobacteria belonging to the *M. tuberculosis* complex and is frequently applied in numerous laboratories to confirm the presence of this organism directly in biological specimens (Thierry et al., 1990). However, several authors found that some *M. tuberculosis* strains failed to hybridize with the IS 6110 probe (Yuen et al., 1993; Thierry et al., 1995) and other authors found that false-positive results may be obtained for clinical samples when some methods based on IS 6110 are used (Lee et al., 1994: Kent et al., 1995). Conversely, the *Rv2108* gene was found to be highly specific for *M. tuberculosis* complex strains. In the PCR-based assay for rapid detection and identification of this mycobacterium (Chevrier et al., 2000), one pair of primers and two oligonucleotide probes were successfully used to amplify and to detect the DNA of strains belonging to the *M. tuberculosis* complex. These primers and probes did not hybridize with DNA from any of the 21 other mycobacterial species tested (*M. avium, M. intracellulare, M. gordonae, M. chelonae, M. xenopi, M. kansasii, M. peregrinum, M. fortuitum, M. marinum, M. flavescens, M. celatum, M. asiaticum, M. malmoense, M. fallax, M. simiae, M. terrae, M. interjectum, M. genavense, M. paratuberculosis, M. szulgaï* and *M. scrofulaceum*) . It is worth noting that the chosen primers and probes hybridize with DNA from the *M. tuberculosis* strain with no IS 6110, furthermore no strain without p27 was found among the 410 strains tested in the study (Chevrier et al., 2000).

Now that many mycobacterium genome have been completely sequenced, the results that *Rv2108* is specific to *Mycobacterium tuberculosis* compex have been confirmed. This name *Rv2108* is those of the gene in the *M. tuberculosis* strain H37Rv. In the *M. tuberculosis* strain CDC1551, the gene number is *MT2167* and in *Mycobacterium bovis*, this gene is called *Mb2132*. No ortholog has been identified in the genome of the closely related *Mycobacterium marinum, Mycobacterium segmatis, Mycobacterium ulcerans* or *Mycobacterium avium subs. paratuberculosis* (Stinear et al., 2008) and those despite some bacteria like *M. marinum* have an higher number of PPE genes than *M. tuberculosis* (106 vs. 69) (Stinear et al., 2008**).**

However an other analysis found a *Rv2108* ortholog in the same strain (Agy99) of *Mycobacterium ulcerans* (Riley et al., 2008). This work presents also that *Rv2108* gene is deleted in the strain C of *Mycobacterium tuberculosis* while it is present in the strains CDC1551, F11, H37Rv and Harlem as in the two strains of *Mycobacterium bovis* tested (BCG stain Pasteur 1173 and AF2122/97). According another study (Gey van Pittius et al., 2006), *Rv2108* have no orthologues in *M. smegmatis, M avium paratuberculosis, M. leprae, M. ulcerans* or *M. marinum.* These results confirm the interest of this gene in terms of diagnostic tool.

M. tuberculosis has become highly specialized for intracellular survival in a very restricted range of mammalian hosts, and several recent studies have shown that lateral gene transfer (LGT) has been a major force in the evolution of the *M. tuberculosis* complex from an environmental *Mycobacterium* (Kinsella et al. 2003; Gutierrez et al., 2005; Rosas-Magallanes et al., 2006; Becq et al., 2007). In fact, *Rv2108* appears to belong to one of the 80 regions (minimal number identified containing 360 Protein coding sequences (CDS)) that have probably been acquired by LGT in *Mtb* (Stinear et al., 2008). Whether acquired by LGT or other means, some of these *M. tuberculosis*-specific regions contain known virulence genes or code for adaptation factors making them pottentially important for bacteria belonging to *Mtb*-complex.

2.2 Genomic organizations

Analysis of the genomic environment of the *Rv2108* gene reveals that it is situated downstream a member of the *pe* gene family, *Rv2107*, coding for the PE22 protein (Fig. 1). These adjacent *Rv2107* and *Rv2108* genes lie in the same orientation. Occasionally, it can be noted that an insertion site IS*6110* is localized between this two genes in the strains H37Rv and CDC1551 (Beggs et al., 2000; Sampson et al., 2001). Genome analysis by the operon/gene cluster method (Strong et al., 2003; Bowers et al., 2004) suggests that the PE and PPE families are functionally linked (Gey van Pittius et al., 2006; Tekaia et al., 1999; Strong et al., 2006; Tundup et al., 2006). That is, the two genes tend to be in close chromosomal proximity on the *Mtb* genome (Strong et al., 2003; Bowers et al., 2004). Based on their short intergenic distance (56 bp) and same transcription direction, *Rv2107* and *Rv2108* were assumed to belong to the same operon (Fig. 1) and so be co-transcribed. In *Mtb* genome, these same-operon PE/PPE pairs comprise less than 10% of the total number of PE and PPE genes (14 pairs of PE and PPE genes are found adjacent – same orientation, minimal intergenic distance – in the genome) (Riley et al., 2008). Genes separated by short intergenic sequences tend to have related function and interact physically (Jacob & Monod, 1961). The structure of a complex of one PE/PPE protein pair was recently characterized (Strong et al., 2006; Tundup et al., 2006). These results indicate that there may be many other instances of interactions between PE and PPE proteins. Like the PE and PPE proteins from the gene *Rv2431c* (PE25) and *Rv2430c* (PPE41) that interact together in vitro as probably *in vivo* (Strong et al., 2006; Tundup et al., 2006), it is stongly probable that PPE36 and PE22 have the same behavior. In fact, computational methods predict that the PE22/PPE36 interaction probability is almost the strongest of all the PE/PPE possible combinations tested (Riley et al., 2008). Furthermore, according to this analysis, this putative complexe is predicted to interact specifically, that is, PPE36 do not appear to interact with PEs other than its operon partner PE22, and vice versa (Riley et al., 2008) but this supposition would need to be experimentaly confirmed. However due to the fact that *Rv2108* is absent in *M. tuberculosis strain C* and *Rv2107* is absent in *M. tuberculosis strain F11*, it is possible that another interacting partner is able to interact with the orphaned gene, possibly restoring the PE/PPE complex's function, or introducing new complexes that help these strains survive in their environmental niches (Riley et al., 2008). A putative interaction PE22/PPE36 is probably under the form of a 1:1 heterodimeric complex (Strong et al., 2003). In their study, they found, as us (Le Moigne et al., 2005), that PPE36 is insoluble when expressed alone. The association with the relative PE protein would lead to a soluble complex: their experiments showed that proteins PE Rv2431c and PPE Rv2430 that are insosuble when expressed on their own are soluble when they are expressed together (Strong et al., 2006; Tundup et al., 2006).

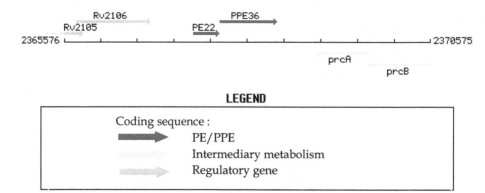

Fig. 1. Genomic environment of *Rv2108* gene. (adapted from TubercuList, http://genolist.pasteur.fr/TubercuList/)

2.3 Regulation expression of *Rv2108*

A fundamental step in understanding the role of *pe* and *ppe* genes is elucidating how their expression is regulated. Although various studies have demonstrated that *pe* and *ppe* genes are expressed under a range of *in vitro* and *in vivo* conditions, they have not revealed any obvious indication of global *pe* and *ppe* gene regulation (Voskuil et al., 2004 (b)). This group of Voskuil and Smith has tested a large variety of diverse conditions to analyse gene expression in *Mtb* (Manganelli et al., 2001; Sherman et al., 2001; Manganelli et al., 2002; Rodriguez et al., 2002; Schnappinger et al., 2003; Voskuil et al., 2003; Voskuil et al., 2004 (a); Voskuil et al., 2004 (b)). Among them, only two conditions induce a variation in *Rv2108* expression (at least two fold): in presence of 0.05% sodium dodecyl sulfate (SDS) 90 min, *Rv2108* expression is repressed (Manganelli et al., 2001) as after 14 days of stationnary phase culture (Voskuil et al., 2004 (a)). Other conditions (Macrophage IFNγ activated, 24 h; diethylenetriamine/nitric oxide adduct (DETA/NO or DNO) 0.5 mM, 40 min; hydrogen peroxide (H_2O_2) 10 mM, 40 min; hypoxia (oxygen from 20% to 0.20%), 2 h (Sherman et al., 2001; Rustad et al., 2008); palmitic acid 50 μm, 4h; non-replicating persistence (NRP) dormancy model 20 days; Iron high vs. low; diamide 5 mM, 1 h; potassium cyanide (KCN) 0.5 mM, 1 h; carbonyl-cyanide 3-chlorophenylhydrazone (CCCP) 0.5 mM, 1 h; ethambutol 10 μm, 24 h; nutrient starvation 24 h (Betts et al., 2002); heat shock (45°C), 30 min (Stewart et al., 2002); acid shock (pH 5.5 vs. 6.9) (Fisher et al., 2002)) do not appear to generate variation (more than 2 fold) in *Rv2108* expression. The associated *pe* gene, *Rv2107* (*pe22*), is found to be induced in macrophage culture of *Mtb* (Schnappinger et al., 2003) and in presence of 0.5 mM DETA/NO (Voskuil et al., 2003).

However, inversely, Park et al. (2003) found that *Rv2108* gene is induced by hypoxia (even if this needs confirmation since standard error deviation is elevated). However, contrarily to the majority of genes powerfully regulated by hypoxia, its induction does not require the putative transcription factor Rv3133/DosR.

Like the majority of other PPE gene (54 of 69), Lsr2, a small basic protein highly conserved in mycobacteria that binds DNA and is implicated in gene regulation, is able to bind Rv2108 sequence (Gordon et al., 2010). The binding of Lsr2 to the majority of *pe/ppe* genes suggests that this factor may negatively affect the expression of these antigenic proteins to modulate interactions with the host.

More generally, *Rv2108* has a low expression in the diverse *M. tuberculosis* strains that have been tested (Gao et al., 2005) and it does not seem that there is a difference of *Rv2108* gene expression between *M. bovis* and *M. tuberculosis* in microarray analysis (Rehren et al., 2007).

Furthermore, a study showed, by high density mutagenesis experiments, that *Rv2108* is not an essential gene for mycobacterial growth (Sassetti et al., 2003). In these experiments, only three of *pe* and *ppe* genes met the criteria for defining growth-attenuating mutations (*Rv1807, Rv3872,* and *Rv3873*). Although mutations in several other *pe* and *ppe* genes appeared to have subtle defects, the fact that such a small fraction are detected in this system suggests either that most of these genes are able to functionally complement each other, or that they are required under conditions that have not been testes. In the same study, the *Mycobacterium leprae* gene ML0411 is presented as an orthologue of *Rv2108*. In the Sanger Institute *Mycobacterium leprae* genome project, *ML0411* is in fact described as being similar to *Rv2108*. ML0411 is coding for a protein 408-amino acid long named as a serine-rich antigen (Sra) that have been largelly described (Vega-Lopez et al., 1993; Rinke de Wit et al., 1993; Macfarlane et al., 2001; Parkash et al.,2006) *Rv2108* belongs the the 27% of genes that are not required for *in vitro* growth having *M. leprae* orthologues while the majority (78%) of the genes that they predict to be required for the optimal growth of *M. tuberculosis* have an orthologue in *M. leprae* genome. Thus, *M. leprae* appears to have selectively conserved the majority of genes that are necessary for optimal growth (Cole et al., 2001).

3. Characterization of P27-PPE36 protein

The *Rv2108* nucleotide sequence encoded for a 243 amino acid length protein. The P27-PPE36 antigen belongs to the PPE protein family, large family of protein present in *Mtb*, which represent ≈3% of the genome of this bacterium (Cole et al., 1998). With the related PE protein family, they account for 10% of the genome. These families appear to have originated in the fast growing mycobacterial species before undergoing extensive expansion

and diversification in certain slow growing species, particularly *M. ulcerans, M. marinum* and members of the *M. tuberculosis* complex (Gey van Pittius et al., 2006). This asparagine or glycine-rich protein family containing 69 members has been termed PPE after the characteristic Pro-Pro-Glu motifs near the N-termini, in position 8-10. The relatively conserved N-terminal domain is about 180 amino acids lenght while C-terminal segments vary in sequence and length. According to this C-terminal region, the PPE proteins are classified into four subfamilies: the first subfamily (24 members), named PPE-SVP, has the well conserved motif Gly–X–X–Ser–Val–Pro—X–X–Trp located approximately at position 350; the second (23 members) constitutes the major polymorphic tandem repeats (MPTR) subfamily and is characterized by the presence of multiple tandem repeats of the motif Asn–X–Gly–X–Gly–Asn–X–Gly; the third subfamily (10 members), named PPE-PPW, is characterized by a highly conserved region comprising Gly–Phe–X–Gly–Thr and Pro–X–X–Pro–X–X–Trp motifs; and the last PPE subfamily (12 members) includes proteins with a low percentage of homology at the C-terminus that are unrelated other than having the PPE motif (Gordon et al., 2001; Adindla & Guruprasad, 2003; Gey van Pittius et al., 2006). P27-PPE36 belongs to this last subfamily. A recent phylogenetic analysis of the 69 *ppe* genes present in the *M. tuberculosis* reference strain H37Rv has uncovered their evolutionary relationships and reveals that they can be divided into 5 sublineages which globally match the subfamilies described above (Gey van Pittius et al., 2006). *Rv2108* is classified in the sublineage III, having the most similarity with *Rv3892c*.

The role of the PPE proteins stills unknown. Firstly, they have been thought to be implicated in increasing antigenic variation and immune evasion due to the highly polymorphic nature of their C-terminal domains (Cole et al., 1998 ; Cole, 1999; Karboul et al., 2008). Concerning this, an interessant study realized by Plotkin et al. (2004) shows that PE/PPE proteins are under strong selection for amino acids substitution. They calculate volatility of codons which is the proportion of their point-mutaions neighbours that encode different amino acids. The volatility of a codon is used to quantify the chance that the most recent nucleotide mutation to that codon caused an amino-acid subtitution. According their calcul, *Rv2108* has a volatility value of 0.1029, which place it at the 594th rank of genes with the higher volatility among the 4099 genes values calculated. Furthermore, in agreement with the theory of an antigenic variation role, it has been observed that many PPE proteins present high levels of polymorphism like for exemple PPE38 (*Rv2352c*), PPE39 (*Rv2353c*) and PPE40 (*Rv2356c*) (McEvoy et al., 2009), PPE34 (*Rv1917c*) (Sampson et al., 2001(a)), PPE42 (Rv2608) (Chakhaiyar et al., 2004), PPE8 (*Rv0355c*) (Srivastava et al., 2006) or PPE18 (*Rv1196*) (Hebert et al., 2007) and sequence variation has been observed between the orthologues of the PE and PPE protein families in *in silico* analyses of the sequenced genomes of *M. tuberculosis* H37Rv, *M. tuberculosis* CDC1551 and *M. bovis* (Gordon et al., 2001; Fleischmann et al., 2002; Garnier et al., 2003). However, this variability can not be extended to all *pe/ppe* family members since some are in fact conserved across strains and species (Cubillos-Ruiz et al., 2008). It has then been suggested that the PPE proteins may play a role in the virulence of *Mtb* (Rindi et al., 1999; Li et al., 2005), in the maintenance of bacterial growth in macrophages (Camacho et al.,1999; Dubnau et al., 2002; Hou et al., 2002; Li et al., 2005; Sassetti et al., 2003) and in the regulation of bacterial iron starvation and oxidative stress responses (Rodriguez at al., 1999; Rodriguez at al., 2002). In addition, PPE might be a target for the protective immune response in experimental mouse models (Skeiky et al., 2000). It has also be emitted the hypothesis that PPE proteins, due to their abundance of asparagine, could have a possible storage function for this amino acid which is one of the preferred nitrogen sources of the tubercle bacilli (Tekaia et al., 1999). Some PPE proteins, like PPE31 (*Rv1807*) could be involved in the protection from antibiotic stress targeting the envelope and help to confer the basal level of Mtb resistance to antibacterial drugs (Provvedi et al., 2009). Many PPE proteins are also known to induce a strong T cell and B cell responses and associate with the cell wall. Following surface exposure, these PPE proteins could act as agonists to various surface receptors of APCs resulting in modulation of the host immune responses (Choudhary et al., 2003; Tundup et al., 2008; Mishra et al., 2008; Chaitra et al., 2008 (a); Chaitra et al., 2008 (b)). Recently, two PPE proteins, PPE18 (*Rv1196*) and PPE34 (*Rv1917c*), were found to specifically interact with the innate immune receptor TLR2 (Nair et al., 2009; Bansal et al., 2010).

Very little is known about the protein encoded by the *Rv2108* gene. Theoretical properties of P27-PPE36 protein are a low pH_i (4.59) and representative amino acid composition is 12% for alanine and 9% for glutamic acid. Predictive secondary structure shows that this protein would be mainly constitued of alpha-helix (58,5%) and the absence of β-feuillet. The resting amino acids (31%) would be in random coil.

3.1 Expression and purification of the PPE36 protein

The *Rv2108* gene was amplified, inserted into bacterial vectors, sequenced, and expressed as a recombinant protein. Either the GST (pGEX-4T-3) in *E. coli* DH5α or the pET (pET15b) in *E. coli* BL21 (DE3) plasmid were used. Induction of the PPPE36 protein by these various expression systems lead to the expression of a protein with an apparent molecular mass of 43 kDa in sodium dodecyl sulfate–polyacrylamide gel electrophoresis (SDS-PAGE) analysis (Fig. 2A and B).

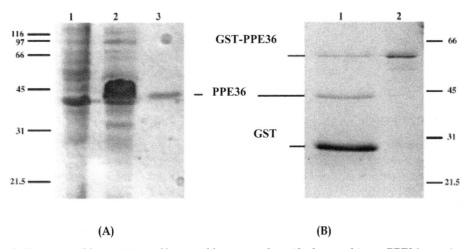

(A) (B)

Fig. 2. Coomassie blue staining of bacterial lysates and purified recombinant PPE36 protein expressed with His-Tag (A) or with GST (B).
(A): Lanes 1 and 2: bacterial extracts of E. coli BL21 (DE3) without or with IPTG induction, respectively. Lane 3: purified PPE36 protein. (B): Lanes 1 and 2: PPE36, GST-PPE36 fusion protein, partially cleaved or not cleaved by thrombin, respectively.

This value was higher than the theoretical mass predicted by its DNA sequence translation of 27 kDa. Mass spectrometric analysis of the expressed protein in the pET system revealed a molecule at 29 kDa, which corresponds to the P27-PPE36 putative protein estimated mass plus 2 kDa for the polyHistidine fusion Tag (Le Moigne et al., 2005). This result was confirmed by partial sequencing of the N-terminal region of the recombinant protein. The reason for this difference may be due to the nature of the P27-PPE36 protein, which belongs to a family of intrinsically unstructured proteins (IUP) with an atypical composition of amino acid sequences (Tompa, 2002). It presents notably a high proportion of Proline dimers (3 for 243 amino acids). These proteins bind less to SDS than most other proteins and their apparent molecular mass is often 1.2–1.8 times higher than the real value calculated from sequence data or measured by mass spectrometry (Dunker et al., 2001). Such a phenomen of electrophoresis abnormal migration has been observed for another protein belonging to the PE protein family of Mtb: the product of the gene Rv1441c has an apparent molecular weight of about 60 kDa instead of a theorical MW of 40,7 kDa (Banu et al., 2002).

Generally, PE and PPE proteins did not express well or expressed in insoluble or unfolded forms (Strong et al., 2006). Our attemps to express P27-PPE36 under the form of a recombinant proteins confirm this rules and lead to the obtention of an insoluble protein (Le Moigne et al., 2005), as confirmed later by an other study (Strong et al., 2006). The lack of apparent transmembrane elements is a possible explanation for their failure to express on their own is that they need protein partners to fold (Strong et al., 2006) like explained above in the *Genomic organization* paragraph.

3.2 Physico-chemical caracteristic of the PPE36 protein

Based on the DNA and protein sequences, the expected pI value of the P27 protein should be 4.8. To determine the PI value of the expressed p27 protein, a two-dimensional gel was applied to the cell lysates from the BCG strain. After gel transfer to a nitrocellulose membrane and blotting with the P27-PPE36-specific antibodies, only one spot with a pI between 4.5 and 5 at the same molecular mass level observed by SDS-PAGE was recognized on the membrane (Le Moigne et al., 2005).

4. Anti-P27-PPE36 antibodies production and localization of P27-PPE36

Very little is known about the cellular localization of the PPE protein family, a 143 kDa PPE protein encoded by the Rv1917c gene (PPE34) was found to be a cell-wall associated protein and probably surface exposed (Sampson et al., 2001) as well as the PPE68 protein (Rv3873 gene) located in the cell envelope (Pym et al., 2002; Okkels et al., 2003; Demangel et al., 2004).

We have generated specific mouse monoclonal and rabbit polyclonal antibodies to P27-PPE36 and used them for the immunochemical characterization and cellular localization of this protein. Specific immunoblot analysis confirmed the presence of the P27-PPE36 antigen in *Mycobacterium bovis* BCG strain and in human clinical isolates of *M. tuberculosis* from infected patients (Fig. 3), but not in other mycobacteria tested which does not belong to the *Mtb* complex (Le Moigne et al., 2005).

Then, after demonstrating that the P27-PPE36 protein was present in the *M. bovis* BCG strain and in clinical isolates of *M. tuberculosis*, we attempted to localize this PPE protein in the BCG strain. To achieve this, bacteria were washed, fixed and ultrathin sections were prepared to be analysed by electron microscopy using immunohistochemistry test with specific anti-P27-PPE36 antibodies. Results generated with monoclonal (Fig. 4 A) and polyclonal antibodies (Fig. 4 B) revealed a peripheral localization of this protein on the cell membrane. Similar results were obtained using western-blot analysis (Fig. 4 D) of the *Mtb* cell fractions with the monoclonal anti-P27-PPE36 antibody indicating that the P27-PPE36 protein is localized in the membrane of the cell (Le Moigne et al., 2005).

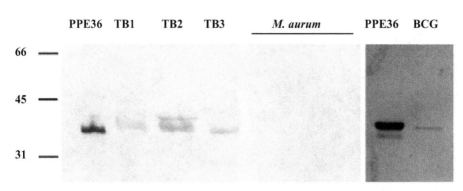

Fig. 3. Western blot analysis of bacterial lysate from different mycobacterial species.
P27-PPE36 is the recombinant PPE36 protein. TB1, TB2 and TB3 are *Mycobacterium
tuberculosis* clinical strains isolated from infected patients. *Mycobacterium aurum* is a fast-
growing mycobacteria, and BCG is the Calmette-Guérin bacillus. The first antibody is a
mouse monoclonal IgG antibody directed against PPE36.

This protein was the third member of its family to be localized at the periphery of the cell
(Sampson et al., 2001; Pym et al., 2002; Okkels et al., 2003; Demangel et al., 2004) and since,
the same localization was assigned to other PPE proteins like for exemple Map3420c and
Map1506 in *Mycobacterium avium* subsp. *paratuberculosis* (Newton et al., 2009). In
Mycobacterium immunogenum, a PPE protein (accessio no. YP_001288073) have been found to
be a cell-membrane-associated antigen (Gupta et al., 2009). In a recent detailed analysis of
the *Mycobacterium marinum* capsule using cryoelectron microscopy in conjunction with
liquid chromatography mass spectrometry (LC-MS) demonstrated that 5 (MM1129,
MM1402, MM0186, MM5047 and MM1497) of the 25 major cell surface proteins were
members of the PPE familie (Sani et al., 2010). Similarly high-throughput proteomics
MALDI-MS and LC-MS approaches have been utilized by Målen et al. (2010) to identify 8
PPEs in the *M. tuberculosis* envelope fractions (PPE18, PPE20, PPE26, PPE32, PPE33, PPE51,
PPE60 and PPE68).

Therefore, these results suggest that cell wall/surface localization is a characteristic of
several PE/PPE proteins although another PPE protein, PPE41, have been shown to be
secreted by pathogenic mycobacteria (Abdallah et al., 2006). So, if for the majority of PE and
PPE proteins are localize to the cell wall, some of them could be secreted into the
extracellular environment.

Like explained above, P27-PPE36 should be, as a disordered protein which need a partner to
fold, associated with the PE protein PE22 (Gey van Pittius et al., 2006; Strong et al., 2006).
Moreover, this putative complex PPE36–PE22 could be associated with a system dedicated
to the secretion of members of the potent T-cell antigen 6-kDa Early Secreted Antigenic
Target (ESAT-6) family (Gey van Pittius et al., 2006). According this last computational
study constructing an evolutionary history of the *pe* and *ppe* genes families, *Rv2107* and
Rv2108 genes are hypothesized to have been duplicated from the ESAT-6 (esx) gene cluster
regions, as they are very homologous to their paralogues within the ESAT-6 (*esx*) gene
clusters and have the same paired genomic orientation. These esx clusters encode the so-

called Type VII or ESX secretion systems, of which there are 5 in *Mtb* (Gey van Pittius et al., 2001). Thus, *Rv2107* and *Rv2108* would derive from ESAT-6 gene cluster Region 2, i.e. from *Rv3893c* (PE36) and *Rv3892c* (PPE69).

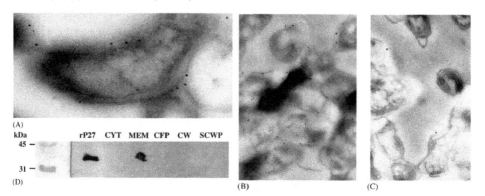

Fig. 4. Localization of P27-PPE36 antigen: Immunogold electron microscopic image (A–C) showing the peripheral localization of the P27-PPE36 protein in cryosectioned *M. bovis* BCG and western-blot on various *M. tuberculosis* cell fractions (D). Incubation was realized either with a mouse monoclonal antibody (A), or rabbit polyclonal anti-P27-PPE36 antibodies (B). Negative control was done using normal rabbit serum (C). (A: ×49 000, B and C: ×23 000). (D): Immunoblot analysis of different cell fractions of *M. tuberculosis* obtained from the Tuberculosis Research Materials and Vaccine Testing Laboratory, Colorado State University using monoclonal anti-P27-PPE36 antibody. Recombinant P27-PPE36 (rP27), cytosol fraction (CYT), cell membrane fraction (MEM), culture filtrate proteins (CFP), cell wall fraction (CW), and SDS-soluble cell wall proteins (SCWP).

5. Serological studies

Diverse reports point out the potential immunodominant nature of PPE proteins. Presence of antibodies against other PPE proteins have been found in mycobacterium infected human or animals: in human against the PPE17 (Rv1168c) (Khan et al., 2008), PPE41 (*Rv2340c*) (Choudhary et al., 2003), PPE42 (*Rv2608*) (Chakhaiyar et al., 2004), PPE55 (*Rv3347c*) (Singh et al., 2005), PPE57 (*Rv3425*) (Zhang et al., 2007), in human and mice against PPE68 (*Rv3873*) (Daugelat et al., 2003), in human (Rindi et al., 2007) and mice (Romano et al., 2008; Bonanni et al., 2005) against the PPE44 (*Rv2770c*), in cattle against PPE68 (*Rv3873*) (Cockle et al., 2002), and against a PPE protein of *Mycobacterium avium subsp paratuberculosis* (Newton et al., 2008). Other studies highlight the capacity of PPE proteins to induce high B cell response in TB patients like PPE41 (*Rv2340c*) (Tundup et al., 2008). Inversely, a study shows that patients with tuberculosis do not develop a strong humoral response against the PPE44 protein (Zanetti et al., 2005). In cattle, no difference is seen in the humoral response to the PPE44 (Rv2770c) between infected and TB-free animals (Molicotti et al., 2008).

The P27-PPE36 expressed protein is immunologically active, and reacts, in western-blot and ELISA, with antibodies from sera of patients infected with *Mtb* (Le Moigne et al., 2005). (Fig. 5).

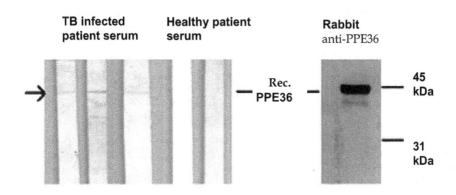

Fig. 5. Western blot analysis of the presence of anti-recombinant PPE36 antibodies in the sera of TB patients in comparison with serum from healthy donors and recombinant PPE36-hyperimmunized rabbit.

So, we then studied PPE36 specific antibody isotype distribution in sera of pulmonary tuberculosis patients and compared them to those in sera from healthy control by enzyme-linked immunosorbent assay (ELISA). Our result showed a significant increase of IgA antibody response in patient's sera, but a less important IgM response accompanied by total absence of IgG2, 3, and 4 responses and a weak IgG1 response in few patients' sera (unpublished results).

The absence of IgG response in the sera of patients allowed verifying for the presence of immune complexes that may inhibit the interaction of antibodies with our antigen on the plate. Using an immunoprecipitation test with goat anti human immunoglobulin antibodies, no immune complex containing P27-PPE36 was present in the patient's sera.

The significance of IgA and IgM is not clear. The IgA response is the more interesting and intriguing results for this protein, because this is the first study showing the presence of IgA alone and the absence of an IgG response against a peptidic antigen. The IgA response is often considered to be local (mucosa and body surface) and non systemic (sera). It has also been reported as a more specific for the non peptidic antigens comparing to the IgG response, which was more reactive (Julián et al., 2005). The IgM response is in general related to the natural auto antibodies found in the sera of healthy and infected peoples and animals, and we couldn't ascribe it a diagnostic value, though we note its augmentation during infection. These antibodies are in general polyspecific with weak affinity for their antigens.

The occurrence of antibodies against the PPE proteins is highly controversial; different studies highlighted the capacity of PPE proteins to induce high B cell response in TB human patients or infected animals (Tundup et al., 2008; Singh et al. 2005). Inversely, a study showed that patients with tuberculosis do not develop a strong humoral response against a PPE protein (Zanetti et al., 2005).

In comparison with other PPE proteins, P27-PPE36 proved to be less useful as a basis for the development of a TB diagnostic test. However, the presence of an IgA response in the absence of an IgG one, could be exploited as an indicator for *Mtb* diagnosis. A large number of sera should be tested to gather further information on the immune responses to this antigen.

6. Immune response against P27-PPE36 by different immunisation ways

We have studied the immune response of mice against the *Mtb* P27-PPE36 protein.

The peripheral localization of the P27-PPE36 protein led to the belief that they might play an important immunological role either in diagnosis or in protection. So, we examined the immune response against the P27-PPE36 protein using different Pathogen associated molecular patterns (PAMPs) as adjuvants and vectors for immunization. PAMPs are expressed only by micro-organisms and are recognized by the eukaryotic cells through the pattern recognition receptors (PRRs) of the innate immune system such as the Toll-like receptors (TLRs) (Medzhitov & Janeway, 2000). The interaction of PAMPs with their corresponding TLRs helps to identify the nature of the PAMP and to guide the adequate adaptive immune response (Medzhitov & Janeway, 2000). Muramyl dipeptides, a major element of the Freund's complete adjuvant, bacterial DNA, and bacterial flagellin are three PAMPs recognized by TLR2, TLR9, and TLR5, respectively.

Different immunization protocols were used to study immunological potential of the P27-PPE36 protein. BALB/c mice were immunized either with the P27-PPE36 recombinant protein in Freund's adjuvant or in phosphate saline buffer (PBS) (classical immunization), with a pcDNA3 plasmid containing the gene encoding the P27-PPE36 protein (DNA immunization), or with the *Escherichia coli* bacteria expressing the P27-PPE36 protein genetically fused into the flagellin (flagellin immunization) (Le Moigne et al., 2008).

We found that P27-PPE36 expressed into the flagellin led to the strongest cellular responses, where we obtained the highest production of IFN-γ (Fig. 6 B) and cell proliferation (Fig. 6 A), an indication of specific Th1-like orientation of the immune response. DNA immunization was less potent in the induction of such responses. We confirmed the role of flagellin in this response by using different immunization combinations (Le Moigne et al., 2008). However, the specific antibody response was weak with either method (Fig. 6 C). On the other hand, classical immunization with the recombinant protein, soluble or incorporated in Freund's adjuvant still yielded the best antibody response (Fig. 6 C). The best cellular and humoral responses were obtained in the group of mice primed with the recombinant protein and boosted by the antigen presented on the modified flagellin (Le Moigne et al., 2008). In general, the P27-PPE36 PPE antigen induced a strong proliferative response accompanied by high production of IFN-γ and low amount of IL-4 (Le Moigne et al., 2008), independently of the PAMP used. The results indicated that this antigen may be involved in the establishment of the host cellular immune responses against the *Mtb*.

Protective anti-mycobacterial immunity is primarily mediated by cellular immune responses (Flynn et al., 1992; Caruso et al., 1999). *Mtb* is rich in antigens that induce IFN-γ secretion, and the presence of such antigens has been reported in purified cell walls, the cytosolic fraction, and short-term culture filtrates (ST-CF) (Mustafa, 2001). The importance of antibodies in tuberculosis is much debated, but it has been suggested that certain antibody specificities against bacterial surface epitopes and with the correct isotype may confer protection against intracellular infections (Glatman-Freedman, 2003; Glatman-Freedman and Casadevall, 1998; Casadevall, 1995).

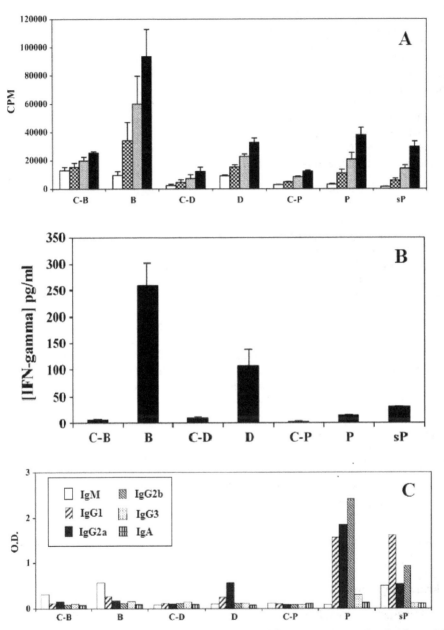

Fig. 6. Immune response generated against P27-PPE36 from mice immunized either with flagellin-modified bacteria (B), DNA plasmid containing the *Rv2108* gene (D) or with the P27-PPE36 recombinant protein associated (P) or not (sP) with Freund's adjuvant. Control groups have been immunized with non-modified bacteria (C-B), the empty pcDNA3 plasmid (C-D) or with PBS in Freund's adjuvant (C-P).

(**A**): Proliferation of splenic cells of immunized mice after incubation *in vitro* with different concentrations ((☐) 0.0 μg/ml, (▨) 1.1μg/ml, (▨) 3.3 μg/ml and (■) 10μg/ml) of purified p27 recombinant protein. The proliferation was monitored by [³H] thymidine uptake at 66 h after stimulation. (**B**): Cytokine secretion by splenic cells of immunized mice. Splenic cells were stimulated *in vitro* by the recombinant P27-PPE36 protein and IFN-γ was quantified in the supernatant after one week of culture. Results are presented as mean cytokine concentrations (±standard errors) compared to a standard curve of purified cytokines. (**C**): Specific anti-P27-PPE36 antibodies responses. Mice sera diluted at 1/500 were tested in ELISA for the presence of anti-P27-PPE36 antibodies of the different isotypes IgG1, IgG2a, IgG2b, IgG3, IgM and IgA one week after the third immunization. The results are presented as the optical density of the different isotypes.

Other PPE proteins have been reported to be strongly immunogenic (Choudhary et al., 2003; Demangel et al., 2004, Okkels et al., 2003; Dillon et al., 1999; Skeiky et al., 2000). Antibodies against PPE41 (*Rv2430c*) are present in TB patients and not in healthy individuals (Choudhary et al, 2003); PPE68 (*Rv3873*) induces IFN-γ production from splenocytes of *M. tuberculosis*-infected mice and from peripheral blood mononuclear cells of TB patients and PPD+ healthy individuals (Demangel et al., 2004, Okkels et al., 2003) and from cattle blood cells (Cockle et al., 2002; Mustafa et al., 2002). Immune responses elicited by PPE18 (*Rv1196*) and PPE14 (*Rv0915c*) have been shown to provide some protection in mice infected with *M. tuberculosis* (Dillon et al., 1999; Skeiky et al., 2000). Together, these studies suggest that several PPE proteins are expressed in vivo. In other mycobacteries, other PPE proteins have been shown to induce immune responses. For exemple in *M. avium subs. paratuberculosis*, two PPE proteins named Map39 and Map41 significantly elicited IFN-γ production in peripheral blood mononuclear cells from infected cattle (Nagata et al., 2005). When immunized in mice, PPE57 (*Rv3425*) and PPE46 (*Rv3018c*) induce also strong humoral and cellular responses (Wang et al., 2008; Chaitra et al., 2007)

7. Conclusion

The P27-PPE36 protein is the third member of its family to be localized at the periphery of the cell (Sampson et al., 2001; Pym et al., 2002; Okkels et al., 2003). Now others PPE have been found to have a similar localization. This may shed some light on its role in the diagnosis and pathogenesis of Mtb.

In conclusion, the P27-PPE36 protein was found to be a specific antigen for the *Mtb* complex and was recognized by sera of tuberculosis patients and localized in the membrane of the bacterial cell.

8. Acknowledgment

We thank Georges Robreau, Jean-Luc Guesdon and Caroline Borot for their help.

9. References

Abdallah, A.M.; Verboom, T.; Hannes, F.; Safi, M.; Strong, M. Eisenberg, D.; Musters, R.J.; Vandenbroucke-Grauls, C.M.; Appelmelk, B.J.; Luirink, J. & Bitter, W.A. (2006).

P27-PPE36 (Rv2108) Mycobacterium tuberculosis Antigen – Member of PPE Protein Family with Surface Localization and Immunological Activities

187

Specific secretion system mediates PPE41 transport in pathogenic mycobacteria. *Mol. Microbiol.*, 62: 667–679.

Adindla, S. & Guruprasad, L. (2003). Sequence analysis corresponding to the PPE and PE proteins in *Mycobacterium tuberculosis* and other genomes. *J Biosci.*, 28: 169-179.

Bansal, K.; Sinha, A.Y.; Ghorpade, D.S.; Togarsimalemath, S.K.; Patil, S.A.; Kaveri, S.V.; Balaji, K.N. & Bayry, J. (2010). Src homology 3-interacting domain of Rv1917c of *Mycobacterium tuberculosis* induces selective maturation of human dendritic cells by regulating PI3K-MAPK-NF-kappaB signaling and drives Th2 immune responses. *J. Biol. Chem.*, 285 (47): 36511-36522.

Banu, S.; Honoré, N.; Saint-Joanis, B.; Philpott, D.; Prevost, M.C. & Cole, S.T. (2002). Are the PE-PGRS proteins of *Mycobacterium tuberculosis* variable surface antigens? *Mol. Microbiol.*, 44 (1) : 9-19.

Becq, J.; Gutierrez, M.; Rosas-Magallanes, V.; Rauzier, J.; Gicquel, B.; Neyrolles, O. & Deschavanne, P. (2007). Contribution of horizontally acquired genomic islands to the evolution of the tubercle bacilli. *Mol. Biol. Evol.*, 24: 1867–1871.

Beggs, M.L.; Eisenach, K.D. & Cave, M.D. (2000). Mapping of IS6110 insertion sites in two epidemic strains of *Mycobacterium tuberculosis*. *J. Clin. Microbiol.*, 38 (8): 2923-2928.

Betts, J.C.; Lukey, P.T.; Robb, L.C.; McAdam, R.A. & Duncan, K. (2002). Evaluation of a nutrient starvation model of *Mycobacterium tuberculosis* persistence by gene and protein expression profiling. *Mol. Microbiol.*, 43 (3): 717–731.

Bonanni, D.; Rindi, L.; Lari, N. & Garzelli, C. (2005). Immunogenicity of mycobacterial PPE44 (Rv2770c) in *Mycobacterium bovis* BCG-infected mice. *J. Med. Microbiol.*, 54 (Pt 5): 443-448.

Bowers, P.M.; Pellegrini, M.; Thompson, M.J.; Fierro, J.; Yeates, T.O. & Eisenberg, D. (2004). Prolinks: a database of protein functional linkages derived from coevolution. *Genome Biol.*, 5 (5):R35.

Camacho, L.R.; Ensergueix, D.; Perez, E.; Gicquel, B. & Guilhot, C. (1999). Identification of a virulence gene cluster of *Mycobacterium tuberculosis* by signature-tagged transposon mutagenesis. *Mol. Microbiol.*, 34: 257-267.

Caruso, A.M.; Serbina, N.; Klein, E.; Triebold, K.; Bloom, B.R. & Flynn, J.L. (1999). Mice deficient in CD4 T cells have only transiently diminished levels of IFN-γ, yet succumb to tuberculosis. *J. Immunol.*, 162 (9): 5407–5416.

Casadevall, A. (1995). Antibody immunity and invasive fungal infections. *Infect. Immun.*, 63: 4211–4218.

Chaitra, M.G.; Nayak, R. & Shaila, M.S. (2007). Modulation of immune responses in mice to recombinant antigens from PE and PPE families of proteins of *Mycobacterium tuberculosis* by the Ribi adjuvant. *Vaccine*, 25 (41): 7168-7176.

(a) Chaitra, M.G.; Shaila, M.S. & Nayak, R. (2008). Detection of interferon gamma-secreting CD8+ T lymphocytes in humans specific for three PE/PPE proteins of *Mycobacterium tuberculosis*. *Microbes Infect.*, 10 (8): 858-867.

(b) Chaitra, M.G.; Shaila, M.S. & Nayak, R. (2008). Characterization of T-cell immunogenicity of two PE/PPE proteins of *Mycobacterium tuberculosis*. *J. Med. Microbiol.*, 57 (Pt 9): 1079-1086.

Chakhaiyar, P.; Nagalakshmi, Y.; Aruna, B.; Murthy, K.J.; Katoch, V.M. & Hasnain, S.E. (2004). Regions of high antigenicity within the hypothetical PPE major polymorphic tandem repeat open-reading frame, Rv2608, show a differential humoral response and a low T cell response in various categories of patients with tuberculosis. *J. Infect. Dis.*, 190 (7): 1237-1244.

Chevrier, D.; Casademont, I. & Guesdon, J.L. (2000). Cloning of a gene from *Mycobacterium tuberculosis* coding for a hypothetical 27 kDa protein and its use for the specific PCR identification of these mycobacteria. *Mol. Cell. Probes*, 14: 241-248.

Choudhary, R.K.; Mukhopadhyay, S.; Chakhaiyar, P.; Sharma, N.; Murthy, K.J.R.; Katoch, V.M. & Hasnain S.E. (2003). PPE antigen Rv2430c of *Mycobacterium tuberculosis* induces a strong B-cell response. *Infect. Immun.*, 71: 6338-6343.

Cockle, P.J.; Gordon, S.V.; Lalvani, A.; Buddle, B.M.; Hewinson, R.G. & Vordermeier, H.M. (2002). Identification of novel *Mycobacterium tuberculosis* antigens with potential as diagnostic reagents or subunit vaccine candidates by comparative genomics. *Infect. Immun.*, 70 (12): 6996-7003.

Cole, S.T.; Brosch, R.; Parkhill, J.; Garnier, T.; Churcher, C.; Harris, D.; Gordon, S.V.; Eiglmeier, K.; Gas, S.; Barry, C.E. 3rd; Tekaia, F.; Badcock, K.; Basham, D.; Brown, D.; Chillingworth, T.; Connor, R.; Davies, R.; Devlin, K.; Feltwell, T.; Gentles, S.; Hamlin, N.; Holroyd, S.; Hornsby, T.; Jagels, K.; Krogh, A.; McLean, J.; Moule, S.; Murphy, L.; Oliver, K.; Osborne, J.; Quail, M.A.; Rajandream, M.A.; Rogers, J.; Rutter, S.; Seeger, K.; Skelton, J.; Squares, R.; Squares, S.; Sulston, J.E.; Taylor, K.; Whitehead, S. & Barrell, B.G. (1998). Deciphering the biology of *Mycobacterium tuberculosis* from the complete genome sequence. *Nature*, 393 (6685): 537-544.

Cole, S.T. (1999). Learning from the genome sequence of *Mycobacterium tuberculosis* H37Rv. *FEBS Lett.*, 452: 7-10.

Cole, S.T.; Eiglmeier, K.; Parkhill, J.; James, K.D.; Thomson, N.R.; Wheeler, P.R.; Honoré, N.; Garnier, T.; Churcher, C.; Harris, D.; Mungall, K.; Basham, D.; Brown, D.; Chillingworth, T.; Connor, R.; Davies, R.M.; Devlin, K.; Duthoy, S.; Feltwell, T.; Fraser, A.; Hamlin, N.; Holroyd, S.; Hornsby, T.; Jagels, K.; Lacroix, C.; Maclean, J.; Moule, S.; Murphy, L.; Oliver, K.; Quail, M.A.; Rajandream, M.A.; Rutherford, K.M.; Rutter, S.; Seeger, K.; Simon, S.; Simmonds, M.; Skelton, J.; Squares, R.; Squares, S.; Stevens, K.; Taylor, K.; Whitehead, S.; Woodward, J.R. & Barrell B.G. (2001). Massive gene decay in the leprosy bacillus. *Nature*, 409 (6823): 1007-1011.

Cubillos-Ruiz, A.; Morales, J. & Zambrano, M.M. (2008). Analysis of the genetic variation in *Mycobacterium tuberculosis* strains by multiple genome alignments. *BMC Research Notes*. vol. 1: article 110.

Daugelat, S.; Kowall, J.; Mattow, J.; Bumann, D.; Winter, R.; Hurwitz, R. & Kaufmann S.H. (2003). The RD1 proteins of *Mycobacterium tuberculosis*: expression in *Mycobacterium smegmatis* and biochemical characterization. *Microbes Infect.*, 5 (12): 1082-1095.

Demangel, C. ; Brodin, P.; Cockle, P.J.; Brosch, R. ; Majlessi, L.; Leclerc, C. & Cole S.T. (2004). Cell envelope protein PPE68 contributes to *Mycobacterium tuberculosis* RD1 immunogenicity independently of a 10-kilodalton culture filtrate protein and ESAT-6. *Infect. Immun.* 72: 2170-2176.

Dillon, D.C.; Alderson, M.R.; Day, C.H.; Lewinsohn, D.M.; Coler, R.; Bement, T.; Campos-Neto, A.; Skeiky, Y.A.W.; Orme, I.M.; Roberts, A.; Steen, S.; Dalemans, W.; Badaro, R. & Reed S.G. (1999). Molecular characterization and human T-cell responses to a member of a novel *Mycobacterium tuberculosis* mtb39 gene family. *Infect. Immun.*, 67: 2941-2950.

Dubnau, E.; Fontan, P.; Manganelli, R.; Soares-Appel, S. & Smith, I. (2002). *Mycobacterium tuberculosis* genes induced during infection of human macrophages. *Infect. Immun.*, 70: 2787-2795.

Dunker, A.K.; Lawson, J.D.; Brown, C.J.; Williams, R.M.; Romero, P.; Oh, J.S.; Oldfield, C.J.; Campen, A.M.; Ratliff, C.M.; Hipps, K.W.; Ausio, J.; Nissen, M.S.; Reeves, R.; Kang, C.; Kissinger, C.R.; Bailey, R.W.; Griswold, M.D.; Chiu, W.; Garner, E.C. & Obradovic, Z. (2001). Intrinsically disordered protein. *J. Mol. Graph. Model.*, 19: 26-59.

Fisher, M.A.; Plikaytis, B.B.; Shinnick, T.M. (2002). Microarray analysis of the *Mycobacterium tuberculosis* transcriptional response to the acidic conditions found in phagosomes. *J. Bacteriol.*, 184 (14): 4025-4032.

Fleischmann, R.D.; Alland, D.; Eisen, J.A.; Carpenter, L.; White, O.; Peterson, J.; DeBoy, R.; Dodson, R.; Gwinn, M.; Haft, D.; Hickey, E.; Kolonay, J.F.; Nelson, W.C.; Umayam, L.A.; Ermolaeva, M.; Salzberg, S.L.; Delcher, A.; Utterback, T.; Weidman, J.; Khouri, H.; Gill, J.; Mikula, A.; Bishai, W.; Jacobs, J.W.R. Jr.; Venter, J.C. & Fraser, C.M. (2002). Whole-genome comparison of *Mycobacterium tuberculosis* clinical and laboratory strains. *J. Bacteriol.*, 184: 5479-5490.

Flynn, J.L.; Goldstein, M.M.; Triebold, K.J.; Koller, B. & Bloom, B.R. (1992). Major histocompatibility complex class I restricted T cells are required for resistance to *Mycobacterium tuberculosis* infection. *P.N.A.S. U.S.A.*, 89 (24): 12013-12017.

Glatman-Freedman, A. (2003). Advances in antibody-mediated immunity against *Mycobacterium tuberculosis*: implications for a novel vaccine strategy. *FEMS Immunol. Med. Microbiol.*, 39: 9-16.

Glatman-Freedman, A. & Casadevall, A. (1998). Serum therapy for tuberculosis revisited: reappraisal of the role of antibody-mediated immunity against *Mycobacterium tuberculosis*. *Clin. Microbiol. Rev.*, 11: 514-532.

Gao, Q.; Kripke, K.E.; Saldanha, A.J.; Yan, W.; Holmes, S. & Small, P.M. (2005). Gene expression diversity among *Mycobacterium tuberculosis* clinical isolates. *Microbiology*, 151 (Pt 1): 5-14.

Gey Van Pittius, N.C.; Gamieldien, J.; Hide, W.; Brown, G.D.; Siezen, R.J. & Beyers, A.D. (2001). The ESAT-6 gene cluster of *Mycobacterium tuberculosis* and other high G+C Gram-positive bacteria. *Genome Biology*, 2 (10): RESEARCH0044.

Gey van Pittius, N.C.; Sampson, S.L.; Lee, H.; Kim, Y.; van Helden, P.D. & Warren, R.M.; (2006). Evolution and expansion of the *Mycobacterium tuberculosis* PE and PPE multigene families and their association with the duplication of the ESAT-6 (esx) gene cluster regions. *B.M.C. Evol. Biol.*, 6, 95.

Garnier, T.; Eiglmeier, K.; Camus, J.C.; Medina, N.; Mansoor, H.; Pryor, M.; Duthoy, S.; Grondin, S.; Lacroix, C.; Monsempe, C.; Simon, S.; Harris, B.; Atkin, R.; Doggett, J.; Mayes, R.; Keating, L.; Wheeler, P.R.; Parkhill, J.; Barrell, B.G.; Cole, S.T.; Gordon, S.V. & Hewinson, R.G. The complete genome sequence of *Mycobacterium bovis*. *Proc. Natl. Acad. Sci. U.S.A.*, 100: 7877-7882.

Gordon, S.V.; Eiglmeier, K.; Garnier, T.; Brosch, R.; Parkhill, J.; Barrell, B.; Cole, S.T. & Hewinson, R.G. (2001). Genomics of *Mycobacterium bovis*. *Tuberculosis (Edinb)*, 81: 157-163

Gordon, B.R.; Li, Y.; Wang, L.; Sintsova, A.; van Bakel, H.; Tian, S.; Navarre, W.W.; Xia, B.; Liu, J. (2010). Lsr2 is a nucleoid-associated protein that targets AT-rich sequences and virulence genes in *Mycobacterium tuberculosis. Proc. Natl. Acad. Sci. U.S.A.,* 107 (11): 5154-5159.

Gupta, M.K.; Subramanian, V. & Yadav, J.S. (2009). Immunoproteomic identification of secretory and subcellular protein antigens and functional evaluation of the secretome fraction of *Mycobacterium immunogenum* a newly recognized species of the *Mycobacterium chelonae- Mycobacterium abscessus* group. *Journal of Proteome Research,* 8 (5): 2319-2330.

Gutierrez, M.C.; Brisse, S.; Brosch, R.; Fabre, M.; Omais, B.; Marmiesse, M.; Supply, P. & Vincent, V. (2005). Ancient origin and gene mosaicism of the progenitor of *Mycobacterium tuberculosis. PloS Pathog.,* 1 (1): e5.

Hebert, A.M.; Talarico, S.; Yang, D.; Durmaz, R.; Marrs, C;F.; Zhang, L.; Foxman, B. & Yang Z. (2007). DNA polymorphisms in the pepA and PPE18 genes among clinical strains of *Mycobacterium tuberculosis*: implications for vaccine efficacy. *Infect. Immun.,* 75: 5798-5805.

Hou, J.Y.; Graham, J.E. & Clark-Curtiss, J.E. (2002). *Mycobacterium avium* genes expressed during growth in human macrophages detected by Selective Capture of Transcribed Sequences (SCOTS). *Infect. Immun.,* 70: 3714-3726.

Jacob, F. & Monod, J. (1961). Genetic regulatory mechanisms in the synthesis of proteins. *J. Mol. Biol.,* 3: 318-356.

Julián, E.; Matas, L.; Pérez, A.; Alcaide, J.; Lanéelle, M.A. & Luquin, M. (2002). Serodiagnosis of tuberculosis: comparison of immunoglobulin A (IgA) response to sulfolipid I with IgG and IgM responses to 2,3-diacyltrehalose, 2,3,6-triacyltrehalose, and cord factor antigens. *J. Clin. Microbiol.,* 40: 3782-3788.

Khan, N.; Alam, K.; Nair, S.; Valluri, V.L.; Murthy, K.J. & Mukhopadhyay, S. (2008). Association of strong immune responses to PPE protein Rv1168c with active tuberculosis. *Clin. Vaccine Immunol.,* 15 (6): 974-980.

Kent, L.; McHugh, T.D.; Billington, O.; Dale J.W. & Gillespie, S.H. (1995). Demonstration of homology between IS6110 of *Mycobacterium tuberculosis* and DNAs of other *Mycobacterium* spp. *J. Clin. Microbiol.,* 33 (9): 2290-2293.

Kinsella, R.J.; Fitzpatrick, D.A.; Creevey, C.J. & McInerney, J.O. (2003). Fatty acid biosynthesis in *Mycobacterium tuberculosis*: Lateral gene transfer, adaptive evolution, and gene duplication. *Proc. Natl. Acad. Sci. U.S.A.,* 100: 10320-10325.

Karboul, A.; Mazza, A.; Gey van Pittius, N.C.; Ho, J.L.; Brousseau, R. & Mardassi, H. (2008). Frequent homologous recombination events in *Mycobacterium tuberculosis* PE/PPE multigene families: potential role in antigenic variability. *J. Bacteriol.,* 190 (23): 7838-7846.

Lee, B.W.; Tan, J.A.; Wong, S.C.; Tan C.B.; Yap, H.K.; Low, P.S.; Chia, J.N. & Tay, J.S. (1994). DNA amplification by the polymerase chain reaction for the rapid diagnosis of tuberculous meningitis. Comparison of protocols involving three mycobacterial DNA sequences, IS6110, 65 kDa antigen, and MPB64. *J. Neurol. Sci.,* 123 (1-2): 173-179.

Le Moigne, V.; Robreau, G.; Borot, C.; Guesdon, J.L. & Mahana, W. (2005). Expression, immunochemical, characterisation and localisation of the *Mycobaterium tuberculosis* protein p27. *Tuberculosis (Edinb),* 85: 213-219.

Le Moigne, V.; Robreau, G. & Mahana, W. (2008). Flagellin as a good carrier and potent adjuvant for Th1 response: Study of mice immune response to the p27 (Rv2108) *Mycobacterium tuberculosis* antigen. *Molecular Immunology,* 45: 2499-2507

Li, Y.; Miltner, E.; Wu, M.; Petrofsky, M. & Bermudez, L.E. (2005). A *Mycobacterium avium* PPE gene is associated with the ability of the bacterium to grow in macrophages and virulence in mice. *Cell. Microbiol.*, 7: 539–548.

Macfarlane, A.; Mondragon-Gonzalez, R.; Vega-Lopez, F.; Wieles, B.; de Pena, J.; Rodriguez, O.; Suarez y de la Torre, R.; de Vries, R.R.; Ottenhoff, T.H. & Dockrell, H.M. (2001). Presence of human T-cell responses to the *Mycobacterium leprae* 45-kilodalton antigen reflects infection with or exposure to *M. leprae*. *Clin. Diagn. Lab. Immunol.*, 8 (3): 604-611.

Mălen, H.; Pathak, S.; Softeland, T.; de Souza, G.A. & Wiker, H.G. (2010). Definition of novel cell envelope associated proteins in Triton X-114 extracts of *Mycobacterium tuberculosis* H37Rv. *BMC Microbiology*, 10: 132.

Manganelli, R.; Voskuil, M.I.; Schoolnik, G.K. & Smith, I. (2001). The *Mycobacterium tuberculosis* ECF sigma factor sigmaE: role in global gene expression and survival in macrophages. *Mol. Microbiol.*, 41 (2): 423-437.

Manganelli, R.; Voskuil, M.I.; Schoolnik, G.K.; Dubnau, E.; Gomez, M. & Smith I. (2002). Role of the extracytoplasmic-function sigma factor sigma(H) in *Mycobacterium tuberculosis* global gene expression. *Mol. Microbiol.*, 45 (2): 365-374.

McEvoy, C.R.E.; van Helden, P.D.; Warren, R.M. & Gey van Pittius, N.C. (2009). Evidence for a rapid rate of molecular evolution at the hypervariable and immunogenic *Mycobacterium tuberculosis* PPE38 gene region. *BMC Evolutionary Biology*, 9: 237.

Medzhitov, R. & Janeway Jr., C. (2000). Innate immune recognition: mechanisms and pathways. *Immunol. Rev.*, 173: 89 - 97.

Mishra, K.C.; de Chastellier, C.; Narayana, Y.; Bifani, P.; Brown, A.K.; Besra, G.S.; Katoch, V.M.; Joshi, B.; Balaji, K.N. & Kremer, L. (2008). Functional role of the PE domain and immunogenicity of the *Mycobacterium tuberculosis* triacylglycerol hydrolase LipY. *Infect. Immun.*, 76 (1): 127-140.

Molicotti, P.; Bua, A.; Ortu, S.; Ladu, M.C.; Delogu, G.; Mura, A.; Sechi, L.A.; Fadda, G. & Zanetti, S. (2008). Heparin binding haemagglutin as potential diagnostic marker of *Mycobacterium bovis*. *New Microbiol.*, 31 (3): 423-427.

Mustafa, A.S. (2001). Biotechnology in the development of new vaccines and diagnostic reagents against tuberculosis. *Curr. Pharm. Biotechnol.*, 2 :157–173.

Mustafa, A.S.; Cockle, P.J.; Shaban, F.; Hewinson, R.G. & Vordermeier, H.M. (2002). Immunogenicity of *Mycobacterium tuberculosis* RD1 region gene products in infected cattle. *Clin. Exp. Immunol.*, 130 (1): 37-42.

Nagata, R.; Muneta, Y.; Yoshihara, K.; Yokomizo, Y. & Mori, Y. (2005). Expression cloning of gamma interferon-inducing antigens of *Mycobacterium avium* subsp. *Paratuberculosis*. *Infec. Immun.*, 73 (6): 3778–3782

Nair, S.; Ramaswamy, P.A.; Ghosh, S.; Joshi, D.C.; Pathak, N.; Siddiqui, I.; Sharma, P.; Hasnain, S.E.; Mande, S.C. & Mukhopadhyay, S. (2009). The PPE18 of *Mycobacterium tuberculosis* interacts with TLR2 and activates IL-10 induction in macrophage. *J. Immunol.*, 183 (10): 6269-6281.

Newton, V.; McKenna, S.L. & De Buck, J. (2009). Presence of PPE proteins in *Mycobacterium avium* subsp. *paratuberculosis* isolates and their immunogenicity in cattle. *Vet. Microbiol.*, 135 (3-4): 394-400.

Okkels, L.M.; Brock, I.; Follmann, F.; Agger, E.M.; Arend, S.M.; Ottenhoff, T.H.M.; Oftung, F.; Rosenkrands, I. & Andersen P. (2003). PPE protein (Rv3873) from DNA segment RD1 of *Mycobacterium tuberculosis*: strong recognition of both specific T-cell epitopes and epitopes conserved within the PPE family. *Infect. Immun.*, 71: 6116–6123.

Park, H.D.; Guinn, K.M.; Harrell, M.I.; Liao, R.; Voskuil, M.I.; Tompa, M.; Schoolnik, G.K. & Sherman, D.R. (2003). Rv3133c/dosR is a transcription factor that mediates the hypoxic response of *Mycobacterium tuberculosis*. *Mol. Microbiol.*, 48 (3): 833-843.

Parkash, O.; Kumar, A.; Nigam, A.; Franken, K.L. & Ottenhoff, T.H. (2006). Evaluation of recombinant serine-rich 45-kDa antigen (ML0411) for detection of antibodies in leprosy patients. *Scand. J. Immunol.*, 64 (4): 450-455.

Plotkin, J.B.; Dushoff, J. & Fraser, H.B. (2004). Detecting selection using a single genome sequence of *M. tuberculosis* and *P. falciparum*. *Nature*, 428 (6986): 942-945.

Provvedi, R.; Boldrin, F.; Falciani, F.; Palù, G.; & Manganelli, R. (2009). Global transcriptional response to vancomycin in *Mycobacterium tuberculosis*. *Microbiology*, 155 (Pt 4): 1093-1102.

Pym, A.S.; Brodin, P.; Brosch, R.; Huerre, M. & Cole, S.T. (2002). Loss of RD1 contributed to the attenuation of the live tuberculosis vaccines *Mycobacterium bovis* BCG and *Mycobacterium microti*. *Mol. Microbiol.*, 46 (3): 709-717.

Rehren, G.; Walters, S.; Fontan, P.; Smith, I. & Zárraga, A.M. (2007). Differential gene expression between *Mycobacterium bovis* and *Mycobacterium tuberculosis*. *Tuberculosis (Edinb.)*, 87 (4): 347-359.

Riley, R.; Pellegrini, M. & Eisenberg, D. (2008). Identifying cognate binding pairs among a large set of paralogs: the case of PE/PPE proteins of *Mycobacterium tuberculosis*. *PLoS Comput. Biol.*, 4 (9): e1000174.

Rinke de Wit, T.F.; Clark-Curtiss, J.E.; Abebe, F.; Kolk, A.H.; Janson, A.A.; van Agterveld, M. & Thole, J.E. (1993). A *Mycobacterium leprae*-specific gene encoding an immunologically recognized 45 kDa protein. *Mol. Microbiol.*, 10 (4):829-38.

Rindi, L.; Lari, N. & Garzelli, C. (1999). Search for genes potentially involved in *Mycobacterium tuberculosis* virulence by mRNA differential display. *Biochem. Biophys. Res. Commun.*, 258: 94–101.

Rindi, L.; Peroni, I.; Lari, N.; Bonanni, D.; Tortoli, E. & Garzelli, C. (2007). Variation of the expression of *Mycobacterium tuberculosis* ppe44 gene among clinical isolates. *FEMS Immunol. Med. Microbiol.*, 51 (2): 381-387.

Rodriguez, G.M.; Gold, B.; Gomez, M.; Dussurget, O. & Smith, I. (1999). Identification and characterization of two divergently transcribed iron regulated genes in *Mycobacterium tuberculosis*. *Tuber. Lung. Dis.*, 79: 287-298.

Rodriguez, G.M.; Voskuil, M.I.; Gold, B.; Schoolnik, G.K. & Smith, I. (2002). IdeR, an essential gene in *Mycobacterium tuberculosis*: role of IdeR in iron-dependent gene expression, iron metabolism, and oxidative stress response. *Infect. Immun.*, 70 (7): 3371-3381.

Romano, M.; Rindi, L.; Korf, H.; Bonanni, D.; Adnet, P.Y.; Jurion, F.; Garzelli, C. & Huygen, K. (2008). Immunogenicity and protective efficacy of tuberculosis subunit vaccines expressing PPE44 (Rv2770c). *Vaccine*, 26 (48): 6053-6063.

Rosas-Magallanes, V.; Deschavanne, P.; Quintana-Murci, L.; Brosch, R.; Gicquel, B. & Neyrolles, O. (2006). Horizontal transfer of a virulence operon to the ancestor of *Mycobacterium tuberculosis*. *Mol. Biol. Evol.*, 23: 1129–1135.

Rustad, T.R.; Harrell, M.I.; Liao, R. & Sherman, D.R. (2008). The enduring hypoxic response of *Mycobacterium tuberculosis*. *PLoS One*, 3 (1): e1502.

P27-PPE36 (Rv2108) Mycobacterium tuberculosis Antigen – Member of PPE Protein Family with Surface Localization and Immunological Activities

193

(a) Sampson, S.L.; Lukey, P.; Warren, R.M.; van Helden, P.D.; Richardson, M. & Everett, M.J. (2001). Expression, characterization and subcellular localization of the Mycobacterium tuberculosis PPE gene Rv1917c. Tuberculosis (Edinb.), 81: 305–317.

(b) Sampson, S.L.; Warren, R.; Richardson, M.; van der Spuy, G. & van Helden, P. (2001). IS6110 insertions in Mycobacterium tuberculosis: predominantly into coding regions. J. Clin. Microbiol., 39 (9): 3423-3424.

Sani, M.; Houben, E.N.; Geurtsen, J.; Pierson, J.; de Punder, K.; van Zon, M.; Wever, B.; Piersma, S.R.; Jiménez, C.R.; Daffé, M.; Appelmelk, B.J.; Bitter, W.; van der Wel, N. & Peters, P.J. (2010). Direct visualization by cryo-EM of the mycobacterial capsular layer: a labile structure containing ESX-1-secreted proteins. PLoS Pathog., 6 (3): e1000794.

Sassetti, C.M.; Boyd, D.H. & Rubin, E.J. (2003). Genes required for mycobacterial growth defined by high density mutagenesis. Mol. Microbiol., 48 (1): 77-84.

Schnappinger, D.; Ehrt, S.; Voskuil, M.I.; Liu, Y.; Mangan, J.A.; Monahan, I.M.; Dolganov, G.; Efron, B.; Butcher, P.D.; Nathan, C. & Schoolnik, G.K. (2003). Transcriptional adaptation of Mycobacterium tuberculosis within macrophages: insights into the phagosomal environment. J. Exp. Med., 198 (5): 693–704.

Sherman, D.R.; Voskuil, M.; Schnappinger, D.; Liao, R.; Harrell, M.I. & Schoolnik G.K. (2001). Regulation of the Mycobacterium tuberculosis hypoxic response gene encoding alpha -crystallin. Proc. Natl. Acad. Sci. U.S.A., 98 (13): 7534-7539.

Singh, K.K.; Dong, Y.; Patibandla, S.A.; McMurray, D.N.; Arora, V.K. & Laal, S. (2005). Immunogenicity of the Mycobacterium tuberculosis PPE55 (Rv3347c) protein during incipient and clinical tuberculosis. Infect. Immun., 73: 5004-5014.

Skeiky, Y.A.; Ovendale, P.J.; Jen, S.; Alderson, M.R.; Dillon, D.C.; Smith, S.; Wilson, C.B., Orme, I.M.; Reed, S.G. & Campos-Neto, A. (2000). T cell expression cloning of a Mycobacterium tuberculosis gene encoding a protective antigen associated with the early control of infection. J. Immunol., 165: 7140–7149.

Srivastava, R.; Kumar, D.; Waskar, M.N.; Sharma, M.; Katoch, V.M. & Srivastava, B.S. (2006). Identification of a repetitive sequence belonging to a PPE gene of Mycobacterium tuberculosis and its use in diagnosis of tuberculosis. J. Med. Microbiol., 55: 1071-1077.

Stewart, G.R.; Wernisch, L.; Stabler, R.; Mangan, J.A.; Hinds, J.; Laing, K.G.; Young, D.B. & Butcher, P.D. (2002). Dissection of the heat-shock response in Mycobacterium tuberculosis using mutants and microarrays. Microbiology, 148 (Part 10): 3129–3138.

Stinear, T.P.; Seemann, T; Harrison, P.F.; Jenkin, G.A.; Davies, J.K.; Johnson, P.D.; Abdellah, Z.; Arrowsmith, C.; Chillingworth, T.; Churcher, C.; Clarke, K.; Cronin, A.; Davis, P.; Goodhead, I.; Holroyd, N.; Jagels, K.; Lord, A.; Moule, S.; Mungall, K.; Norbertczak, H.; Quail, M.A.; Rabbinowitsch, E.; Walker, D.; White, B.; Whitehead, S.; Small, P.L.; Brosch, R.; Ramakrishnan, L.; Fischbach, M.A.; Parkhill, J. & Cole, S.T. (2008). Insights from the complete genome sequence of Mycobacterium marinum on the evolution of Mycobacterium tuberculosis. Genome Res., 18 (5): 729-741.

Strong, M.; Mallick, P.; Pellegrini, M.; Thompson, M.J. & Eisenberg, D. (2003). Inference of protein function and protein linkages in Mycobacterium tuberculosis based on prokaryotic genome organization: a combined computational approach. Genome Biol., 4 (9): R59.

Strong, M.; Sawaya, M.R.; Wang, S.; Phillips, M.; Cascio, D. & Eisenberg, D. (2006). Toward the structural genomics of complexes: crystal structure of a PE/PPE protein complex from *Mycobacterium tuberculosis*. *Proc. Natl. Acad. Sci. U.S.A.*, 103: 8060–8065.

Tekaia, F.; Gordon, S.V.; Garnier, T.; Brosch, R.; Barrell, B.G. & Cole, S.T. (1999). Analysis of the proteome of *Mycobacterium tuberculosis* in silico. *Tuber. Lung. Dis.*, 79: 329–342.

Thierry, D.; Cave, M.D.; Eisenach, K.D.; Crawford, J.T.; Bates, J.H.; Gicquel, B. & Guesdon, J.L. (1990). IS6110, an IS-like element of *Mycobacterium tuberculosis* complex. *Nucleic Acids Res.*, 18 (1): 188.

Thierry, D.; Chavarot, P.; Marchal, G.; Le Thi, K.T.; Ho, M.L.; Nguyen, N.L.; Le, N.V.; Ledru, S.; Fumoux, F. & Guesdon, J.L. (1995). *Mycobacterium tuberculosis* strains unidentified using the IS6110 probe can be detected by oligonucleotides derived from the Mt308 sequence. *Res. Microbiol.*, 146: 325–328.

Tompa, P. (2002). Intrinsically unstructured proteins. *Trends Biochem. Sci.*, 27: 527–533.

Tundup, S.; Akhter, Y.; Thiagarajan, D. & Hasnain, S.E. (2006). Clusters of PE and PPE genes of *Mycobacterium tuberculosis* are organized in operons: evidence that PE Rv2431c is co-transcribed with PPE Rv2430c and their gene products interact with each other. *FEBS Lett.*, 580 (5): 1285-1293.

Tundup, S.; Pathak, N.; Ramanadham, M.; Mukhopadhyay, S.; Murthy, K.J.; Ehtesham, N.Z. & Hasnain, S.E. (2008). The co-operonic PE25/PPE41 protein complex of *Mycobacterium tuberculosis* elicits increased humoral and cell mediated immune response. *PLoS One*, 3: e3586.

Voskuil, M.I.; Schnappinger, D.; Visconti, K.C.; Harrell, M.I.; Dolganov, G.M.; Sherman, D.R. & Schoolnik, G.K. (2003). Inhibition of respiration by nitric oxide includes a *Mycobacterium tuberculosis* dormancy program. *J. Exp. Med.*, 198 (5): 705–713.

(a)Voskuil, M.I.; Visconti, K.C. & Schoolnik, G.K. (2004). *Mycobacterium tuberculosis* gene expression during adaptation to stationary phase and low-oxygen dormancy. *Tuberculosis (Edinb)*, 84 (3-4): 218-227.

(b)Voskuil, M.I.; Schnappinger, D.; Rutherford, R.; Liu, Y. & Schoolnik, G.K. (2004). Regulation of the *Mycobacterium tuberculosis* PE/PPE genes. *Tuberculosis (Edinb.)*, 84 (3-4): 256-262.

Wang, J.; Qie, Y.; Zhang, H.; Zhu, B.; Xu, Y.; Liu, W.; Chen, J. & Wang H. (2008). PPE protein (Rv3425) from DNA segment RD11 of *Mycobacterium tuberculosis*: a novel immunodominant antigen of *Mycobacterium tuberculosis* induces humoral and cellular immune responses in mice. *Microbiol. Immunol.*, 52 (4): 224-230.

Yuen, L.K.; Ross, B.C.; Jackson, K.M. & Dwyer, B. (1993). Characterization of *Mycobacterium tuberculosis* strains from Vietnamese patients by Southern blot hybridization. *J. Clin. Microbiol.*, 31: 1615–1618.

Zanetti, S.; Bua, A.; Delogu, G.; Pusceddu, C.; Mura, M.; Saba, F.; Pirina, P.; Garzelli, C.; Vertuccio, C.; Sechi, L.A. & Fadda, G. (2005). Patients with pulmonary tuberculosis develop a strong humoral response against methylated heparin-binding hemagglutinin. *Clin. Diagn. Lab. Immunol.*, 12: 1135-1138.

Zhang, H.; Wang, J.; Lei, J.; Zhang, M.; Yang, Y.; Chen, Y. & Wang, H. (2007). PPE protein (Rv3425) from DNA segment RD11 of *Mycobacterium tuberculosis*: a potential B-cell antigen used for serological diagnosis to distinguish vaccinated controls from tuberculosis patients. *Clin. Microbiol. Infect.*, 13 (2): 139-145.

Permissions

The contributors of this book come from diverse backgrounds, making this book a truly international effort. This book will bring forth new frontiers with its revolutionizing research information and detailed analysis of the nascent developments around the world.

We would like to thank Dr. Pere-Joan Cardona, for lending his expertise to make the book truly unique. He has played a crucial role in the development of this book. Without his invaluable contribution this book wouldn't have been possible. He has made vital efforts to compile up to date information on the varied aspects of this subject to make this book a valuable addition to the collection of many professionals and students.

This book was conceptualized with the vision of imparting up-to-date information and advanced data in this field. To ensure the same, a matchless editorial board was set up. Every individual on the board went through rigorous rounds of assessment to prove their worth. After which they invested a large part of their time researching and compiling the most relevant data for our readers. Conferences and sessions were held from time to time between the editorial board and the contributing authors to present the data in the most comprehensible form. The editorial team has worked tirelessly to provide valuable and valid information to help people across the globe.

Every chapter published in this book has been scrutinized by our experts. Their significance has been extensively debated. The topics covered herein carry significant findings which will fuel the growth of the discipline. They may even be implemented as practical applications or may be referred to as a beginning point for another development. Chapters in this book were first published by InTech; hereby published with permission under the Creative Commons Attribution License or equivalent.

The editorial board has been involved in producing this book since its inception. They have spent rigorous hours researching and exploring the diverse topics which have resulted in the successful publishing of this book. They have passed on their knowledge of decades through this book. To expedite this challenging task, the publisher supported the team at every step. A small team of assistant editors was also appointed to further simplify the editing procedure and attain best results for the readers.

Our editorial team has been hand-picked from every corner of the world. Their multi-ethnicity adds dynamic inputs to the discussions which result in innovative outcomes. These outcomes are then further discussed with the researchers and contributors who give their valuable feedback and opinion regarding the same. The feedback is then collaborated with the researches and they are edited in a comprehensive manner to aid the understanding of the subject.

Apart from the editorial board, the designing team has also invested a significant amount of their time in understanding the subject and creating the most relevant covers. They scrutinized every image to scout for the most suitable representation of the subject and create an appropriate cover for the book.

The publishing team has been involved in this book since its early stages. They were actively engaged in every process, be it collecting the data, connecting with the contributors or procuring relevant information. The team has been an ardent support to the editorial, designing and production team. Their endless efforts to recruit the best for this project, has resulted in the accomplishment of this book. They are a veteran in the field of academics and their pool of knowledge is as vast as their experience in printing. Their expertise and guidance has proved useful at every step. Their uncompromising quality standards have made this book an exceptional effort. Their encouragement from time to time has been an inspiration for everyone.

The publisher and the editorial board hope that this book will prove to be a valuable piece of knowledge for researchers, students, practitioners and scholars across the globe.

List of Contributors

Toshi Nagata
Department of Health Science, Hamamatsu University School of Medicine, Hamamatsu, Japan

Yukio Koide
Department of Infectious Diseases, Hamamatsu University School of Medicine, Hamamatsu, Japan

Rhea N. Coler, Susan L. Baldwin, and Steven G. Reed
Infectious Disease Research Institute (IDRI) Seattle, USA

Fei Chen, Yanfeng Gao and Yuanming Qi
Department of Bioengineering, Zhengzhou University, Zhengzhou, China

Armando Acosta, Yamile Lopez, Nadine Alvarez and Maria Elena Sarmiento
Instituto Finlay, La Habana, Cuba

Norazmi Mohd Nor
School of Health Sciences, Universiti Sains Malaysia, Kelantan, Malaysia

Rogelio Hernández Pando
Experimental Pathology Section, National Institute of Medical Sciences and Nutrition, Mexico City, Mexico

Rajko Reljic
Clinical Sciences Division, St George's, University of London, GB

Juraj Ivanyi
Clinical and Diagnostic Sciences Department, Kings College London, Guy's Campus of Kings College London, GB

Cristina Vilaplana and Pere-Joan Cardona
Unitat de Tuberculosi Experimental, Fund. Institut Germans Trias i Pujol, Catalonia, Spain

Diana G. Dlugovitzky, Cynthia Stanford and John Stanford
Cátedra de Microbiologia, Virologia y Parasitologia, Facultad de Ciencias Medicas, Universidad Nacional de Rosario, Santa Fe Rosario, Argentina
Centre for Infectious Diseases & International Health, Windeyer Institute of Medical Sciences, University College London, London, UK

Elinos-Báez Carmen Martha
Departamento de Medicina Genómica y Toxicología Ambiental, Edificio C, 2° piso Instituto
de Investigaciones Biomédicas, Circuito Exterior, UNAM, Universidad Nacional Autónoma
de México, Ciudad Universitaria, México, D.F., Mexico

Ramírez González
Departamento de Farmacología, Facultad de Medicina, UNAM, Ciudad Universitaria, México, D.F., México

**María T Milanés-Virelles, Roberto Suárez-Méndez, Magalys Valdés-Quintana, Norma
Fernández-Olivera and Isis Cayón-Escobar**
"Benéfico Jurídico" Hospital, Havana, Cuba

Yamilet Santos-Herrera
"Amalia Simoni" Hospital, Camagüey, Cuba

Gladys Abreu-Suárez
Pediatric Hospital of Centro Habana, Havana, Cuba

**Idrian García-García, Pedro A López-Saura, Carmen M Valenzuela-Silva and Lidia
González- Méndez**
Center for Genetic Engineering and Biotechnology, Havana, Cuba

Wahib Mahana
Université de Bretagne Occidentale, France
Endotoxines, IGM, Université Paris sud, Orsay, France

Vincent Le Moigne
Université de Bretagne Occidentale, France

Printed in the USA
CPSIA information can be obtained
at www.ICGtesting.com
JSHW011401221024
72173JS00003B/382